REPAIR AND RENEWAL

JOURNEY THROUGH THE MIND AND BODY

TIME®
LIFE
BOOKS

Other Publications:
WEIGHT WATCHERS® SMART CHOICE RECIPE COLLECTION
TRUE CRIME
THE AMERICAN INDIANS
THE ART OF WOODWORKING
LOST CIVILIZATIONS
ECHOES OF GLORY
THE NEW FACE OF WAR
HOW THINGS WORK
WINGS OF WAR
CREATIVE EVERYDAY COOKING
COLLECTOR'S LIBRARY OF THE UNKNOWN
CLASSICS OF WORLD WAR II
TIME-LIFE LIBRARY OF CURIOUS AND UNUSUAL FACTS
AMERICAN COUNTRY
VOYAGE THROUGH THE UNIVERSE
THE THIRD REICH
THE TIME-LIFE GARDENER'S GUIDE
MYSTERIES OF THE UNKNOWN
TIME FRAME
FIX IT YOURSELF
FITNESS, HEALTH & NUTRITION
SUCCESSFUL PARENTING
HEALTHY HOME COOKING
UNDERSTANDING COMPUTERS
LIBRARY OF NATIONS
THE ENCHANTED WORLD
THE KODAK LIBRARY OF CREATIVE PHOTOGRAPHY
GREAT MEALS IN MINUTES
THE CIVIL WAR
PLANET EARTH
COLLECTOR'S LIBRARY OF THE CIVIL WAR
THE EPIC OF FLIGHT
THE GOOD COOK
WORLD WAR II
HOME REPAIR AND IMPROVEMENT
THE OLD WEST

*For information on and a full description of any of
the Time-Life Books series listed above, please call*
1-800-621-7026 *or write*:
Reader Information
Time-Life Customer Service
P.O. Box C-32068
Richmond, Virginia 23261-2068

REPAIR AND RENEWAL

JOURNEY THROUGH THE MIND AND BODY

BY THE EDITORS OF TIME-LIFE BOOKS
ALEXANDRIA, VIRGINIA

CONSULTANTS:

SIMON J. ARCHIBALD currently researches nerve regeneration at Duke University Medical Center, where he also serves as assistant research professor in the Division of Neurosurgery.

DEAN BOK is professor of anatomy and cell biology at the School of Medicine, University of California, Los Angeles. His work focuses on the eye at a molecular level, examining inherited gene defects that lead to degenerative eye conditions.

JUDITH CAMPISI is a senior scientist and group leader for carcinogenesis and radiation biology at the Lawrence Berkeley Laboratory, University of California, Berkeley.

LARAINE FIELD, an internist practicing in northern Virginia, specializes in preventive cardiology.

SHAKTI P. KAPUR, whose research emphasis is bone biology, holds the directorship of the Cell Biology and Histology Program at Georgetown University School of Medicine in Washington, D.C.

NAOMI KLEITMAN is located at The Miami Project to Cure Paralysis, where much of her work centers on neuronal regeneration. She is director of education and editor of the foundation's newsletter, *The Project*.

ROBERT M. LAVKER teaches at the University of Pennsylvania School of Medicine in Philadelphia, with an area of concentration in skin and hair-follicle stem cells.

THOMAS MACIAG's work explores how growth factors signal cells to divide. He is department head of molecular biology at the American Red Cross Holland Laboratory in Rockville, Maryland, and holds a teaching position at George Washington University in Washington, D.C.

BRUCE A. MAST has been published extensively in the field of wound-healing research, particularly in scarless fetal healing. A fully trained general surgeon, Dr. Mast is completing training in plastic and reconstructive surgery at the University of Pittsburgh.

DAVID A. WILLIAMS's research specialty is stem cells and blood cell development. He lectures at the Indiana University School of Medicine in Indianapolis.

ISAAC L. WORNOM III splits his time between a busy clinical practice—covering all aspects of reconstructive and cosmetic plastic surgery—and a teaching position at the Medical College of Virginia in Richmond.

JOURNEY THROUGH THE MIND AND BODY

Time-Life Books is a division of
Time Life Inc.

PRESIDENT AND CEO: John M. Fahey Jr.
EDITOR-IN-CHIEF: John L. Papanek

TIME-LIFE BOOKS

MANAGING EDITOR: Roberta Conlan

Executive Art Director: Ellen Robling
Director of Photography and Research:
John Conrad Weiser
Senior Editors: Russell B. Adams Jr., Dale
M. Brown, Janet Cave, Lee Hassig,
Robert Somerville, Henry Woodhead
Director of Technology: Eileen Bradley
Director of Editorial Operations: Prudence G.
Harris
Library: Louise D. Forstall

PRESIDENT: John D. Hall

Vice President, Director of Marketing:
Nancy K. Jones
Vice President, New Product Development:
Neil Kagan
Vice President, Book Production: Marjann
Caldwell
Production Manager: Marlene Zack

SERIES EDITOR: Robert Somerville
Administrative Editor: Judith W. Shanks

Editorial Staff for *Repair and Renewal*

Art Directors: Dale Pollekoff, Barbara M.
Sheppard, Fatima Taylor
Picture Editor: Kristin Baker Hanneman
Text Editors: Jim Watson (principal), Darcie
Conner Johnston
Associate Editors/Research and Writing: Ruth
Goldberg, M. Kevan Miller, Mark Rogers
Senior Copyeditor: Donna D. Carey
Editorial Assistant: Kris Dittman
Picture Coordinator: Paige Henke

Special Contributors:
George Constable, Juli Duncan, Sharon
Groth, Doug Harbrecht, Steven Mirsky,
Peter Pocock (text); Nancy Blodgett, Elaine
Friebele, Anna Gedrich, Stephanie Sum-
mers Henke, Maureen McHugh (research);
Barbara L. Klein (index); John Drummond
(design).

Correspondents:
Elisabeth Kraemer-Singh (Bonn); Christine
Hinze (London); Christina Lieberman (New
York); Maria Vincenza Aloisi (Paris); Ann
Natanson (Rome). Valuable assistance was
also provided by Trini Bandrés (Madrid);
Elizabeth Brown, Daniel Donnelly (New
York); Mary Johnson (Stockholm).

**Library of Congress
Cataloging-in-Publication Data**
Repair and renewal: journey through the
mind and body/by the editors of
Time-Life Books.
p. cm.— (Journey through the mind
and body)
Includes bibliographical references
and index.
ISBN 0-7835-1048-9
1. Regeneration (Biology). 2. Human
growth. 3. Wound healing. 4. Neuro-
plasticity. I. Time-Life Books. II. Series.
QP90.2.R47 1994
612'.022—dc20   94-18844

This volume is one of a series that
explores the fascinating inner universe
of the human mind and body.

CONTENTS

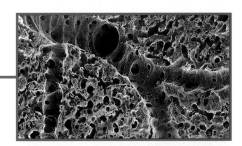
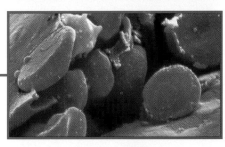
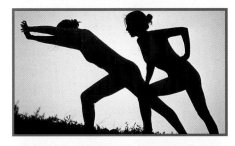
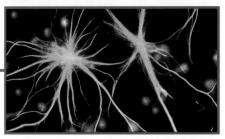

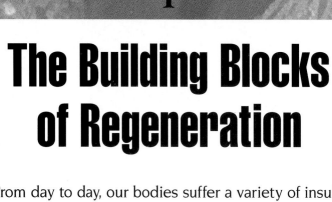

1

The Building Blocks of Regeneration

From day to day, our bodies suffer a variety of insults that are, for the most part, familiar and mundane: A child falls and scrapes her knee; a man cuts himself shaving. Some injuries are more dramatic, or even life-threatening—a skier's broken leg, an accident victim's punctured lung. Either way, though, people tend to take their healing for granted. After a week or two, we notice that bruises and cuts have disappeared; a broken bone mends eventually. In similar fashion, we accept as unremarkable the growth of our fingernails and hair, getting out the nailclipper or scheduling a haircut as a matter of course. We watch a summer suntan peel away with regret but not astonishment.

Yet the way that damaged bones, tissues, and organs patch themselves up is nothing short of miraculous. And if we stopped to think about it, we would find the quiet regeneration of skin and hair and nails—and other parts of the body as well—profoundly astonishing: It goes on 24 hours a day, week in and week out, literally remaking us, biochemically speaking, many times during the course of our lives.

The body's methods of repair and renewal might be likened to the repaving of streets or the construction of multistory buildings: Materials are specific to the task

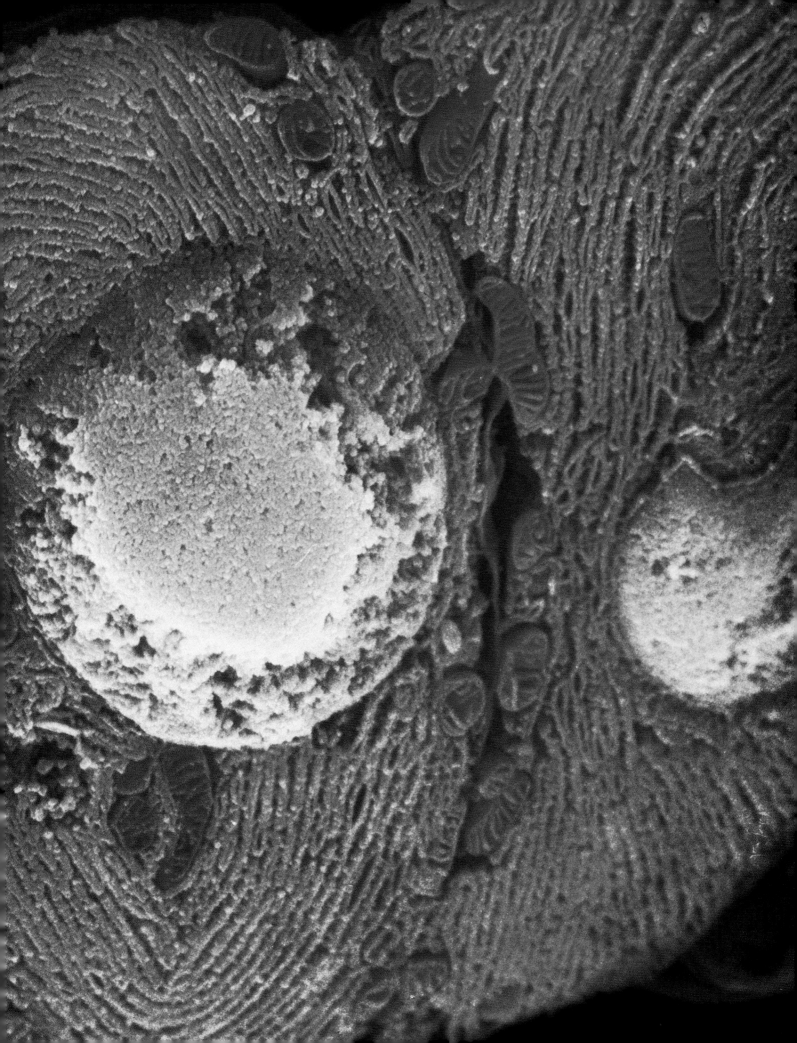

PRECEDING PAGE: This image of human liver cells, magnified 10,000 times, shows the nucleus *(yellow)* surrounded by material in the cytoplasm—including mitochondria *(red)*, the source of each cell's energy. Liver cells typically grow and divide at a slow rate but have the remarkable ability to step up the pace— by as much as a factor of 10—when liver tissue is damaged and must be restored.

and appear on site as required. In the body, however, notification that repairs are needed comes not from an external supervisor but, in effect, from the very materials in need of fixing—as if a pothole sent out an SOS for more asphalt *(pages 54-63)*.

The process is initiated by an elaborate interplay of cellular signals that scientists have only recently begun to decode. Indeed, mastering the complex language of cells is an ambitious task, but the potential rewards are enormous. By learning how cells respond to injury, perform routine maintenance, and work in concert to sustain one another, researchers continue the ceaseless effort to pierce two of humankind's most enduring conundrums: the mystery of life and the inevitability of death. Advances in cell and molecular biology, for example, have shed new light on the mechanism that prompts cells to divide again and again for a period of time—then suddenly stop. Scientists are also zeroing in on what causes damaged or faulty cells to self-destruct. In years to come, these and other findings may lead to changes in the way doctors practice medicine, providing new methods for fighting cancer, for instance, or slowing the aging process.

The simplest forms of life, such as amoebas and bacteria, are one-celled units that propagate merely by dividing in two. Offspring of these organisms emerge as replicas of the parent. Higher life forms resemble cellular cities made up of many types of inhabitants. Scientists estimate that the number of cells in the average human adult ranges somewhere between 10 trillion and 100 trillion, which come in more than 200 distinct varieties.

Despite their differences, which can be extensive, cells do share several characteristics. Each is a small compartment filled with a fluid called cytoplasm, a number of specialized molecules, and, in most cases, a nucleus, the cell's center of operations. The whole affair is surrounded by a pliant membrane, which, besides providing a protective "skin," serves as a kind of molecular message board, allowing the cell to receive signals from other cells. Finally, virtually every cell in the human body has one thing in common with its neighbors: 23 pairs of chromosomes made up of DNA code containing all of that person's genetic information. The DNA not only tells each cell that it is part of a human being and not part of, say, a turtle, but it also serves as a blueprint for the specialized functions of all that person's cells.

Once portions of the DNA molecule are turned on or off during embryonic development, each cell is assigned an identity—as a skin cell, for instance, or as a bone cell. Most adult cells are differentiated, meaning they have distinct roles and behave as if their basic character is irreversible. These cells often retain their specialized traits even when uprooted from their original environment and moved, in effect, to foreign cellular soil. For example, if living skin cells from the tail of a rat are transplanted onto the animal's kidney, they continue growing as if they were skin cells, even to the extent of forming hair follicles.

Such devotion to function is the norm, but researchers have found that some cells can modify themselves when they are subjected to certain environmental cues. For instance, scientists have been able to provoke a role change, in the laboratory at least, among smooth epithelial cells from the underside of a rat's tongue. When placed in a culture with tissue from the appropriate sensory nerves, the epithelial cells organize themselves into tiny clusters of taste buds, structures that are normally formed only from cells on the top surface of the tongue. When the nerve tissue is removed, the induced taste buds break down and disappear.

In most circumstances, however, cells retain their identity throughout their lives, and when a cell of a certain kind dies, one of its kin fills the vacancy. Some cells do this through

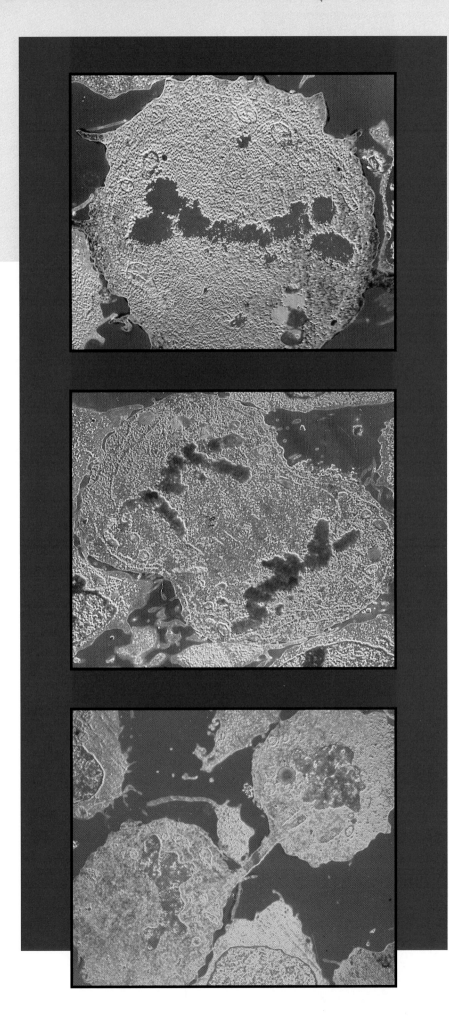

PHASES OF MITOSIS. Caught in the act, a single lymph cell splits in two during the process of cell division, or mitosis, in these false-color images. In the so-called metaphase *(top)*, the cell's 46 chromosomes *(pink)*, each having already duplicated itself, line up along the center of the cell. As the cell begins to pull apart during anaphase *(middle)*, the two copies of each chromosome separate and begin migrating toward opposite ends of the cell. Division nears completion during telophase *(bottom)*, when new nuclei start forming in the daughter cells.

simple division—splitting in two like one-celled amoebas. This type appears to have a vast capacity for renewal, seemingly able to continue multiplying as long as the organism remains alive to provide nutrients and the appropriate chemical signals. Among this type are the endothelial cells that line the walls of blood vessels, from the largest arteries and veins to the tiniest capillaries. Endothelial cells can go for months or even years without dividing. But if a blood vessel is damaged, neighboring cells suddenly go into a reproductive frenzy, churning out new growth and stopping at nothing to get the job done. For example, when surgeons use plastic tubing to replace a damaged blood vessel, newly created endothelial cells often coat the inside of the tubing like barnacles covering the hull of a ship.

Such simple-duplication cells, as they are known, tend to vanish into their own progeny and appear not to die at all, although scientists have determined that their reproductive capabilities do in fact diminish with age. Other cells in the body, by contrast, do die and are replaced by the offspring of a kind of understudy, known as a stem cell, that waits in the wings until pressed into service.

Simple Cell Division

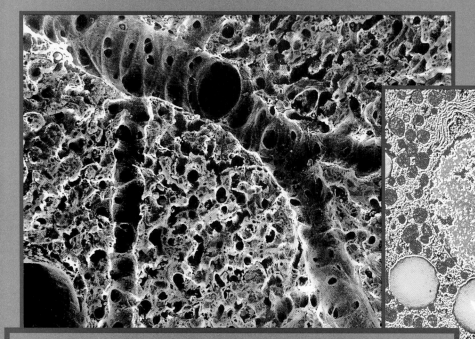

A Trio of Cell Types

In one way or another, most of the body's tissues refurbish themselves in their myriad struggles against injury, disease, the environment, and even time itself. Many stay healthy and functional by growing new cells as others die. In blood vessels and certain organs, including the liver, simple cell division— the process by which a single parent cell divides into two daughter cells—provides a regular means of renewal. Such components as new bone, blood, and lung cells, on the other hand, are formed by stem cells, which are undifferentiated but programmed to create specialized cells. Their only task is to generate replacements as needed, a service they perform quickly and efficiently. However, some of the body's cells— most notably those in the heart and the lens of the eye, as well as the neurons of the brain and spinal cord—never turn over and cannot be replaced once they die, often because a continual change of players would hamper functioning in these complex systems. Examples of all three types of tissues appear here and on the following pages.

Stem cells, which have neither stems nor any other salient characteristic, have no specific function until they are called into action. They are common in tissues of the body that suffer direct and damaging exposure to a harsh environment. One example is the skin. Another is the small intestine, whose lining is covered with tubular structures called villi, which absorb nutrients and convey digested foods through the gut with a kind of rhythmic, wavelike motion.

At the base of the villi, beneath the surface of the intestine, lie deep crypts occupied by legions of stem

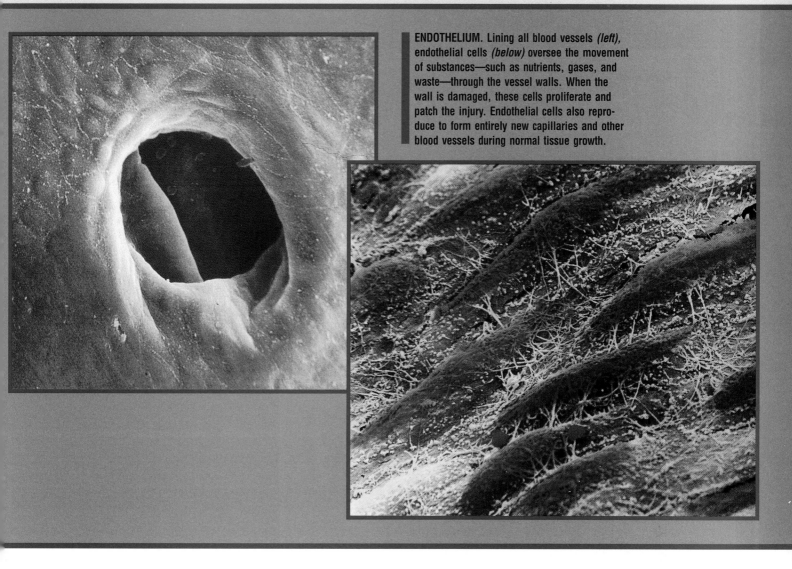

ENDOTHELIUM. Lining all blood vessels *(left)*, endothelial cells *(below)* oversee the movement of substances—such as nutrients, gases, and waste—through the vessel walls. When the wall is damaged, these cells proliferate and patch the injury. Endothelial cells also reproduce to form entirely new capillaries and other blood vessels during normal tissue growth.

cells. These little factories work unceasingly to manufacture replacements for the tiny cells that make up the walls of the villi themselves. Over a period of about five days, freshly minted cells work their way up into portions of the villi that project from the intestine wall, where they are in turn destroyed or carried away in the rough-and-tumble of digestion.

In the skeletal muscles, such as those of the arms and legs, healthy cells sometimes make up for those cells that die or are damaged by simply growing bigger and stronger, so that each can take on a larger share of the burden. Increased work load on the muscles causes cells to boost production of the internal protein fibers that give them strength. This hypertrophy, as the condition is called, is what enables bodybuilders to bulk up, and in the skeletal muscles it generally serves a useful purpose, allowing cells to adjust their abilities to meet new demands.

This adjustment goes both ways. When muscles are not used for a long time, such as when a fractured limb is immobilized by a cast, they shrink, or atrophy, leading to a reduction in the supply of proteins within the cells that are usually used in muscle contraction. A similar wasting of cells, called denervation atrophy, occurs in muscles that lose connection with the nerves that normally activate them.

Besides growing or shrinking according to demand, skeletal muscles also have stem cell backups that can

Stem Cell Division

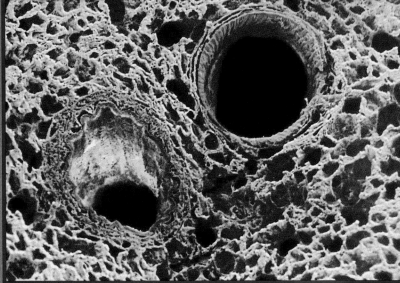

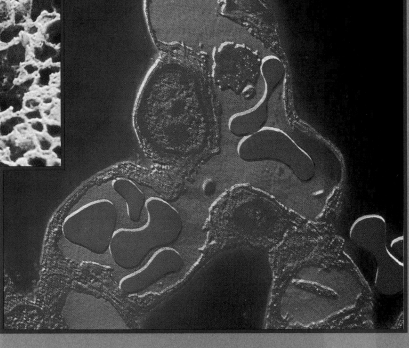

LUNG. Woven throughout lung tissue *(above)* are countless blood vessels that take in oxygen for delivery to the body. Because interruption of the organ's work for more than a matter of minutes is usually fatal, destruction of lung tissue must be remedied immediately—a service performed by stem cells such as those shown in pink in the image of a lung capillary at right.

be transformed into new cells when the need arises. These muscle stem cells, called myoblasts, are the original source of all muscle tissue. In a developing embryo, myoblasts proliferate actively, then begin to congregate to form muscle cells. However, some myoblasts remain as small, flattened, undifferentiated cells hugging the outer membranes of muscle cells. Damage to the skeletal muscles signals these standbys to begin reproducing just as they did in the embryo. The numerous progeny then fuse to each other or with existing muscle fibers to rebuild injured muscle tissue.

Myoblasts are most numerous at birth, but over the course of a lifetime the body's ability to replenish muscle tissue diminishes. In adults, the proportion of stem cells to actual muscle cells drops to a tiny fraction, and the stem cells nearly vanish in old age.

Scientists who have studied the aging process have been intrigued by the seeming correlation between growing old and the gradual reduction in the number of stem cells, on one

hand, and the decline in a cell's ability to divide. In recent years, evidence has emerged suggesting that life expectancy itself is programmed into the cell. In laboratory experiments, fibroblasts—the family of cells that produce connective tissue in most organs—taken from a human fetus have been shown to divide about 50 times before they reach senescence, or old age. As the person grows older, the number of divisions plummets: Fibroblasts from adults multiply an average of 30 times, whereas those from elderly people divide only 10 or 20 times. Researchers have found that

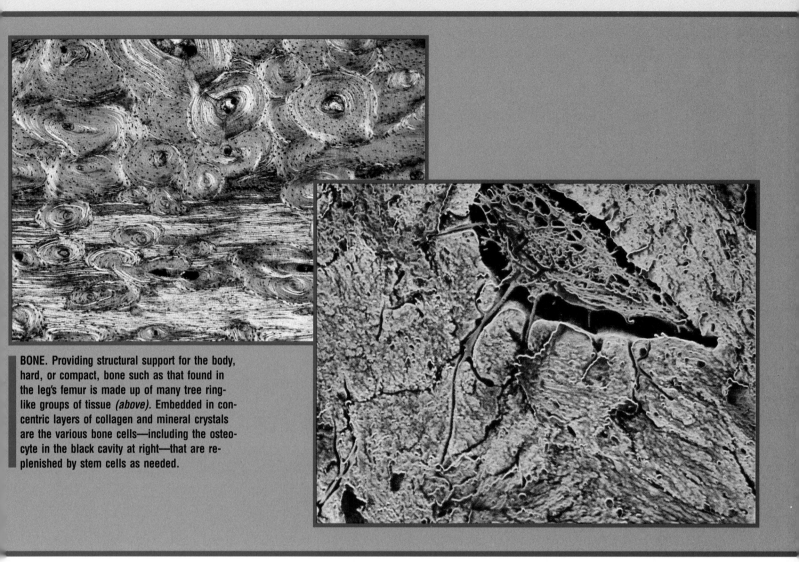

BONE. Providing structural support for the body, hard, or compact, bone such as that found in the leg's femur is made up of many tree ring-like groups of tissue *(above)*. Embedded in concentric layers of collagen and mineral crystals are the various bone cells—including the osteocyte in the black cavity at right—that are replenished by stem cells as needed.

cells from long-lived animals, such as elephants, divide more times than do cells from creatures with short life spans, indicating that each cell has an internal counting mechanism of some kind that remembers how many times it has divided and halts the process after a set number.

This cellular memory even defies attempts to trick cells into forgetting. For example, when fibroblasts from human embryos are frozen in liquid nitrogen after 20 divisions and later thawed, they will undergo 30 more doublings and then stop. If they have undergone 10 divisions before being frozen, they will divide 40 more times after thawing out. With clocklike consistency, the cells seem to count up to 50 divisions and then stop. Even cells frozen for as long as 13 years have retained the memory of how many divisions they have already undergone.

Scientists now think the cellular clock lies deep within the nucleus, embedded in the coded segments of DNA. When a cell gets the signal to divide, the 23 pairs of chromosomes in its nucleus duplicate themselves and split into two strands, each with the same number of pairs. The original nucleus disappears, and the strands migrate to opposite sides of the cell, where each grouping forms a new nucleus. Soon the entire cell, which has also doubled its entire contents, pulls apart to form two identical cells.

Researchers have found that a cell's chromosomes have tails at both ends that shrink slightly every time the cell

Permanent Cells

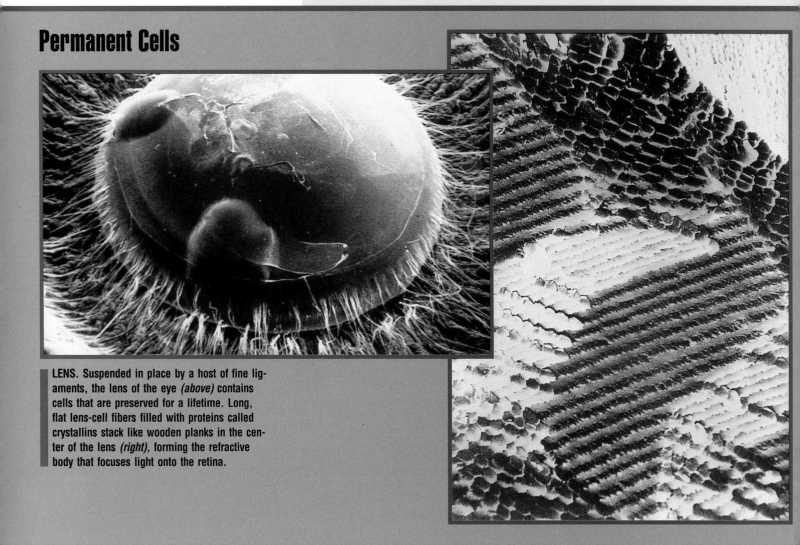

LENS. Suspended in place by a host of fine ligaments, the lens of the eye *(above)* contains cells that are preserved for a lifetime. Long, flat lens-cell fibers filled with proteins called crystallins stack like wooden planks in the center of the lens *(right)*, forming the refractive body that focuses light onto the retina.

divides. These tails, called telomeres (derived from the Greek words for "end" and "part"), contain thousands of segments of dummy DNA—that is, they hold no vital genetic information. Researchers think these nonsense sequences may act as protective caps of sorts, helping to stabilize the tips of chromosomes and to keep the chains from breaking apart and hooking back together in abnormal, possibly dangerous, combinations. With every division, telomeres lose from 50 to 200 of these sequences, a consistency that scientists have found makes the length of the telomeres an amazingly accurate predictor of a cell's age and division potential.

Telomeres have recently been cited as important players in the spread of cancer, which arises when aberrant cells, somehow impervious to the normal effects of aging, proliferate out of control. After a certain number of divisions, when their telomeres are significantly shortened, normal cells lapse into senescence and usually die. Cancer cells apparently avoid this fate by activating a dormant gene that works to prevent the telomeres from shedding. This gene triggers the production of an enzyme called telomerase, which actually adds more DNA material to the telomeres every time they divide, thus extending the life of the cell indefinitely. When the enzyme is blocked, however, the cell quickly loses its immortality. Researchers are now trying to develop drugs that directly inhibit telomerase and, as one expert put it, "remortalize" cancer cells to halt the spread of the disease.

One fact of human life that has long puzzled scientists is that some of the

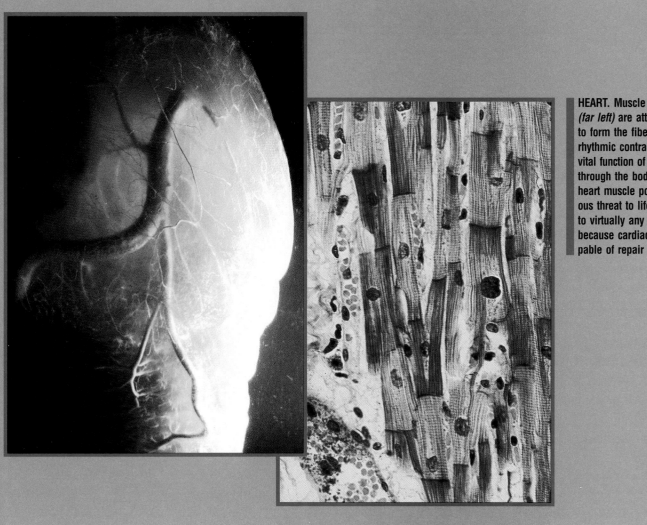

body's most essential organs and tissues are made up of cells that do not replace themselves, whether by division or by stem cell progeny. During embryonic development, each of us is equipped with a given complement of cells for the brain, the heart, and the nervous system; their numbers are huge but finite, and these so-called permanent cells must last a lifetime. Meanwhile, cells in other organs such as the spleen—which the body does not even need to survive—have an apparently unlimited capacity for replacement and growth.

So far, no good explanation has emerged for this seeming paradox, although researchers have advanced a number of theories. In the case of permanent neurons in the brain, for example, scientists believe regeneration would create more problems than it would solve, since it would be extremely difficult for newly formed cells to retrace the intricate pattern of connections that linked the original neurons to their neighbors. Or it may be that permanent cells evolved as a way to protect the organism against high rates of mutation. The more often a cell divides, the greater the chances that a tear or mistake will occur in the DNA as chromosomes are repeatedly pulled apart. When this occurs in sperm or egg cells, the mutation can be passed along to offspring; when it occurs in other cells of the body, any change in genetic expression affects only that individual.

Two scientists working independently have come up with a theory that suggests the common goal of all body cells is not so much to prolong the life of an individual organism but to ensure survival of the species as a whole. Thomas B. L. Kirkwood, a gerontologist at the Medical Research Council in London, and molecular biologist Richard G. Cutler at the National Institute on Aging, a branch of the National Institutes of Health (NIH) located in Baltimore, insist that cells in the body are designed to last only as long as it takes to pass the organism's genes along to the next generation; what happens after that, biologically speaking, is irrelevant. One-celled life forms, according to this argument, must be able to replicate or risk the species dying out. In humans, by contrast, the nonreproductive cells of the body must last just long enough for the individual to contribute to the gene pool by mating and raising offspring, perhaps no more than 40 years. At that point, say Kirkwood and Cutler, most of the cells in the body are expendable; as they lose the ability to respond to environmental stress, the person eventually dies.

On September 5, 1913, an article appeared on page 8 of the New York Times under a headline that read simply, "The Fountain of Youth." Despite its vague title and modest placement —alongside a notice about an upcom-

ing golf tournament—the article went on to describe an earthshaking medical achievement. Readers that day were greeted with news of a scientific breakthrough that, as was reported nonchalantly near the end of the article, "may prove the most significant made in the history of medicine."

Alexis Carrel, a surgeon and biologist at the Rockefeller Institute for Medical Research, had made a startling discovery. A specialist in grafting blood vessels and organs, the French-born scientist had managed, in his words, to "activate artificially the process of repair" in animal wounds by applying dressings made from various animal tissues and organs. In one experiment, he used a pulp made from a canine thyroid gland to treat wounds on a dog. Not only did these extracts increase the healing process in the animals "marvelously," as the New York Times put it, but they also accelerated—by as much as 40 times the normal rate—the growth of connective tissue isolated in glass jars. Carrel did not know it at the time, but he had proved the existence of a group of proteins now known as growth factors.

Carrel was no stranger to celebrity. A year earlier, he had earned widespread acclaim when he won the 1912

Nobel Prize for research in medicine. In a famous experiment, he had kept a fragment of a chicken's heart alive and beating in a lab dish for 120 days, marking the first time anyone had sustained living tissue outside the body. His later success at spurring growth in animal tissue came after long hours of experimentation with different solutions and dressings designed to make cells divide. In the course of his research, Carrel found that each type of tissue grew faster and for longer periods of time when immersed in a certain artificial culture—what he called "an optimum medium"—than in the body's own natural environment.

It was as if Carrel had confirmed the starry-eyed notions of medieval alchemists and their attempts to concoct magical healing elixirs, or had given credence to the musings of explorer Juan Ponce de León, who believed that soothing, magical waters could restore wasted tissues. But by establishing a link between the rate of cell growth and the biological medium that surrounds cells, Carrel launched a new era of medical research: He unearthed the first clues to how human cells communicate with each other for repairing and renewing the body.

In his writings, Carrel speculated that one day the effects of these substances on cell growth and death would be "investigated profitably."

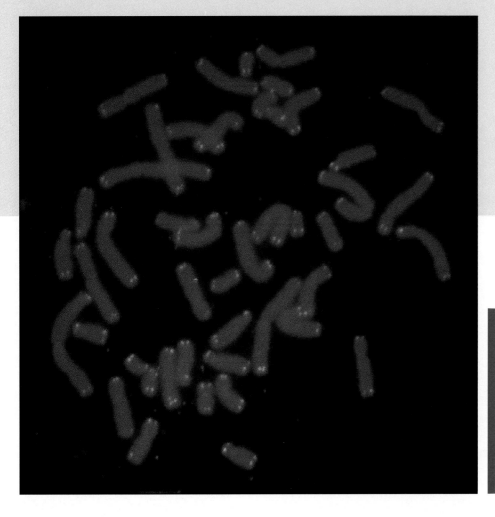

Aglow with the aid of fluorescent dye, segments of DNA known as telomeres *(yellow)* dot the ends of human chromosomes. Telomeres serve as a kind of protective cap, in that they prevent coded genetic information from being lost from the ends of chromosomes, and exposed genetic material can lead to damage or death of a cell. Researchers speculate that telomeres limit the life spans of cells by shortening with each cell division.

Little did the scientist know that his area of research would balloon into a multibillion-dollar industry bent on producing growth factors to do everything from helping the body heal faster to coaxing bone marrow to produce greater quantities of disease-fighting cells, such as in cases where a patient's immune system has been weakened by chemotherapy.

Decades after his prizewinning achievement, Carrel continued his scientific excursions into the chemical communications system among cells. In one series of experiments, the scientist had noticed that blood clots mysteriously broke down in the pres-

ence of minced tumor tissue. After more research, he was able to isolate certain substances in tumors that act to dissolve clotting proteins. It turns out that when new blood vessels are needed in the body—say, after a severe wound—cells that line the inside walls of existing vessels secrete these protein-dissolving enzymes. These chemicals digest their way through vessel walls and allow the cells to grow out into wound areas to supply the damaged tissues with blood.

While working with blood clots, Carrel found that these clusters of coagulating blood have growth-inducing properties of their own: When fibroblasts from chick embryos were placed next to blood clots in a laboratory dish, the cells began multiplying at a rapid clip. Clearly, he thought, some

substance in the clots was sending a signal to the fibroblasts to reproduce.

Although Carrel did not have techniques sophisticated enough to isolate and identify these substances, his work laid the foundation for a new generation of scientists examining the complex behavior of cells. In the years that followed, researchers experimenting with human serum— blood that has been stripped of its red blood cells and other proteins as a result of clotting—found that substances in the serum also caused cells in laboratory dishes to divide and multiply. In other words, growth enhancers were seemingly everywhere,

Self-Restoring Cells
That Protect Vision

Although the body's permanent cells cannot reproduce, most of them possess unique abilities to restore some of their own parts—a feat dramatically illustrated by the photoreceptor cells called rods that are found at the back of the eyeball in the retina. Rods—so named for their long, thin shape—are responsible for visual acuity during the dim evening hours. (Another group of photoreceptors, called cones, perceive color and fine detail.)

Certain components of the rod cell, including its nucleus and inner segment (*below*), remain relatively unchanged throughout a person's lifetime. However, the outer segment of each cell is in constant flux. This region consists of a stack of about 1,000 disks, each containing visual pigments necessary for the proper absorption of light. New disks forming at the bottom of the segment push older disks toward the top at such a rapid rate that all 1,000 disks are replaced in just 10 days (*far right*). As the older disks reach the tip of the outer segment, they are removed by cells in the epithelial layer.

Experts believe that the process of disk renewal helps protect photoreceptors from long-term injury. Because the eye is the most oxygenated area of the body, it is at risk for damage caused when light interacts with oxygen, creating unstable, toxic oxygen molecules known as free radicals. But as long as the disk-restoration mechanism remains active, the rod cells may well last a lifetime.

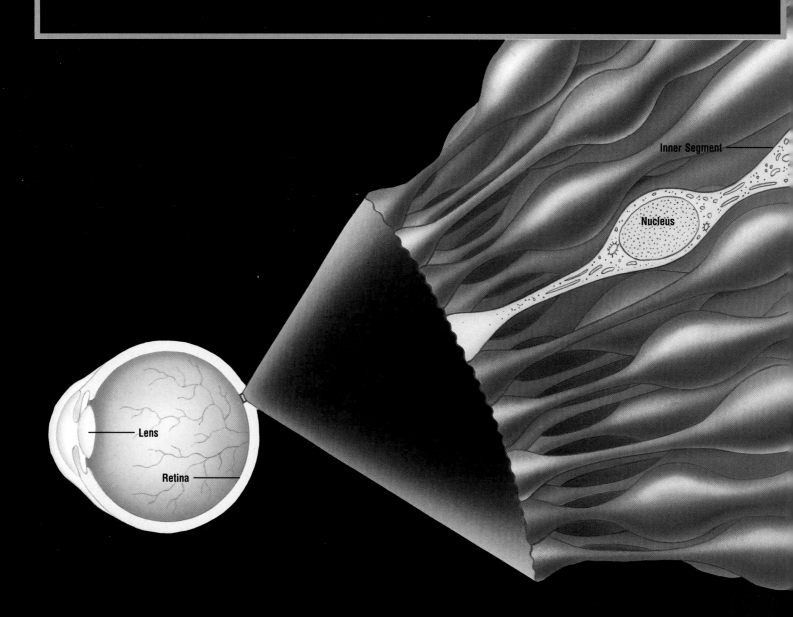

Inner Segment

Nucleus

Lens

Retina

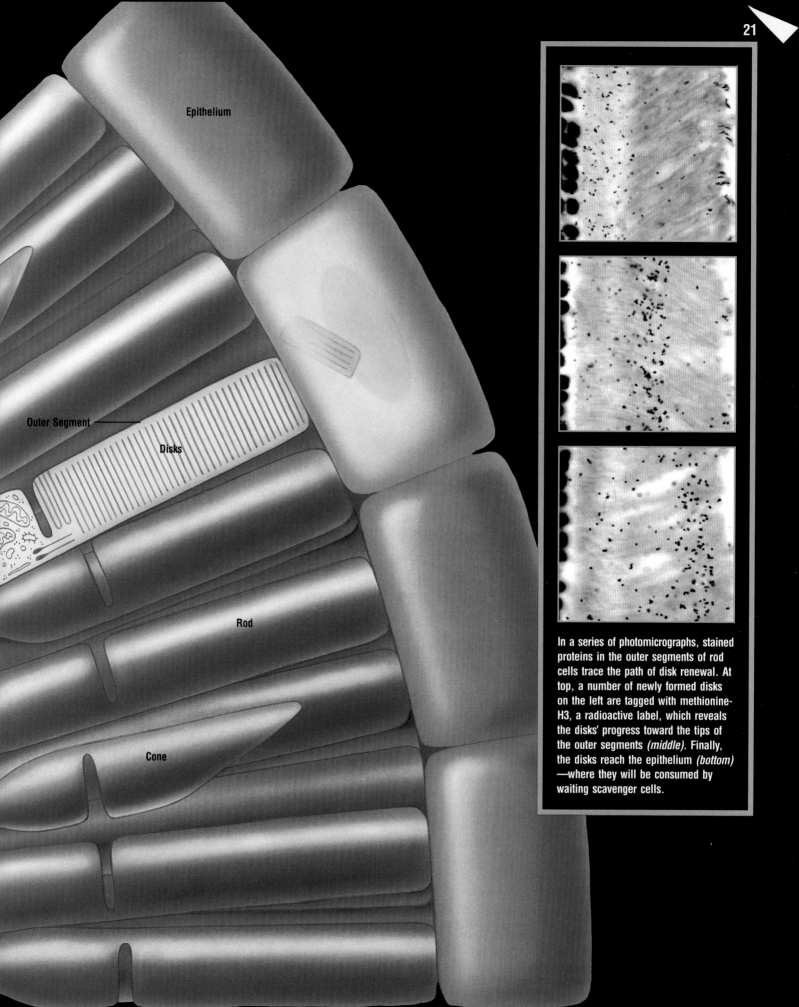

Epithelium

Outer Segment

Disks

Rod

Cone

In a series of photomicrographs, stained proteins in the outer segments of rod cells trace the path of disk renewal. At top, a number of newly formed disks on the left are tagged with methionine-H3, a radioactive label, which reveals the disks' progress toward the tips of the outer segments *(middle)*. Finally, the disks reach the epithelium *(bottom)* —where they will be consumed by waiting scavenger cells.

not just in the tissues and organs.

One of the most significant revelations in the field occurred in 1950, when a cell biologist named Rita Levi-Montalcini, working in the laboratory of neuroembryologist Viktor Hamburger of Washington University in St. Louis, deduced that there must be a substance that attracts nerves to body tissues. In an effort to learn more about how nerves develop, she had been conducting experiments grafting tumors from mice onto chick embryos. Eight days after transplanting the tumors, she placed a slide of tissue under a microscope for a look. As she later wrote, "The scenario that presented itself to my eyes was so extraordinary that I thought I might be hallucinating." A thick network of nerve fibers had sprouted in the embryo, spreading tentacle-like not just into the developing organs of the animal but into the tumor itself.

Levi-Montalcini presented her findings at a conference of the New York Academy of Sciences in 1951 to mixed reviews. While one prominent colleague pronounced hers the "most exciting discovery of the year," other researchers were skeptical about her descriptions of a "nerve growth-promoting agent" in mouse tumors. Nonetheless, she had no other explanation for what she described as a "halo" of nerves cascading from the chick embryo. So she pressed ahead,

determined to find further evidence to bolster her theory that an unknown chemical in the tissues had induced the growth of nerve fibers.

Because the labs at Washington University were not equipped for the type of experiments she wanted to perform, Levi-Montalcini traveled to the Biophysics Institute in Rio de Janeiro to work with Hertha Meyer, an expert in cell culture. Their key experiment was similar to Levi-Montalcini's earlier tests, but this time, instead of using whole embryos, the scientists cultured mouse tumors with ganglia, or clumps of nerve cells, taken from the spines of embryonic chicks. The results came even more quickly and more convincingly than before. Within 10 hours, a dense fringe of nerve fibers had erupted from each of the ganglia, extending outward like myriad rays of the sun. At last, Levi-Montalcini had the proof she needed. The experiment showed not only that nerve fibers could be coaxed to grow, but also that the growth agent was produced in the tumor tissue, not in the embryo itself.

In 1953 Levi-Montalcini returned to St. Louis and teamed up with Stanley Cohen, a young biochemist newly hired at Washington University. To-

gether, with the support of Viktor Hamburger, they began trying to trace the exact chemical structure of the growth-promoting substance, which they dubbed nerve growth factor. Cohen had only vague notions about the nervous system, but he was an expert at isolating biochemicals. After more than a year of painstaking work, he managed to zero in on the growth agent in the mouse tumor. He ultimately identified the chemical as a protein, but at first he suspected that it was a viruslike complex made up of nucleic acids and proteins. At a colleague's suggestion, Cohen decided to test his analysis by exposing embryonic chick ganglia to growth-promoting factor that had been treated with snake venom, which contains an enzyme that breaks down such nucleic acids.

The results were startling. Instead of dissolving the nucleoproteins and stopping the proliferation of nerve fibers in the ganglia, as Cohen expected it would, the snake venom produced the opposite result. It actually enhanced the growth of nerve cells. Evidently the venom contained a factor endowed with the same nerve growth-stimulating properties found in the mouse tumors.

Armed with these new revelations, Cohen—who transferred to Vanderbilt University in the early 1960s—embarked on a search for growth factors in the salivary extracts of other crea-

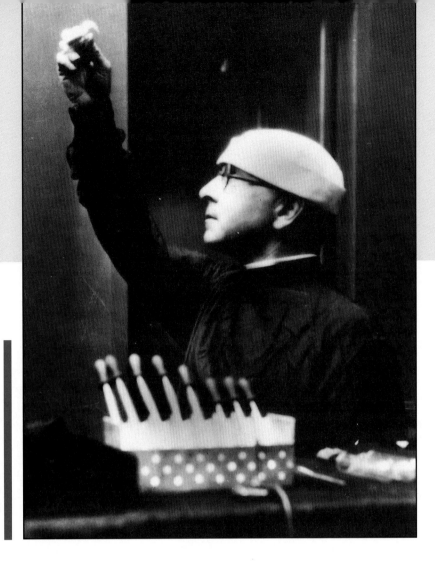

Biologist Alexis Carrel, shown here in the 1930s, carried out pioneering research in tissue grafting and wound healing that earned him the 1912 Nobel Prize in medicine. Carrel's experiments with animal tissues kept alive outside the body—in his own specially brewed media—proved that the health of a cell depends on substances in its environment.

tures. He wondered if animals, which often lick their wounds, might be conferring some kind of natural healing agent to the damaged tissue. To test his hypothesis, Cohen injected newborn mice with mouse salivary extracts. Young mice normally grow teeth eight to 10 days after they are born and open their eyes after 12 or 14 days. Amazingly, though, the animals that received Cohen's saliva injections sprouted teeth five to six days after birth and opened their eyes after only six or seven days.

Cohen identified the stimulating substance as another protein, and he labeled this one an epidermal growth factor after discovering it had a powerful proliferative effect on the epidermal, or skin, cells as well as on the cells that make up connective tissue in mice. Later, he discovered the same growth-stimulating chemical in human urine. This finding suggested that a protein similar to epidermal growth factor might be commonly cast off as a waste product by tissues.

Some three decades after their pioneering work, Stanley Cohen and Rita Levi-Montalcini shared the 1986 Nobel Prize in physiology and medicine for discovering the first two growth factors. Today, researchers using techniques developed by the two scientists continue to unlock new secrets about the actions of growth factors. The study of these remarkable proteins has, in fact, become one of the richest and most promising in all of biology, for it gives scientists an unprecedented opportunity to eavesdrop on the body's complex cellular dialogue. Some experts are already drawing parallels between the medical impact of growth factors and that of antibiotics a half-century ago.

Judging by what has been learned about these chemical messengers, the comparison does not seem too far-fetched. Growth factors have been found to regulate not only cell proliferation but also a broad range of cell activities, from inflammation and tissue repair to differentiation and survival. They also can stimulate the pro-

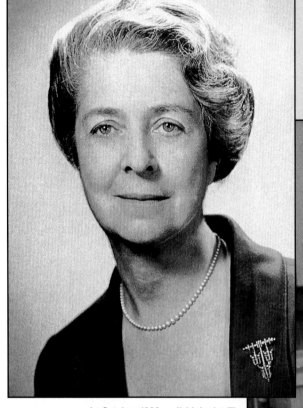

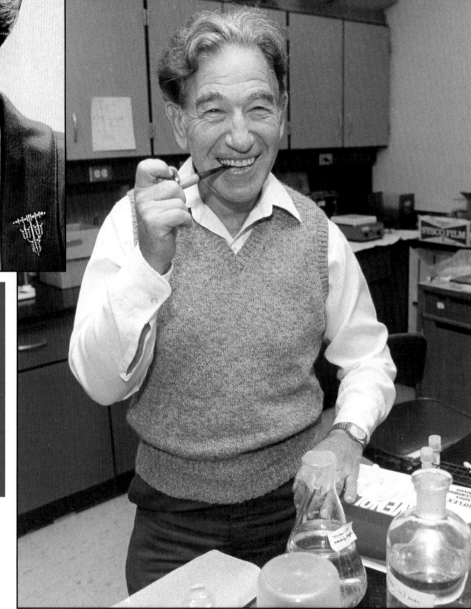

In October 1986, cell biologist Rita Levi-Montalcini *(above)* shared the Nobel Prize in medicine with biochemist Stanley Cohen, shown at right in his lab at Vanderbilt University after learning the news. Levi-Montalcini had worked with Cohen at Washington University in the 1950s, when they began the research that would lead them to identify the first growth factors.

duction of proteins needed to restore the extracellular matrix, the mesh of elastic material that holds cells in place throughout the body. Of equal interest to researchers is that growth factors, which are clearly essential to cell division and development, also have a dark side. Sometimes, for reasons unknown, they go haywire, turning healthy cells into malignant ones that multiply out of control.

Since Cohen and Levi-Montalcini's groundbreaking discovery, the number of known growth factors has soared to almost 100, due largely to an explosion in recombinant DNA biotechnology, techniques that allow researchers to isolate the responsible genes and then manufacture large quantities of the chemicals artificially in the laboratory. Scientists disagree on whether all of the body's growth factors have been identified; some "discoveries," in fact, have turned out to be no more than combinations of already-identified growth factors working in tandem.

The practical applications of growth factors seem boundless, and in some cases this promise has already blossomed into reality. In Japan, for instance, people hoping to cure stomach ulcers are gulping down doses of tissue-enhancing epidermal growth factor; doctors in Italy prescribe the same substance for patients with eye injuries. The use of growth factors in

the United States is developing more slowly, mostly because of concerns expressed by the Food and Drug Administration that these substances could spur abnormal cellular growth. Even so, in 1989 the FDA approved for clinical use the growth factor erythropoietin, which stimulates the bone marrow to produce greater quantities of red blood cells. This property makes the drug useful for kidney dialysis patients or for people with chronic anemia who otherwise would require frequent blood transfusions.

In years to come, medications derived from the human body's own stores of cellular growth enhancers may help to smooth out wrinkles or even battle cancer. One class of growth factors, those called colony-stimulating factors, bolsters the immune system by increasing production of disease-fighting white blood cells. Injections of these substances allow people to tolerate stronger doses of chemotherapy, especially in cases where the levels of radiation or chemicals necessary to kill cancerous tumors would damage the immune system. Soon, scientists predict, growth factors will play a major role in everyday medicine, enlisting the body's community of cells to mend

broken bones, say, or to patch the skin of burn victims—even to coax new growth from severed nerves.

In one of the most promising applications of growth factors—and arguably the most bizarre—scientists are looking at ways to trick the body, in effect, into growing replacement organs alongside those that are beyond medical treatment. The efforts began with experiments in the late 1980s by molecular biologist Thomas Maciag of the American Red Cross and biochemist John Thompson with a protein called fibroblast growth factor. FGF-1, as it is known, is one of the substances responsible for triggering the intense cell proliferation that turns a fertilized egg into a fetus. The cells of most adults harbor little of the protein, and it shows up only when cellular cleanup crews discharge it in the area of a cut or other wound.

In 1987 Thompson conducted some intriguing experiments with FGF-1 while he was working at the National Heart, Blood, and Lung Institute of NIH in Bethesda, Maryland. He and some co-workers soaked surgical sponges in the growth factor and implanted them into animals. Later, when he peered inside, he discovered that the chemical had apparently triggered a frenzy of blood vessel growth. The sponges dissolved after two weeks, however, and the new blood vessels began to collapse.

Cell Growth

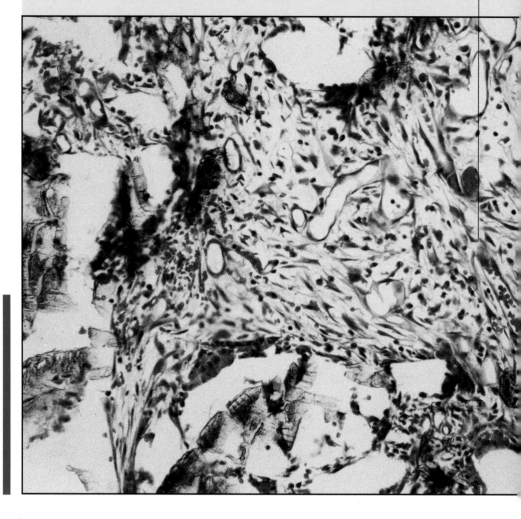

This microscopic view shows the results of a feat of biological engineering, in which strands of the synthetic fiber Gore-Tex were soaked in collagen and growth factor and then implanted near a rat's liver. A mass of tissue composed of growing cells formed around the fibers. This so-called organoid was linked to the liver by blood vessels but developed no specific function. However, some researchers believe they may one day be able to grow useful organs and tissue for humans in this way.

Thompson got in touch with Maciag at the American Red Cross's laboratory in Rockville, Maryland, and also with Christian Haudenschild, a pathologist at Boston University. The three men, who had met during a conference years earlier, agreed to work together on the problem. The scientists decided to try the same experiments but this time using Gore-Tex, a synthetic material often used to make waterproof sporting and outdoor apparel. Unlike surgical sponges, which are designed to break down quickly in the body, Gore-Tex does not dissolve; luckily, Gore-Tex also does not cause an immunological reaction.

After sterilizing the synthetic fibers, the researchers dipped them in growth factor and implanted them next to the liver of a laboratory rat. When they examined the area several weeks later, they were astonished by what they saw. Not only were newly formed blood vessels emanating from the rat's liver, but they were nourishing a growing cellular mass on the Gore-Tex patch. Haudenschild dubbed the mass an organoid. Although the embryonic structure had not yet assumed a specialized function, it was equipped with such a variety of cell types that the researchers believed it could develop, eventually, into a mature organ. In this case, however, development of the organoid was cut short because the growth factor remained active in the rat's body for only a limited time.

Today scientists on the cutting edge of biotechnology are exploring how organoids can be put to practical use. Before long, surgeons might be able to replace damaged or diseased blood vessels in the body with networks of veins, arteries, and capillaries that have all been grown in such pseudo-organs. Thompson, who now teaches at the University of Alabama in Birmingham, predicts that within

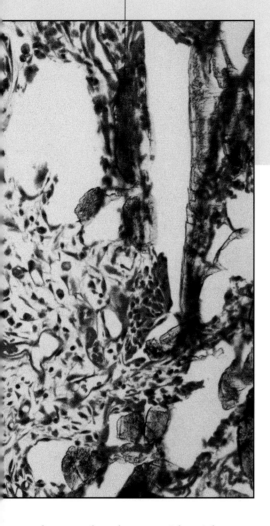

Gore-Tex Fibers

the next decade organoids might even be induced to take the final steps toward specialization, serving as backup spleens or livers, for example, when their natural counterparts fail.

For most of this century, scientists believed that growth factors such as FGF-I belonged to a unique family of body substances biochemically distinct from hormones, the chemical message bearers of the endocrine system. Because of this perceived distinction, hormone research and the

study of growth factors proceeded along separate tracks. In fact, however, the two are functionally similar, differing only in their origin and the distances they travel. Hormones are secreted by specialized cells in certain glands and organs; they typically cover great distances in the body and take effect relatively slowly. Growth factors, for their part, are produced by almost all the tissues in the body and tend to have a more localized effect.

The distinction was proved false in the 1970s. First, cell biologists Gordon Sato and Isumi Hayashi of the University of California at San Diego showed that endocrine glands—the thyroid, adrenal, and pituitary glands—produce chemicals that cause fibroblast cells to multiply, a phenomenon characteristic of growth factors. Shortly after, a decade or so before he helped create the first organoid, Thomas Maciag demonstrated that even the parts of the brain that rule the endocrine system and the autonomic nervous system produce factors that influence growth in a wide variety of cells.

Today some scientists speculate that the endocrine and autonomic nervous systems are the regulators of the body's renewal and repair efforts. Both systems are governed by the hypothalamus, an olive-size structure in the center of the brain, which carries on a constant dialogue with the cerebral cortex and the limbic system, the

seats of higher thought and emotion, respectively. The hypothalamus also communicates with the nearby pituitary gland through a bridge called the pituitary stalk.

On orders from higher brain centers, the hypothalamus signals the pituitary gland to increase or suppress the release of growth factors into the bloodstream. During an infection or invasion by disease-causing microorganisms, for example, the hypothalamus rallies bodily defenses through the familiar response known as fever. In the first stages of fever, scavenger cells called macrophages near the affected area release growth factors into the bloodstream that activate the immune system. These chemicals also make their way to the hypothalamus, which responds by raising the brain's thermostat. Suddenly, the body feels cold. Shivering and chills result, which in turn stimulate a broad range of other defensive responses.

Such precise choreography requires that each cell population—blood cells, muscle cells, and nerve cells, for example—be able to call on its neighbors at a moment's notice and to respond to the requirements of others with equal dispatch. To help make communication more immediate, growth factors secreted by one set of cells are often absorbed rapidly by other cells in the vicinity. This property also confines the body's natural healing response to a local area, rather than triggering activity all over the body. For example, epidermal growth factor secreted by connective tissue and certain other types of cells prompts skin cells to multiply—but only in the area of a wound.

Growth factors and hormones act on cells in two basic ways. Some, such as steroid and thyroid hormones, pass right from the bloodstream into the cell through the cellular membrane and activate special proteins inside the cell itself. Others work by hooking up with molecules known as receptors that protrude by the hundreds of thousands from the cell's surface. When growth factors brush up against a cell's surface, they latch onto certain receptors in much the same way as keys fit into specific locks. Each receptor transfers the signal from the outside to the inside of the membrane, where chains of messenger proteins wait to shuttle the signal deeper into the cell. Special messenger proteins translate the message into a type of cellular code and pass the contents to the nucleus, thus activating genes that enable the cell to carry out the appropriate response.

Sometimes after a growth factor has attached to a cell surface receptor, the whole complex is swallowed by the target cell: A coated vesicle, or tiny cellular cyst, engulfs the complex and escorts it toward the nucleus. In this way, once a cell has had contact with a growth factor, the number of available receptors on the cell surface decreases—a mechanism, scientists believe, that may prevent cells from overproliferating. It also could be a way to shift concentrations of specific receptors to new locations on the cell.

Although growth factors are clearly a vital catalyst for cell division, they can turn deadly when the process goes awry. In the case of cancer, the genes that carry instructions for growth factor receptors on the outside of cells and for messenger proteins on the inside undergo mutations that can transform healthy cells into malignant ones. These abnormal cells disobey the usual constraints on cell division, and their wild proliferation can form tumors. The mutant genes sometimes even order the host cell to produce faulty receptors, which then behave as if growth factors are constantly hooked up and present.

In other cases, healthy cells can react to an overabundance of growth factor and become "frozen" in a heightened state of stimulation. Per-haps the best example of this is heart disease, the most prevalent cause of death in Western civilization. The problem arises when growth factors derived from platelets—essential clotting agents in the blood—direct the construction of an excessive, sticky latticework of connective tissue and fatty deposits inside the walls of blood vessels. These deposits are the principal villain in atherosclerosis, better known as hardening of the arteries (*pages 72-85*).

As even Alexis Carrel recognized nearly a century ago, without some regulating system, cells activated by growth factors would quickly proliferate out of control. If cells were allowed to reproduce without restraint, he said, "the organs and tissues would lose their relative size and morphology, and the whole body would become monstrous." Since Carrel's day, scientists have confirmed that the body does have ways to counteract or halt the effects of growth enhancers—but the mechanisms of growth inhibition are not as well understood as those of growth stimulation.

When the skin is cut, cells at the margin of the wound are prompted to divide and spread over the damaged surface until they have laid down a new layer of growth. At that point, the rapid proliferation and movement abruptly stops. Epithelial cells cultivated in a lab dish will do the same,

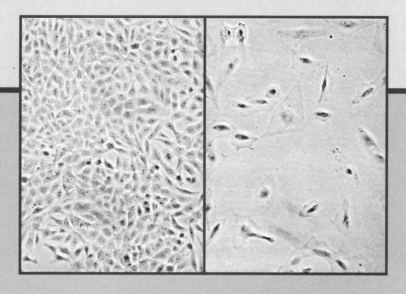

A New Industry: Seeking Uses for Growth Factors

Stanley Cohen and Rita Levi-Montalcini's 1954 discovery of the first growth factor sent barely a ripple through the scientific community. Some 30 years later, however, the advent of recombinant DNA technology inspired a new generation of researchers—and biotechnology firms—to explore whether these miracle proteins could be manufactured and then used to cure diseases, heal cuts and bruises, and even slow the aging process.

Growth factors are a group of proteins in the body that monitor cell development and proliferation. Some encourage cell production; epidermal growth factor, for instance, is used to produce new skin for grafts on burn victims. Other growth factors act as inhibitors, arresting cell division. In the images above, human lung-cell division—normally prolific (left)—ceases after an application of an inhibiting factor (right). Researchers are investigating whether inhibitors may stifle the uncontrolled multiplying of cells that characterizes cancer.

By the mid-1990s, three types of artificially produced factors had already been approved by the U.S. Food and Drug Administration, one for use with severe anemia, the other two for cancer. Waging war on such lethal diseases with naturally occurring agents is an attractive alternative to the devastating effects some chemical therapies can have. Unfortunately, growth factors can also disrupt vital body processes. The same factor that arrests lung-cell division has been identified as the culprit in a kidney condition in which the kidney's filtration units become blocked by an excess of surrounding tissue.

In any case, researchers are finding it easier to locate genes that produce specific factors than to identify uses for those factors. Scientists experimenting with growth factor "cocktails," for example, have run into a fair measure of complexity. They have discovered that some effective applications depend on interactions among a variety of substances in addition to the factors themselves. One crucial element for the future is whether manufacturers intent on mass commercial production of growth factors will be able to prove that once they have turned these factors on, they have a way to turn them back off.

dividing to form a single-cell layer until they come in contact with neighboring cells. Then they stop dividing.

At first, scientists thought growth was halted due to a so-called contact inhibition; the cells presumably sent chemical signals to each other when they touched. But later experiments revealed that cells divide more rapidly in a freshly prepared medium than they do in a solution that has just bathed other cells—suggesting that cells compete for small amounts of growth factor and cease dividing when the chemical fuel is depleted. This competition appears to prevent cells from proliferating beyond a certain population density.

But limiting the supply of growth factors is only one strategy for regulating cell proliferation. Recent evidence has shown that the body also produces growth inhibitors, or a set of "off" proteins that counteract the "on" signals issued by growth enhancers. In fact, it has become clear that cancer is not just a result of excessive growth factors or mutant genes forcing cells to divide. Tumors can also come about from the failure of cells to express or respond to growth inhibitors.

As it happens, the same molecules that inhibit growth in some cells actually promote growth in others, and reaction to a common signaling molecule can differ greatly from one type of cell to the next. For example, the protein interleukin-1, which prompts the proliferation of infection-fighting T cells, also retards the growth of endothelial cells necessary to heal wounds. Similarly, transforming growth factor beta, a growth stimulator for a number of tumor cells in the body, severely inhibits the proliferation of many types of epithelial cells and curbs the production of lymphocytes in the blood.

Scientists think a particular chemical's effect may depend on the target cell's internal signaling machinery as well as on the kind of receptors it has on its surface. But while some progress has been made in decoding many aspects of the extracellular communication, the internal goings-on are still shrouded in mystery. For example, researchers have identified certain internal enzymes that counteract the activity of the proteins that translate and deliver messages to the cell nucleus; at this point, however, they can only speculate on how growth inhibitors binding to the cell's surface activate these enzymes and somehow shut off the signal to divide.

In any event, as is true of almost everything else that goes on in the body, growth factors and growth inhibitors do not work in isolation but can be understood only within the larger context. For example, many growth factors and inhibitors are collected and then released in the body through the complex of proteins and polysaccharides that makes up the extracellular matrix. Various kinds of molecular bonds in the matrix create tissues of different strength, flexibility, and permeability, thereby lending shape to everything from the teeth and tendons to the transparent cornea of the eye.

Scientists long regarded the matrix as little more than an inert scaffolding for bone and connective tissue. Recently, however, researchers have found the extracellular matrix to be an essential part of wound healing, acting as choreographer and controller of cell behavior. Soon after a cut, gash, or scrape occurs, the extracellular matrix in the injured region binds up fibroblast growth factor in high concentrations, thus signaling nearby cells to begin multiplying.

The matrix then directs the healing process by guiding skin and fibroblast cells toward the target zone and providing binding sites for the cells in the injured area. When the cells are alerted to a crisis, they change the chemical structure of special protein receptors called integrins on their outer surface; the altered integrins help the cells, in effect, skate along the matrix until they arrive at the wound site.

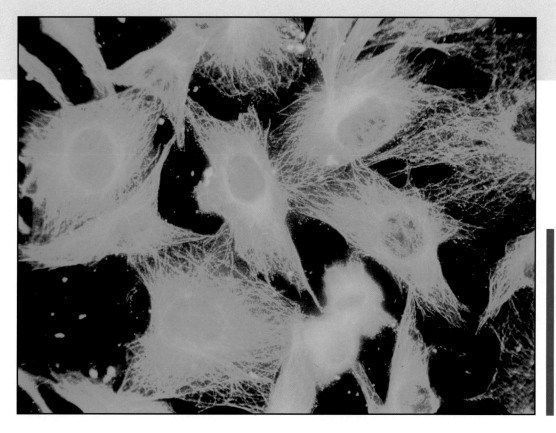

Microscopic fibers—stained with a dye that fluoresces green in ultraviolet light—make up these mammalian kidney cells' intricate cytoskeletons. A network of microtubules and special filaments, the cytoskeleton conducts growth factors and other important proteins between the cell's cytoplasm and its nucleus.

The integrins then change composition again, helping the cells to anchor themselves in the matrix. By producing certain dissolving enzymes, the cells can take shortcuts through the extracellular matrix, burrowing their way through scabs, for example, for quick access to the wound site.

In instances of damage or loss, the body's cellular army often responds by generating fresh reinforcements; surviving cells begin multiplying to fill out their ranks. But injured cells also can act to prevent damage from persisting in the body. Sometimes, for reasons that are not clearly understood, cells simply destroy themselves—when supplies of a particular hormone run low, for instance, or when some types of immune cells come in contact with certain harmful invaders. Cells also shut down when they are exposed to sudden extreme heat, mild poisoning, or too much ultraviolet radiation.

Such external shocks can seriously damage a cell's genetic storehouse, and what is in effect cellular suicide may be a way to keep damaged DNA from accumulating in the body and to prevent the transfer of possibly al-tered genes to future cell generations.

When cells self-destruct, the nucleus and cytoplasm shrink and fragment, and the remains are absorbed by other cells. This process is called apoptosis, a word derived from the Greek for "falling off." Evidence suggests that cell suicide, which appears to be common among most animals, may be controlled by signals from other cells, and that failure of damaged cells to die can lead to the abnormal growth of tumors.

But not every cell does itself in at

Holding Cells Together: The Extracellular Matrix

The body's various tissues and organs are not composed of cells alone. They get their structure from what is known as the extracellular matrix, an intricate mesh— of several different substances—that binds the tissue cells together. In the case of connective tissue such as that making up tendons and cartilage, the extracellular matrix actually forms a greater proportion of the tissue than do the cells themselves.

Extracellular matrix is produced by cells, and its characteristics vary with cell types. For example, bone cells secrete a specific mix of substances that creates a relatively inflexible extracellular web, giving bone its rigidity. Cells of other tissues may generate very elastic or even aqueous versions of the matrix.

The matrix typically consists of polysaccharides (a carbohydrate) and proteins. The former provide a gel-like base for other matrix components, and the latter give the matrix its structure and given degree of elasticity.

the first sign of trouble. Damaged cells are also capable of mounting a formidable defense in a crisis. When cells are subjected to assault, they increase production of certain molecules that buffer them from harm. This reaction—whether in the tissues of feverish children stricken with disease, in the organs of heart-attack victims, or in the cells of cancer patients receiving chemotherapy—is called the cell stress response, and, like many scientific breakthroughs, it came to light almost by accident.

In the early 1960s, scientists hoping to learn more about the function of genes in animal development concentrated much of their attention on the tiny fruit fly *Drosophila melanogaster.* The reason had to do with a unique feature of the insect's genetic makeup: Cells from the fruit fly's salivary glands have a cluster of chromosomes that contain thousands of times the usual amount of DNA. The chromosomes, grouped side by side, are so huge that they show up clearly under an ordinary light microscope. Furthermore, when certain genes are activated, distinct regions of the chromosomes puff out. Thus, they make perfect models for the study of gene expression. Geneticist F. M. Ritossa of the International Laboratory of Genetics and Biophysics in Naples noticed that ambient temperatures slightly higher than normal for the flies pro-

voked a unique pattern of puffing in these chromosomes. Researchers later found that this heat-induced puffing was accompanied by the production of what became known as heat-shock proteins, or stress proteins.

Eventually it became clear that the enlarged section of chromosome marked the sites where the cell's genetic machinery was creating the messenger RNA that would carry the instructions for synthesizing these

proteins. Cell biologists were particularly intrigued by several aspects of this cell stress response. The newly created proteins not only helped the cells break up and dispose of chemicals damaged by heat, they actually assisted in the production of replacement chemicals.

More intriguing, perhaps, was the fact that the proteins remained present in cells long after the initial shock had passed. Follow-up research suggested that the lingering proteins had a kind of immunizing effect. In laboratory experiments, animal cells that were given a mild heat shock with-

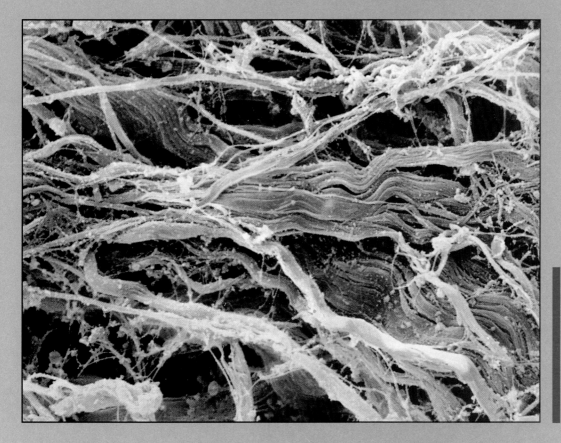

Fibers of collagen and elastin weave and cross in the extracellular matrix of connective tissue, shown in false color in this scanning electron micrograph. The two proteins help organize cells enveloped in the matrix and also determine its resilience.

stood a subsequent dose of stress from any number of agents—whether heat or something seemingly unrelated, such as heavy-metal poisoning— more readily than cells that had not been previously exposed to heat. Furthermore, in recent years, the genes responsible for these heat-induced proteins have been found to be almost identical from one species to another, leading scientists to believe that this genetic legacy proved so

beneficial that it has been passed down through evolution to the cells of every living organism.

Other survival strategies have evolved as well. When damage to a cell's genetic master code is relatively minor, cellular suicide is not necessary. Instead of destroying its DNA (and consequently itself), the cell can carry out a repair job on the injured segment. In this way, cells can counteract the steady low-level assault by chemicals, radiation, and other harmful forces in the environment. Within the nucleus of every cell, crews of maintenance enzymes continuously

patrol the chromosomes looking for trouble spots and reconstructing bits of torn genetic material. Making the job possible is the fact that the cell keeps two identical copies of its DNA code, one in each strand of the double helix. In simple DNA repair (when only one strand is damaged), special cleanup enzymes snip away debris from the broken section and prepare the site for another group of enzymes, which fill in the gaps by copying infor-

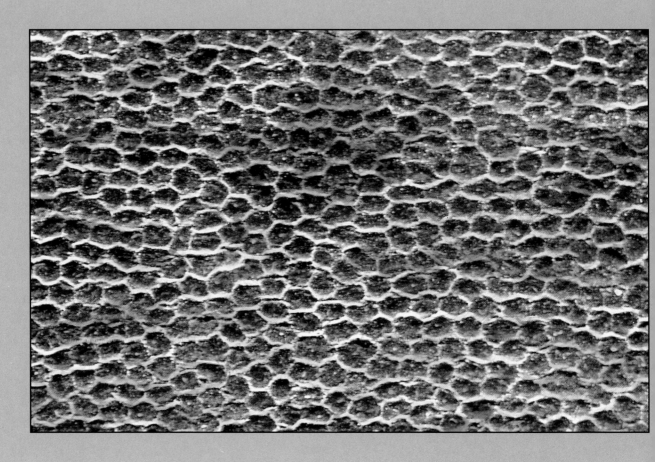

mation from the undamaged portion. Later, yet another set of enzymes arrives to finish the job by sealing up the patch. (Some cells can fix their DNA when both strands are damaged, but scientists do not fully understand how this process works.)

While it is not surprising that cells have to fend off assaults from the outside environment, they are also sometimes prey to enemies from within their own protective membranes. Among their more common internal assailants are rampaging oxygen molecules known as free radicals, which can be the by-product of normal cell metabolism, for example, or can be created when cells are exposed to sunlight or x-rays.

Such a molecule, equipped with an unpaired—and thus highly reactive—electron is dangerously unstable. To stabilize its unpaired electron, the free radical steals an electron from another molecule, which in turn becomes unstable and combines too easily with still another. The resulting chain reaction of molecular bonding can trigger the creation of abnormal proteins, membranes, and even DNA.

Free radicals do not usually run rampant for long, however. Some eventually decay on their own. And for those that linger, cells have developed a defense system made up of proteins called antioxidants, which seek out and hook up with the volatile molecules, neutralizing them. Among the antioxidants that have been identified by scientists are vitamins C and E, beta carotene, and a naturally produced enzyme called superoxide dismutase, or SOD for short. These substances prevent most de-

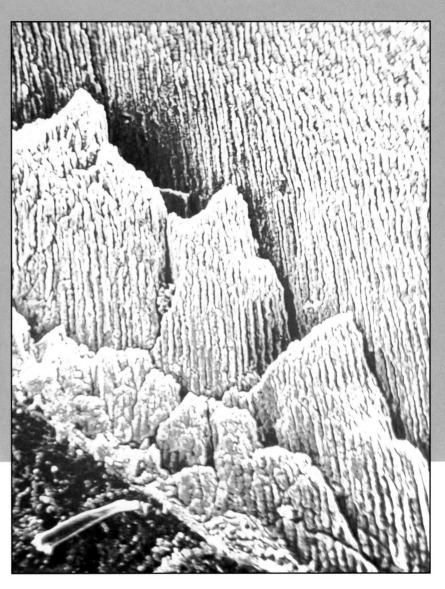

CORNEA. Many layers of flat and transparent cells *(left)* make up the honeycomb structure of the cornea of the eye. In order for the eye to function properly, the matrix that holds corneal cells together in such well-ordered ranks must be see-through as well.

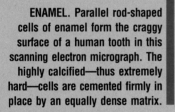

ENAMEL. Parallel rod-shaped cells of enamel form the craggy surface of a human tooth in this scanning electron micrograph. The highly calcified—thus extremely hard—cells are cemented firmly in place by an equally dense matrix.

struction by free radicals, but not all of it: As the damage mounts, so do deteriorating tissues and organs—symptoms of the advance of old age.

The theory that free radicals slowly erode the cells of the human body, first proposed in 1987 by biologist Denham Harman at the University of Nebraska, has set off a modern-day quest for wonder drugs that will fight the aging process. Studies with fruit flies have shown that inserting extra copies of the gene responsible for the SOD antioxidant into fly cells can extend the insects' lives by as much as five to 10 percent.

Such findings have raised hopes that if we cannot halt or reverse the process of human aging we can—by adding antioxidants as nutrients to cells in the body—at least slow it down. Successful methods for doing so have yet to be developed, however. Ingesting the substances appears to have no effect; the digestive system simply breaks down the enzymes before they can reach the cells. And when antioxidant vitamins are introduced directly into tissues in laboratory experiments, the cells shut down production of their own defensive chemicals, thus offsetting any boost that the vitamins may have added.

Perhaps not unlike Ponce de León in his long search for magical healing waters, today's scientists refuse to give up their quest for the secrets of longevity. But the body is a stubborn subject, adamantly predisposed to wearing down and, eventually, wearing out. Despite all countervailing efforts, aging cells gradually lose the ability to divide. They also become less able to produce stress proteins and to restore breaks in the genetic code. By the time we reach the age of 60, for example, our ability to repair DNA has dropped 30 percent below that of someone half as old.

Since damaged DNA has been linked to diseases such as cancer, which mostly affects the elderly, scientists are beginning to explore whether artificially raising and lowering the levels of stress proteins in cells might give an additional measure of protection to injured tissues and organs. In a number of experiments, scientists have shown that increasing the temperature of tissues causes certain types of tumors to regress; this find-

ing suggests that tumor cells are more sensitive to heat than cells in normal tissue. The task now facing scientists is to figure out how to render tumor cells vulnerable by preventing them from defending themselves with stress proteins.

One exciting area of research currently under way centers on the role that stress proteins play in fighting infectious disease. Every living organism produces these chemicals—and often, as scientists have recently discovered, for reasons other than self-defense. For example, some stress proteins have been shown to participate in cell metabolism, for example, while others seem to influence the molecules that regulate cell growth and differentiation. Nonetheless, immunologists have found that microbes such as those responsible for tuberculosis and malaria emit stress proteins into the bloodstream and that these substances are the first indication to the human immune system that an invasion is occurring.

Although they are manufactured by the body itself, stress proteins act, in effect, like flags of the invader, appearing on the horizon even before the enemy itself has been spotted. Scientists hope eventually to find a way to produce these proteins in the laboratory, then use them as a kind of safe vaccine that would cause the body to build up its natural defenses

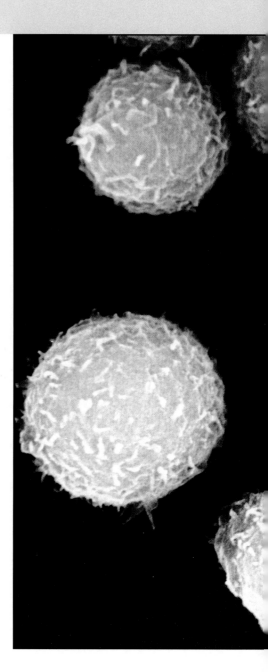

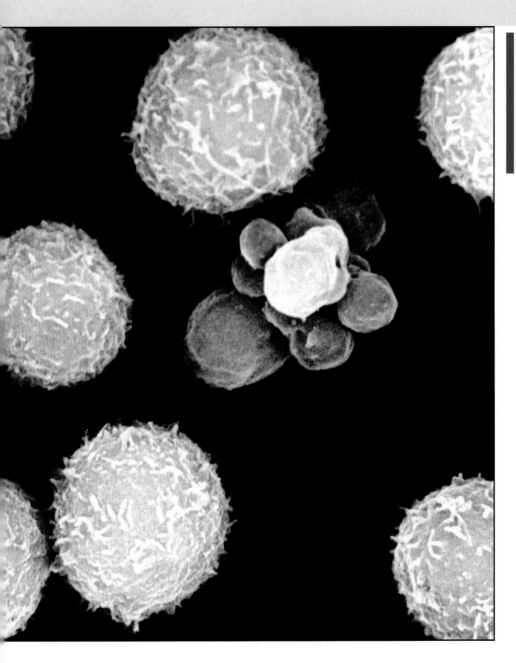

Surrounded by healthy companions, a human myeloid cell fragments in a suicidal process known as apoptosis. During such programmed cell elimination, the genetic material in the nucleus clumps together as the nucleus itself dissolves. Eventually the cell breaks apart, and scavenging white blood cells absorb the debris.

before the enemy actually arrives.

As these developments suggest, science and medicine have been moderately successful at prolonging life, while leaving unchanged the inevitability of death. The telomeres at the tip of every chromosome in every cell continue to keep track of how many of the cell's allotted number of divisions have been carried out and how many remain; when the magic number is reached, the cell simply dies, and—for now, at least—nothing can be done to alter that.

Still, the surety of death does not mean that the body's remarkable system of repair and renewal is flawed. It may be that death's role is to safeguard cells from mutations in the genetic code, or to signal the end of the body's reproductive usefulness. Scientists' understanding of the human body's healing mechanisms is fragmentary at best and so far, as molecular biologist Thomas Maciag has put it, "We cannot improve on the system designed by Mother Nature."

2

Ways and Means: Restoration at Work

As a self-tending system, the human organism is prodigiously resourceful, especially in times of adversity. A person who cuts a finger with a kitchen knife or breaks a bone in a football game may bemoan how long the injury takes to heal. But the reconstruction challenges are enormous—equivalent to the difficulties facing a city struck by a mighty earthquake. In microview, a cut presents a vista of ruin: cells devastated perhaps by the millions; transport channels for nutrients torn asunder and spewing forth their contents; vulnerable inner tissues beset by invading legions of bacteria. A broken bone is worse. The fracture not only tears apart a section of the elaborate crystalline strut work that gives mechanical strength to the body, it also savages the delicate web of blood vessels needed to keep bone tissue alive, damages precious marrow, and bruises or severs associated muscles, tendons, and ligaments.

Yet a cell-level view also reveals the body's extraordinary preparedness for trouble—as though a city struck by an earthquake turned out to be populated by whole armies of cleanup workers, masons, plumbers, electricians, and other experts at reconstruction. When skin is cut, cells of several kinds rush to the wound to remove contaminants and microbes; fibrous material is

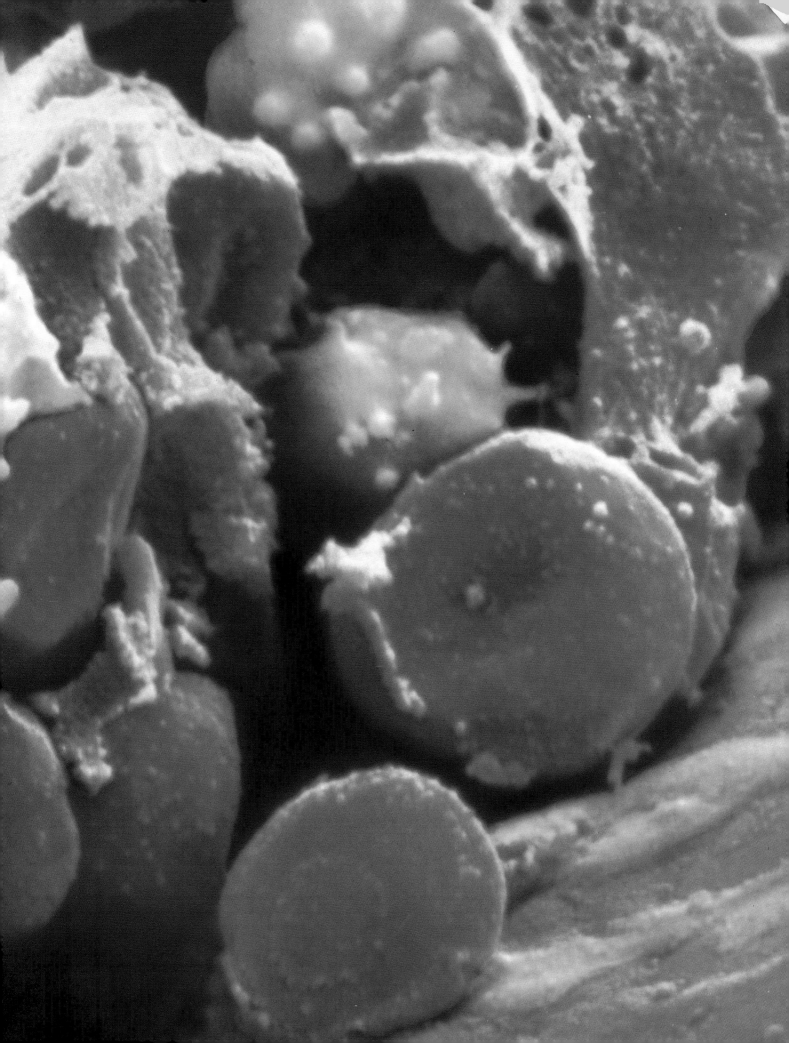

PRECEDING PAGE: Immediately after injury, a lacerated artery *(brown and pink)* spills its contents into surrounding tissue. Red and white blood cells waste no time initiating the repair process: Upon release, they signal other cells to migrate to the area and begin mending the damaged blood vessel and tissue. Red blood cells also form a clot *(bottom center)* to stop blood from flowing out of the artery.

deposited to shore up the repair site; new capillaries sprout from surviving vessels nearby; and, like a paving crew, cells emerge from the edges of the wound to smooth over the lesion —often so perfectly that virtually no sign of the mishap remains.

Similarly, a broken bone quickly musters various agents that remove the debris around the injury site, then proceeds to splint itself, grow a new network of blood vessels, lay down fresh minerals to form a hardened matrix, and shape this material for optimal support. The bone emerges from the reconstruction process every bit as sturdy as the original, if not more so. Although the bone may take several months to remake itself, hardly an instant is lost in the repair process.

As with any major construction project, healing must be carefully orchestrated, with the appropriate sets of cells going into action at exactly the right time and others retiring from the scene in orderly fashion. But dealing with injury represents only a fraction of the organism's efforts at remaking itself. Far more extensive are the body's many versions of renovation, the process of retiring old components and putting new ones in their place. People are aware of some of these ongoing activities—the growing and shedding of hair, for example, or the lengthening of nails. But most of the renewal processes go unnoticed,

even when their scale is numerically stupendous. Every day, more than 200 billion red blood cells are replaced: Worn cells, battered by months of traveling 60,000 miles of arteries, veins, and lesser vessels, are digested by the liver and spleen as a fresh supply is created in the bone marrow.

Every day, nearly a billion skin cells are sloughed off as new ones emerge from below, the rate of turnover depending on whether that portion of the body gets hard usage. Every one to three days, the entire complement of the much-abraded cells lining the intestine are also retired from their nutrient-absorbing duties and replaced by battle-ready newcomers. The same happens with the cells that line the 300 million tiny, balloonlike alveoli of each lung. In the course of a year, even after the attainment of adulthood and a full-size skeletal system, about five percent of the body's bone mass is rebuilt, and certain heavily stressed areas of bone are remodeled every four months.

The body has several ways of creating and installing these replacement parts. One procedure is straightforward cloning: A worn cell is divided to produce two vigorous offspring, whose shared genetic blueprint ex-

actly matches that of the parent cell.

This process is, in fact, the magic behind one of the body's most impressive regenerative feats—the ability of the liver to restore itself to its original size even after most of its mass has been destroyed or removed. Weighing about three pounds, the liver is the body's heaviest internal organ. The liver is extremely versatile, performing as many as 500 distinct functions, which include producing bile for digestion, helping to maintain proper glucose levels in the blood, storing essential vitamins, converting fats into carbohydrates, detoxifying poisons in the blood, and disposing of worn-out blood cells.

Although a great deal is known about what the liver does, the precise mechanism behind its restorative abilities remains somewhat murky. In tests with rats, scientists have shown that, under normal conditions, only about one percent of all liver cells are dividing at any given time. But when part of the organ is surgically removed, cells in the remaining portion go into a reproduction frenzy. Within two days, as many as 10 percent of the cells in the remnant are making copies of themselves. Just two weeks after surgery, rat livers grow back to their original size and cell number, even in cases where 70 percent or more of the organ has been removed.

Scientists think this massive recon-

struction effort may be controlled by growth factors and growth-inhibiting chemicals that send "on" and "off" signals to liver cells. Apparently the growth spurt is triggered by a chemical imbalance brought on by the removal of liver tissue. Each liver cell secretes a chemical messenger known as a chalone, which in normal concentrations appears to check the rate of reproduction among neighboring cells. When part of the liver is taken away, overall chalone levels plummet, creating a deficiency that prompts remaining cells to start dividing. Gradually, as the organ rebuilds itself, chalone levels return to normal and the rate of cell division slows down.

Various other body tissues compensate for loss through simple cell division, but more often cell replacement operates through the action of stem cells, the nonspecialized precursor cells that can, under certain circumstances, take on a specialized identity. Promotion to the new status is not always immediate. In some cases, first-generation offspring of the precursors are little different from their parents, and several more divisions may be necessary to produce descendants that can carry out the destined duties. However, the cell line is now irre-

versibly committed to a new role.

All of this transformation is orchestrated by biochemical signals. For example, a low level of oxygen in the blood will induce the kidneys and liver to secrete a hormone that commands stem cells in the bone marrow to begin adding to the body's supply of oxygen-carrying red blood cells. This process may begin mere minutes after oxygen levels drop, and the new cells will enter the bloodstream about five days later. An infectious illness will cause blood-producing stem cells to receive a completely different set of biochemical signals, leading them to create particular types of white blood cells to deal with the problem.

While some of the body's cells are free-floating loners, most work in fixed groupings that are made up of a number of different cell types, together performing some particular task such as secreting digestive acids or responding to light. Such differentiated patterns of cells are known as tissue, and they represent a kind of middle level of complexity in the body's architecture. In turn, tissues of several types form more elaborate structural elements—a hand, perhaps, or an organ that carries out some complex function such as extracting wastes from the bloodstream. At a still higher level are the organism's various systems, consisting of structures that are broadly distributed

through the body and operate together for some overarching purpose, such as exchanging gases with the atmosphere (the respiratory system), transporting the gases as well as nutrients and wastes (the circulatory system), or transmitting DNA to future generations (the reproductive system).

All renovation and repair work must respect this multilevel architecture, and indeed the body has numerous mechanisms to ensure that boundaries, connections, and other organizational features are maintained. For example, certain cells may preferentially adhere to one another. Others may cease growing when their allotted space is filled, or they may die if they stray too far from some important growth factor. In a successful repair, the layout of blood vessels, nerves, and other features does not precisely replicate that of the predecessor tissue, but it is close enough so that the tissue works in the same way and honors the form and function of higher-level structures. Behind each repair lies a kind of blueprint inscribed in the genes; improvisation is forbidden.

For one reason or another, producing a functional replica during reconstruction work is not always possible. Such is the case with damage to carti-

lage—the tough, elastic connective tissue that absorbs impact, smooths contact between bones, and lends shape and support throughout the body. Unlike bone, cartilage has no vessels delivering blood or lymphatic fluid. Instead, it draws nutrients from neighboring tissues by diffusion through a dense web of molecules known as the extracellular matrix.

Since cartilage has no natural supply routes for bringing in cleanup crews from the bloodstream, all repair work must be carried out by resources available at the site. And yet by themselves, cartilage cells lack the ability to make effective repairs. They cannot divide in sufficient quantities, nor are they able to use the fibrous structure of blood clots as a scaffold for rebuilding tissue. This is why damage involving cartilage alone usually heals poorly, if at all. Repairs are generally more successful when the damage extends beyond the cartilage and into adjacent bone or tissue. In such cases, cells from ruptured blood vessels migrate into the cartilage, triggering an inflammatory response among local cells that promotes healing.

The body's inability to fix some types of damage is also evident in cases of severe lacerations or burns, when skin tissue may be unable to regenerate itself and instead fills in much of the injured area with scar tissue—fibrous connective material that for the most part lacks cells and capillaries. Scar tissue is extremely strong and serves as an excellent barrier against bacteria, but it typically has no glands, sensory neurons, or hair; at best, it is a patch.

Organs, too, can be scarred. For example, the liver—despite its exceptional powers of regeneration—may become clogged with fibrous tissue because of protracted exposure to alcohol or other toxins. The condition, known as cirrhosis, leaves little room for normal liver cells to grow even after the poisons are eliminated. Damage to heart muscle almost always results in scarring, since the cells of that tissue are entirely lacking in regenerative ability. The consequences may be dire: In time, the scar tissue shrinks, which may impair the flow of blood through the heart; or the scarring may prevent the heart muscle from contracting normally.

Repair work can go wrong in other ways. Sometimes bacteria overwhelm the body's defenses, traveling ever deeper into tissue, causing blood vessels to leak, killing cells wholesale. The result may be a spreading ulcer or the massive tissue death known as gangrene. Or the body may harm itself in the course of a repair. For instance, the circulatory disease known as atherosclerosis begins with fat deposits and small lesions in the lining of arteries. Although the exact nature of the process is uncertain, the secretion of growth factors appears to stimulate inappropriate cell proliferation at the site. The excess cells thicken the walls of the blood vessel and, along with the deposited debris, can restrict blood flow—sometimes with catastrophic results (*pages 78-83*).

In renovation and repair, the human organism plainly has priorities as well as limits. For instance, both bone and cartilage are important for proper mechanical functioning of the body, but bone is the more essential of the two; evolution has reflected this ranking in its repair programs. As for nonessentials, the body sometimes does not bother to rebuild. When a hair root is destroyed, it is gone forever; a filler of collagen takes its place, since survival of the organism is not an issue.

Scientists have just begun to comprehend the biochemical workings of the body's reconstruction programs —intricate to a degree undreamed of only a few decades ago. But the physical mechanisms of repair and renewal make up only part of the research frontier. The mind, too, can be a powerful player in these matters.

Before the modern era, healing was thought to involve forces that lay outside the familiar physical realm.

Today, body and mind are increasingly seen as partners in the healing process.

Among many tribal peoples, shamans conducted elaborate ceremonies in the hope of gaining the aid of the spirits. In some Asian cultures, an illness or injury was treated by methods that aimed at correcting the flow of invisible energies in the body.

In premodern Europe, healers relied heavily on magical charms, incantations, prayers, and elaborate rituals to dispel a host of maladies, most of them thought to be the work of fairies, evil spirits, and other supernatural forces. To treat wounds inflicted in battle, some early physicians concocted an ointment using a recipe that called for two ounces of moss taken from a buried skull, a half-ounce of embalmed human flesh, two ounces of human fat, and a small amount of the patient's own blood. One group of healers insisted that the ointment be applied not only to the wound but also to the weapon that caused it. Through a mystical process of animal magnetism, they believed, the technique promoted healing by reuniting the wound with the "vital spirits" in the congealed blood on the weapon —a transfer that could take place over distances as great as 30 miles.

The art of magical healing was not limited to wizards and other "cunning folk," as medical practitioners were sometimes called. Indeed, among history's most conspicuous healers were members of the European royalty, who were thought to be endowed with supernatural curative powers. During solemn religious ceremonies, sufferers waited in long lines to kneel before the monarch, who would gently stroke their faces and hang gold pieces around their necks. Faith in the royal touch was deep and widespread, as evidenced by the number of subjects who sought it. During his reign in the mid-17th century, for example, England's Charles II reportedly ministered to 90,798 people; remarked one observer, the monarch touched "near half the nation." Although the king's blessing did not likely have any effect on the biological roots of the disease, it did provide a large measure of hope, a psychological boost that in itself served as an uplifting tonic for the sick.

Behind all such procedures, in Europe and elsewhere, lay a belief that the tangible, material realm and the invisible, magical realm were overlapping realities, and both had to be addressed in treatments. With the rise of science, rites and spells receded, but one intangible factor in healing has held its ground: Skilled physicians of the ancient world suspected that the outlook of the patient figured importantly in health, and today's physicians have confirmed this many times over. Indeed, their respect for the power of their patients' emotions and expectations is rapidly growing.

Today, body and mind are increasingly seen as partners in the healing process. Medical researchers are exploring many ways of ensuring that these fundamental components of the self work together to promote healing. Some physicians are teaching their patients techniques of relaxation, meditation, or biofeedback to deal with pain or anxiety. Some recommend hypnosis or visualization techniques as effective ways of sending messages from mind to body. Some are focusing on relationships—positive, trust-building interactions between doctor, patient, and family. Some seek to rouse self-healing energies with touch, a fixture of the ancient healing arts. No single approach has won universal acceptance, and a few have been strongly challenged. But there is little doubt that attention to emotions and other mental attributes will be as much a part of tomorrow's medicine as promoting proper action on the cellular level. Jointly, body and mind make up what has been called "the doctor within," and they are indissoluble.

WELLSPRINGS OF NEW CELLS

Throughout life, the human body is a work in progress, continuously replacing many of its cellular building materials. Some types of cells renew and maintain their populations by splitting in two again and again. Others rely on small pools of understudies called stem cells to churn out replacements. Although their relative rarity and physical simplicity make these generic versions difficult to pick out among a mix of cell types, scientists are finding new ways to isolate and study them.

The destiny of stem cells is thought to be genetically predetermined, but they show a certain versatility along the way. In response to chemical signals indicating a need for replacements, stem cells may split into one new stem cell and one cell that will eventually become specialized. Or they may divide several times first. For example, only after numerous divisions do blood stem cells become mature red blood cells by ejecting their nuclei (*right*).

The advantage of such versatility becomes most apparent after an injury, when stem cells can double themselves many times over to generate armies of replacements for cells that have been destroyed or damaged. But even in their everyday tasks of renewing such components as blood, skin, hair, and nails, these prolific cell factories are among the body's most miraculous talents.

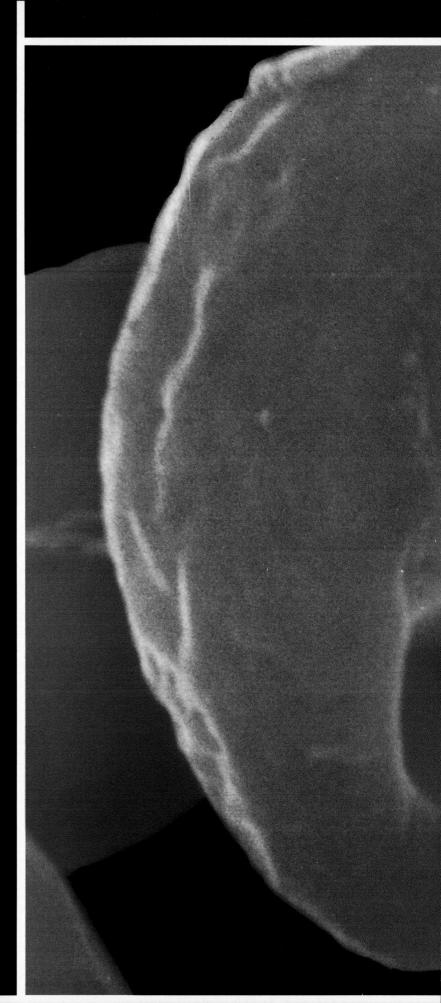

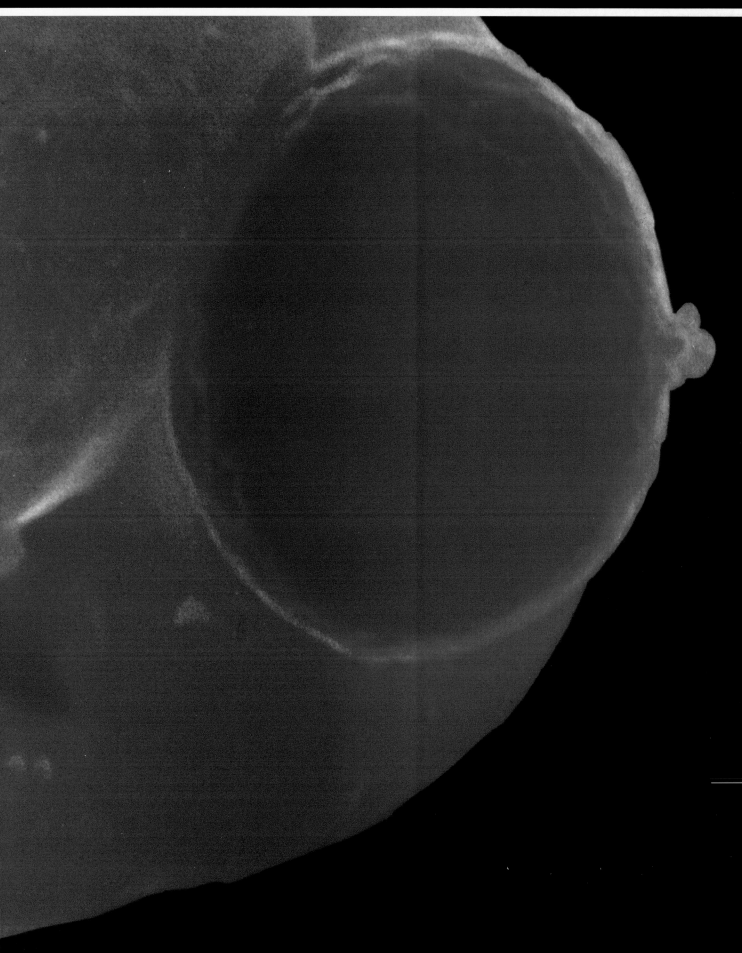

FROM SO SIMPLE A BEGINNING: BLOOD

The blood that courses through our veins and arteries is a fluid of somewhat surprising complexity. The body of the average adult contains about 10 pints of blood, half of whose total volume is plasma—mostly water and important substances such as proteins, salts, sugars, vitamins, hormones, and antibodies. The rest is a blend of at least eight cell types, each of which is essential to the maintenance of life and health. In addition to masses of red blood cells, blood also consists of six kinds of so-called white blood cells, which ward off disease, and platelets—actually fragments of larger cells—which help stanch bleeding by forming clots.

Because many of these cells last only a matter of hours, the body must always be replacing them. The source for all types of blood cells is a relatively small community of stem cells residing in the bone marrow. Making up as few as one in every 100,000 cells in the bone marrow, these cells nevertheless manage to produce three million new red blood cells every second—some 260 billion each day—in addition to large numbers of every other blood cell type.

Various growth factors and other chemicals not only signal stem cells to begin the transformation process but also may play a role in determining which of the eight types is produced. However, because stem cells tend to look the same for a while after they start to differentiate, scientists cannot be entirely sure of the transition's precise details.

A CASCADE OF POSSIBILITIES. The illustration below shows three ways in which a stem cell (right) may divide to become one of the eight types of blood cell. In each case here, one of the two still-joined daughter cells is a copy of the original cell (red); the other is either a precursor of a B cell (green) or T cell (purple), or a kind of stem cell (pink) that will become one of the six other blood cell types. Many divisions later, fully differentiated versions prepare to enter a capillary (bottom).

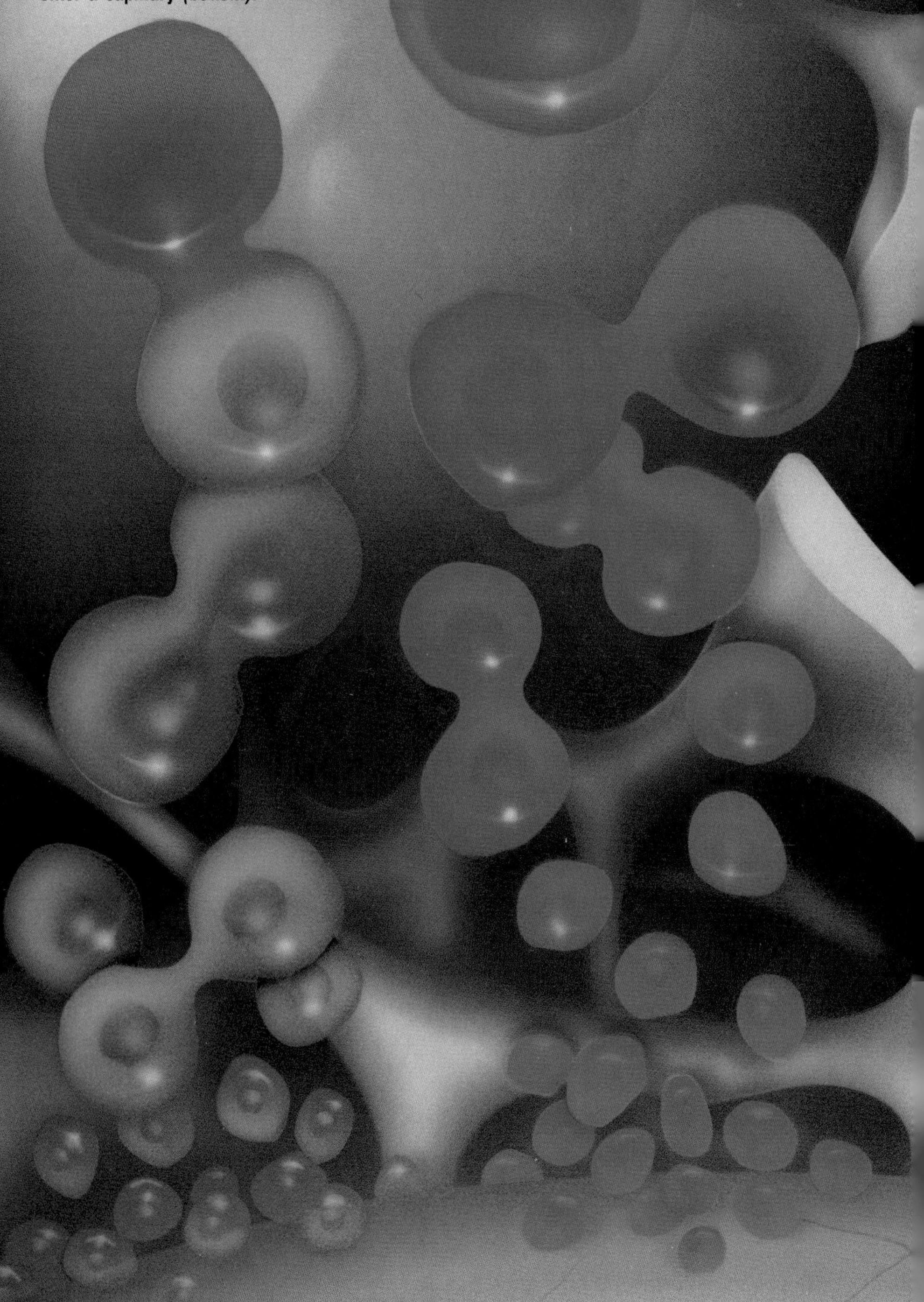

B CELLS are types of immune cells that recognize specific sorts of invaders and eventually mature in the bloodstream or tissues into antibody-producing plasma cells.

PRE-T CELLS travel to the thymus, where they mature into T cells—another type of immune cell that learns to spot, then destroy, virus-infected or cancer cells.

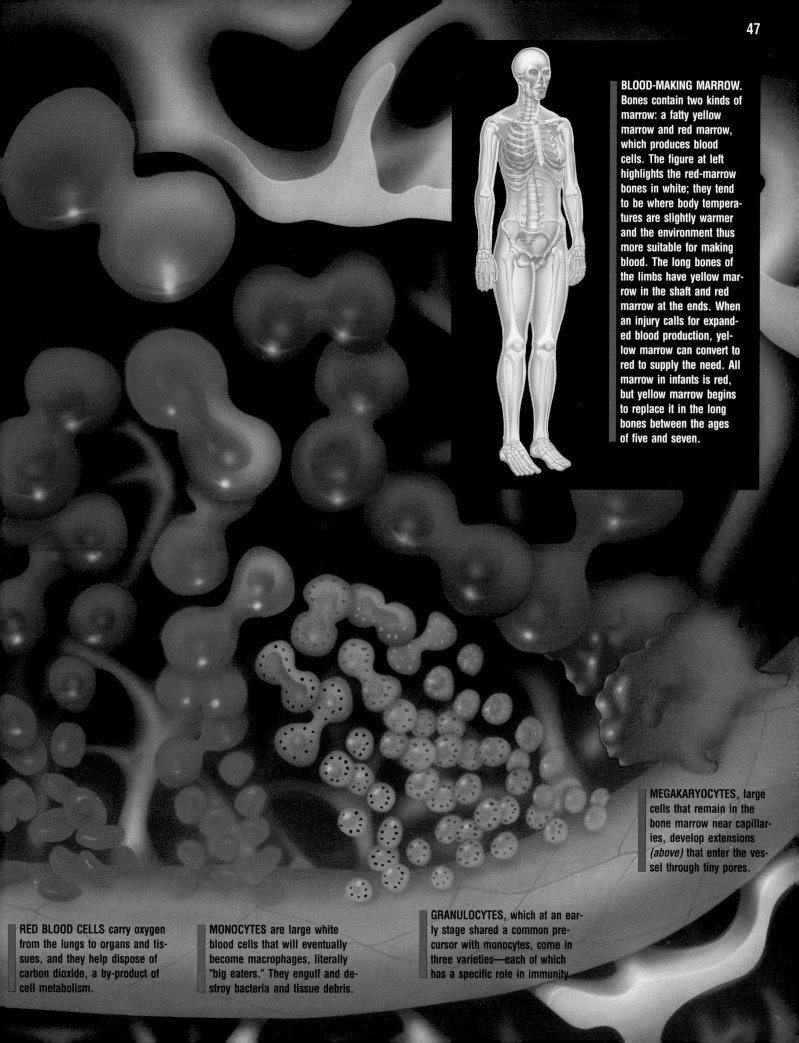

BLOOD-MAKING MARROW. Bones contain two kinds of marrow: a fatty yellow marrow and red marrow, which produces blood cells. The figure at left highlights the red-marrow bones in white; they tend to be where body temperatures are slightly warmer and the environment thus more suitable for making blood. The long bones of the limbs have yellow marrow in the shaft and red marrow at the ends. When an injury calls for expanded blood production, yellow marrow can convert to red to supply the need. All marrow in infants is red, but yellow marrow begins to replace it in the long bones between the ages of five and seven.

MEGAKARYOCYTES, large cells that remain in the bone marrow near capillaries, develop extensions *(above)* that enter the vessel through tiny pores.

RED BLOOD CELLS carry oxygen from the lungs to organs and tissues, and they help dispose of carbon dioxide, a by-product of cell metabolism.

MONOCYTES are large white blood cells that will eventually become macrophages, literally "big eaters." They engulf and destroy bacteria and tissue debris.

GRANULOCYTES, which at an early stage shared a common precursor with monocytes, come in three varieties—each of which has a specific role in immunity.

IN THE MARROW, THE LAST STAGES OF BLOOD CELL PRODUCTION

At varying rates and to varying degrees, blood cells mature in the spongy structure of red marrow. Both precursor and more fully developed cells tend to congregate in spaces formed by a weblike network of bony extensions running through the marrow, shown in the illustration here in gray. Red cells cluster around macrophages, which snag the nuclei that the red cells eject in the final stage of their maturation (below).

All blood cells eventually migrate to the capillaries that snake through the red marrow. As mature blood cells press against the capillary wall, the wall's lining of endothelial cells thins and develops tiny pores through which the new blood cells pass; the pores then close behind them.

Not all the details of how different cell types develop are so well established. For example, the precursors of white cells in the red marrow outnumber those of red cells by about three to one, but in the bloodstream itself, red cells outnumber white by close to 600 to one. These numbers partly reflect the longer life span of mature red cells in the bloodstream, but researchers also believe the figures show that white cells take longer to go through the stages of maturity they complete in the red marrow.

RED BLOOD CELLS MATURE. Before they enter the bloodstream, red blood cells complete their development by jettisoning their nuclei (below); they will now go through no further divisions. The ejected nuclei are cleaned up by nearby scavenging macrophages (right).

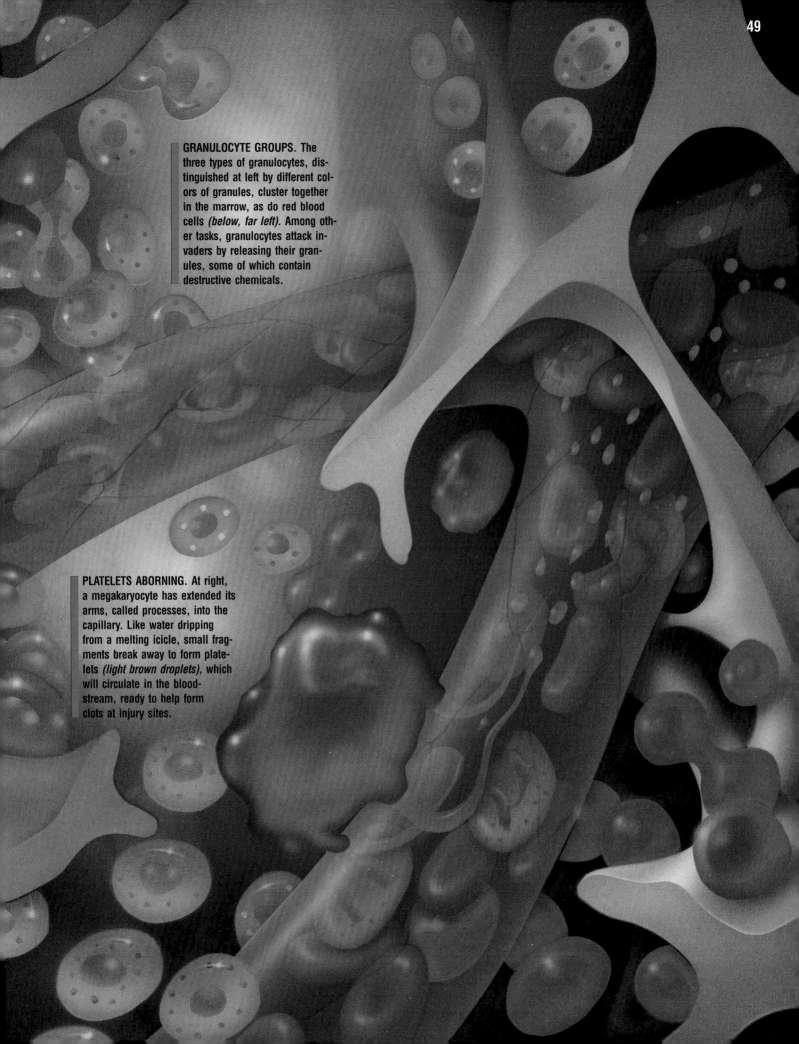

GRANULOCYTE GROUPS. The three types of granulocytes, distinguished at left by different colors of granules, cluster together in the marrow, as do red blood cells *(below, far left)*. Among other tasks, granulocytes attack invaders by releasing their granules, some of which contain destructive chemicals.

PLATELETS ABORNING. At right, a megakaryocyte has extended its arms, called processes, into the capillary. Like water dripping from a melting icicle, small fragments break away to form platelets *(light brown droplets)*, which will circulate in the bloodstream, ready to help form clots at injury sites.

SKIN: THE BODY'S SELF-RENEWING ARMOR

Covering more than 20 square feet and weighing some 10 pounds, the skin is the body's largest organ—and among the most versatile. It not only serves as a shield against microorganisms and ultraviolet light but also prevents dehydration and manufactures vitamin D. And, like blood, it constantly renews itself.

The skin's primary features are a thin top layer, the epidermis, and the thicker underlying dermis, the two of which meet in a series of peaks and valleys. The dermis (*below*) includes various components, from blood vessels and nerves to hair follicles. The main action of regeneration, however, takes place in the epidermis.

As shown at right, the very structure of the epidermis reflects how its primary cells, the keratinocytes, develop. The bottom layer includes a scattering of stem cells that, by dividing and differentiating, give rise to all keratinocytes. As they mature, individual keratinocytes migrate upward from this basal layer, forming new layers as their features change. One of the more significant developments occurs at the granular layer, where the protein keratin begins to replace all cellular components. This process results in several sheets of tough dead cells (the cornified layer) that eventually slough off at the surface—ever to be replaced by new cells from below.

CELLS OF THE EPIDERMIS. In addition to several layers of keratinocytes at different stages of development, the epidermis also consists of three other distinct types of cells. In the basal layer, melanocytes *(brown)* produce the pigment melanin, which shields the nuclei of keratinocytes from ultraviolet radiation and, in different amounts, gives skin its many possible colors. Also in this layer are Merkel cells *(purple)*, touch receptors that convey information to nerves. Langerhans' cells *(blue)* attack intruders and initiate responses by other immune cells.

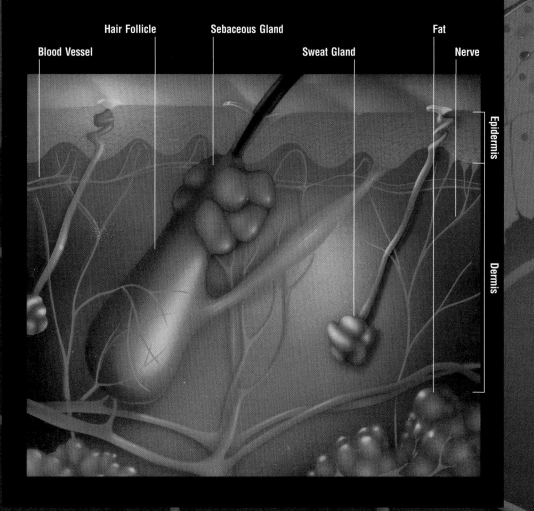

Blood Vessel · Hair Follicle · Sebaceous Gland · Sweat Gland · Fat · Nerve · Epidermis · Dermis

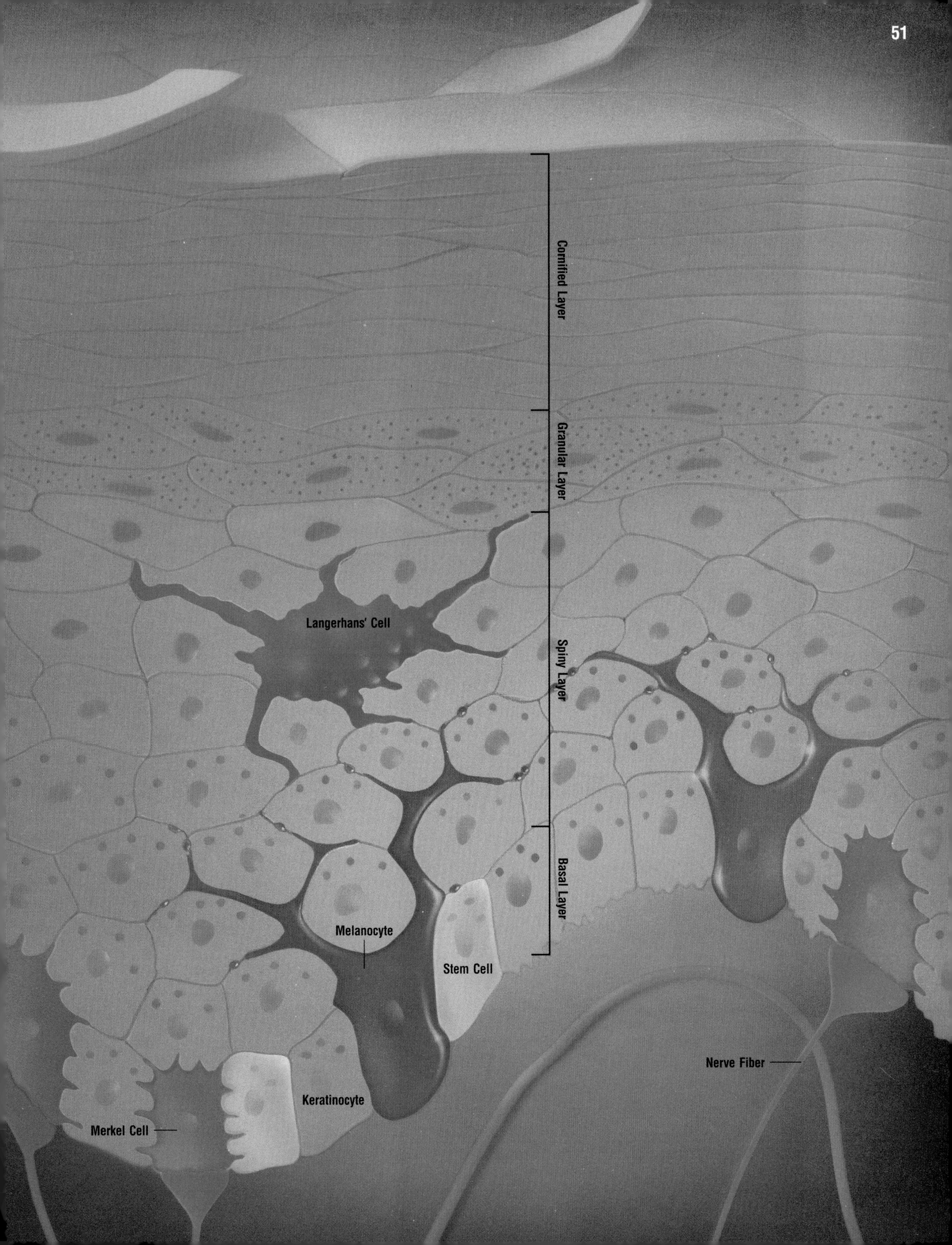

Cornified Layer

Granular Layer

Spiny Layer

Basal Layer

Langerhans' Cell

Melanocyte

Stem Cell

Keratinocyte

Nerve Fiber

Merkel Cell

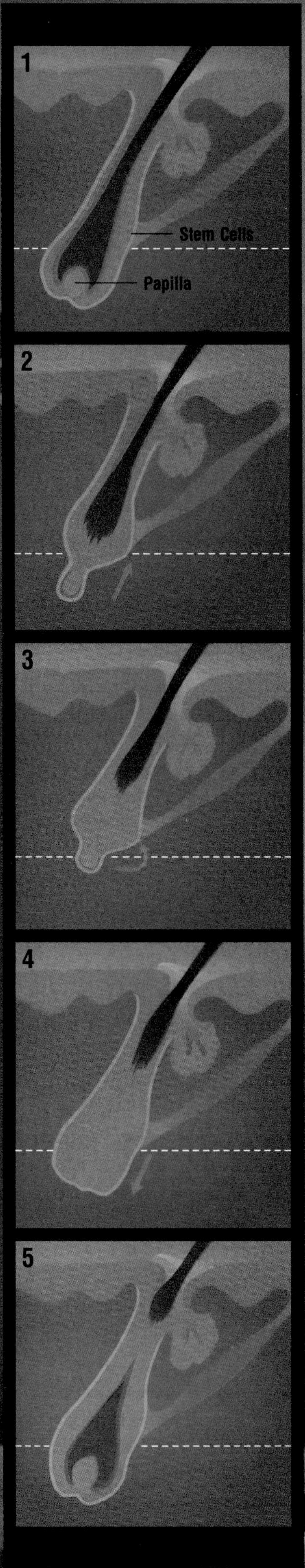

1

Stem Cells

Papilla

2

3

4

5

STIMULUS FOR GROWTH. The sequence at left illustrates one theory of how hairs grow. In the first stage *(1)*, a fully grown hair remains attached for a time to the papilla, and stem cells *(orange dots)* in an area known as the bulge are inactive. The hair then detaches from the papilla *(2)*, and the shrinking follicle moves the papilla up toward the bulge *(arrow)*. The papilla stimulates stem cells in the bulge to divide *(3)*, and as they grow they push the papilla back down *(4)*. Daughters of the stem cells then form the hair matrix around the papilla, and a new hair starts growing *(5)*.

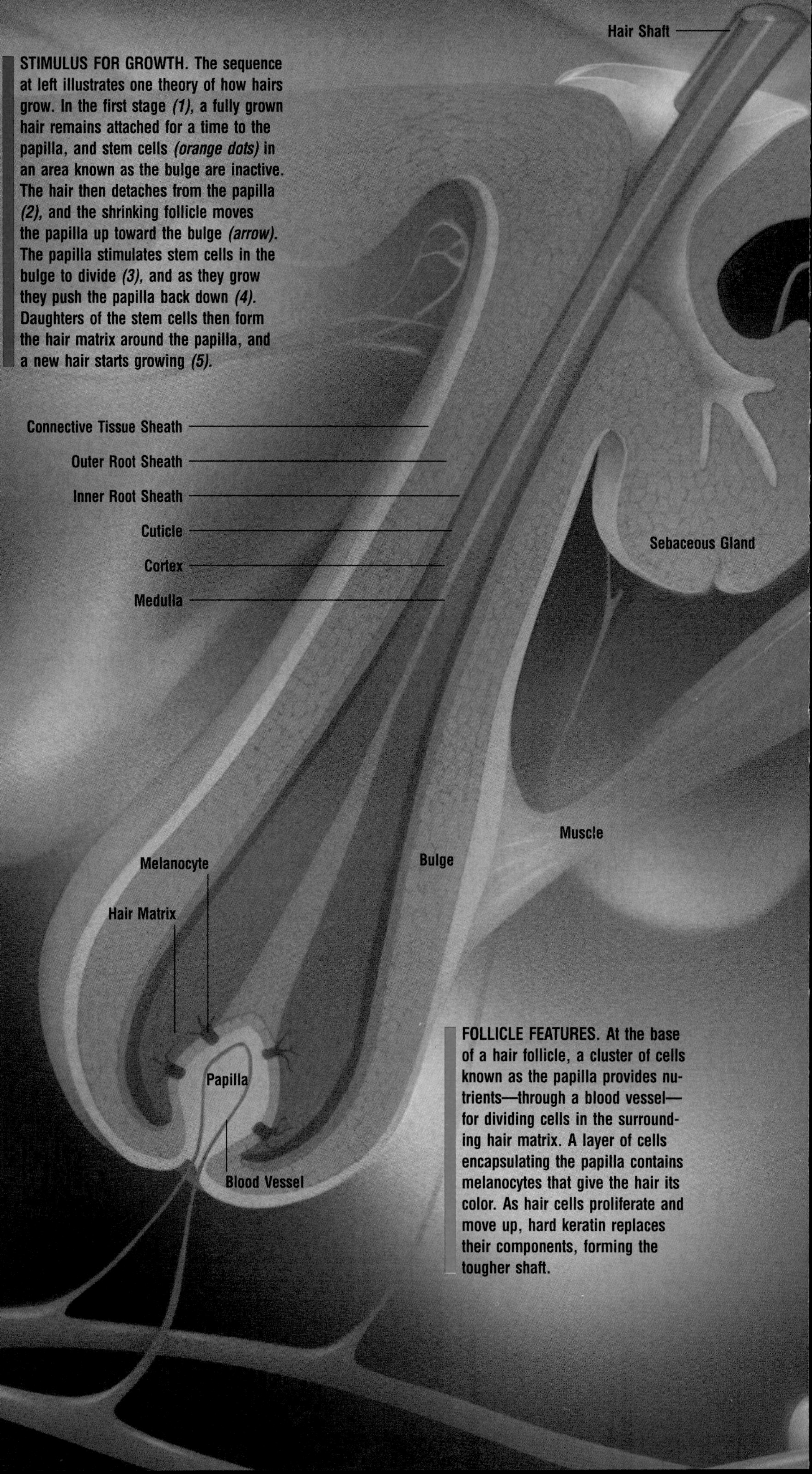

Hair Shaft

Connective Tissue Sheath

Outer Root Sheath

Inner Root Sheath

Cuticle

Cortex

Medulla

Sebaceous Gland

Muscle

Bulge

Melanocyte

Hair Matrix

Papilla

Blood Vessel

FOLLICLE FEATURES. At the base of a hair follicle, a cluster of cells known as the papilla provides nutrients—through a blood vessel—for dividing cells in the surrounding hair matrix. A layer of cells encapsulating the papilla contains melanocytes that give the hair its color. As hair cells proliferate and move up, hard keratin replaces their components, forming the tougher shaft.

GROWING FROM THE ROOTS: HAIR AND NAILS

Nowhere are the body's regenerative powers more visible than in the nonstop growth of hair and nails. Although they appear to be entirely different from the skin, both hair and nails also originate from epidermal cells, grow and develop through the activity of stem cells, and undergo a process of keratinization that results in a tough mantle of dead cells. One major difference is that hair and nail cells contain another form of keratin that makes for a harder texture.

Like the skin, nails keep growing without interruption, but hairs go through a cycle in which one hair grows—for as long as 10 years—and is then replaced by an entirely new hair. The continual turnover means that an average adult, with some 100,000 hairs on the scalp, loses any-where from 50 to 150 hairs every day.

Hair growth occurs entirely within the hair follicle, an indentation in the skin's surface that holds the hair in place. The visible part of the hair, called the shaft, consists only of dead, keratin-filled cells.

Some researchers think that the bulbous part of the hair at the base of the follicle contains the originating stem cells and is thus solely responsible for hair growth. Indeed, a region of rapidly dividing cells known as the hair matrix, from which almost all new cells arise, is found here. Another theory, illustrated by the sequence of diagrams at far left, suggests instead that the stem cells reside elsewhere and that the growth process entails a more complex relationship between several other follicle components.

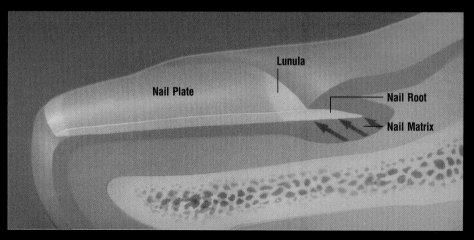

CELLS AS HARD AS NAILS. Unlike hair, nails grow continuously, but the cellular process is much the same. Beneath the nail root, which lodges the nail securely in the skin, new cells proliferate in the nail matrix, pushing older cells outward (arrows). These ultimately form the hard, visible part of the nail known as the nail plate, where nail-cell components have been entirely replaced by hard keratin. At the base of the nail, a whitish crescent called the lunula (visible in most people on the thumb) is thought to be caused by the relatively thick matrix blocking out the pinkish color that the underlying blood supply gives to the rest of the nail. Nails grow at varying rates: faster in summer than in winter, and faster both on the dominant hand and on the longer fingers and toes. The average rate of growth is about one and a half inches a year for fingernails, and a half to one inch for toenails.

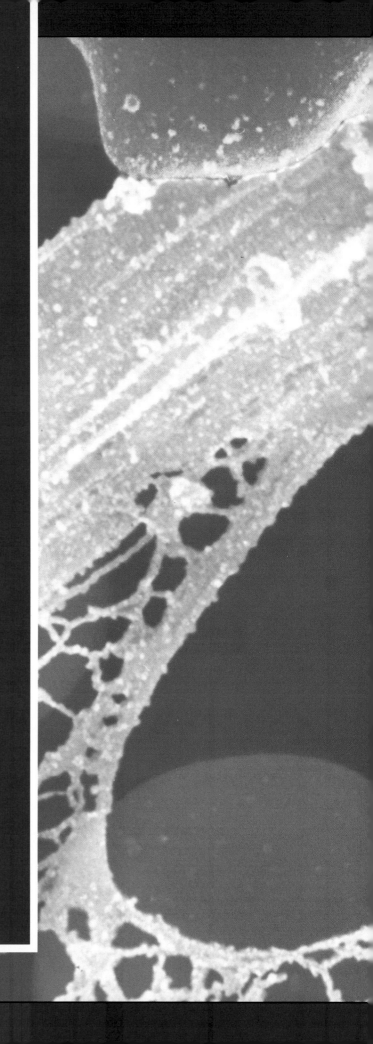

A WOUND ON THE MEND

A scratch from a thorn, a small cut from a kitchen knife, a scraped knee —such minor wounds usually heal so quickly and completely that we tend to take for granted the body's remarkable ability to mend itself. Even in cases that might require bandaging or stitches, the body remains the prime agent of healing, setting in motion an intricate and elegant process of damage control, defense, and repair.

Wound healing typically necessitates the coordinated actions of cells, tissues, and other substances. For example, the crucial task of blood clotting involves a series of agents and events that lead to red blood cells being trapped in a web of protein called fibrin (*right*). Among the most important players are enzymes and other proteins known collectively as factors, each of which signals specific targets in the tissues around the wound when the time comes for them to take their part in responding to the injury.

The many elements of the process are best understood in the skin, as illustrated on the following pages. Rapid response to a skin injury is particularly essential, not only to repair the damaged tissue but also to defend against dangerous foreign matter that might enter by the wound and lead to further trouble.

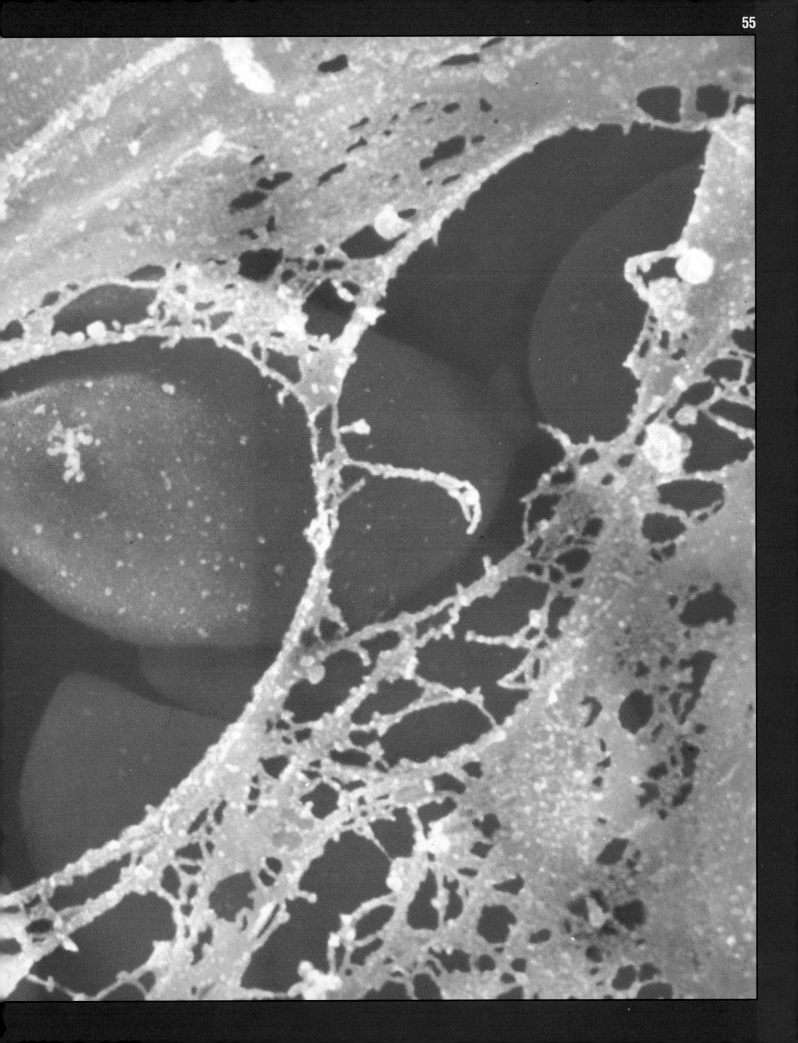

STOPPING THE BLEEDING

Even a relatively shallow laceration damages several types of tissue, which work together to heal the wound. Damage control begins at the moment of injury, when blood from severed vessels spills into the surrounding tissue and moves through the cut to the surface. Platelets in the blood trigger the initial stage of healing, known as hemostasis (arrest of bleeding). These small particles, ordinarily contained within the vessel by its thin lining of endothelial cells, come in contact with collagen, a fibrous protein that gives shape to the blood vessel wall and to nearby connective tissue. Platelets adhere to the collagen and release chemicals that cause other platelets to accumulate, forming a plug that seals the wound.

At the same time, the injured endothelial cells exude another chemical called tissue factor, initiating a series of reactions that contribute to the clotting of the spilled blood. One component of blood plasma—the fluid part of blood—is converted to the protein thrombin, which in turn transforms another plasma protein into insoluble fibrin. Threads of fibrin form a crisscross pattern as they adhere to the surrounding tissue, snaring blood cells, platelets, and plasma.

Within minutes, the fibrin threads begin to contract as platelets and other blood cells pull on them. Blood fluid minus clotting proteins is squeezed out, but the cells are trapped even more tightly. Platelets within the clot also release factors that strengthen, compress, and stabilize it. Closing the wound, the clot provides a scaffold for the next wave of cells arriving to work at the wound site.

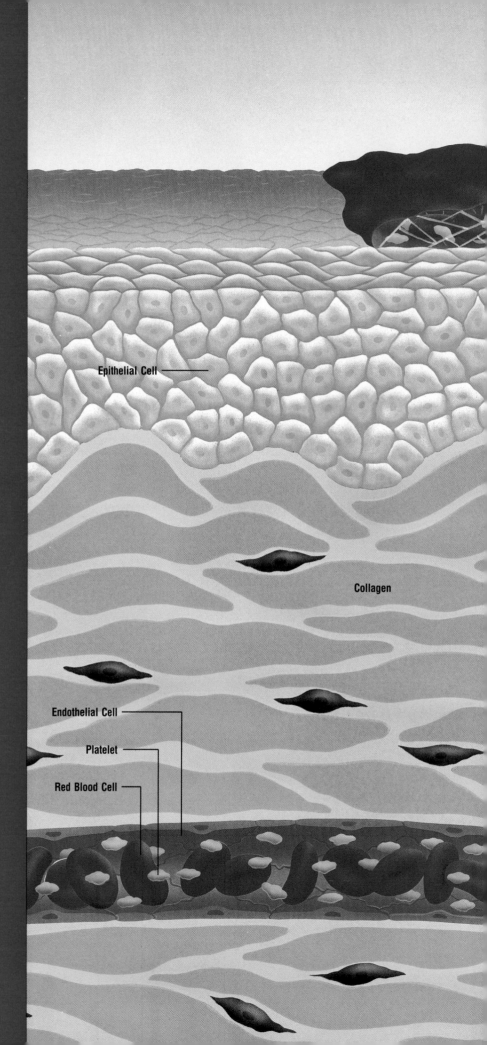

Epithelial Cell

Collagen

Endothelial Cell

Platelet

Red Blood Cell

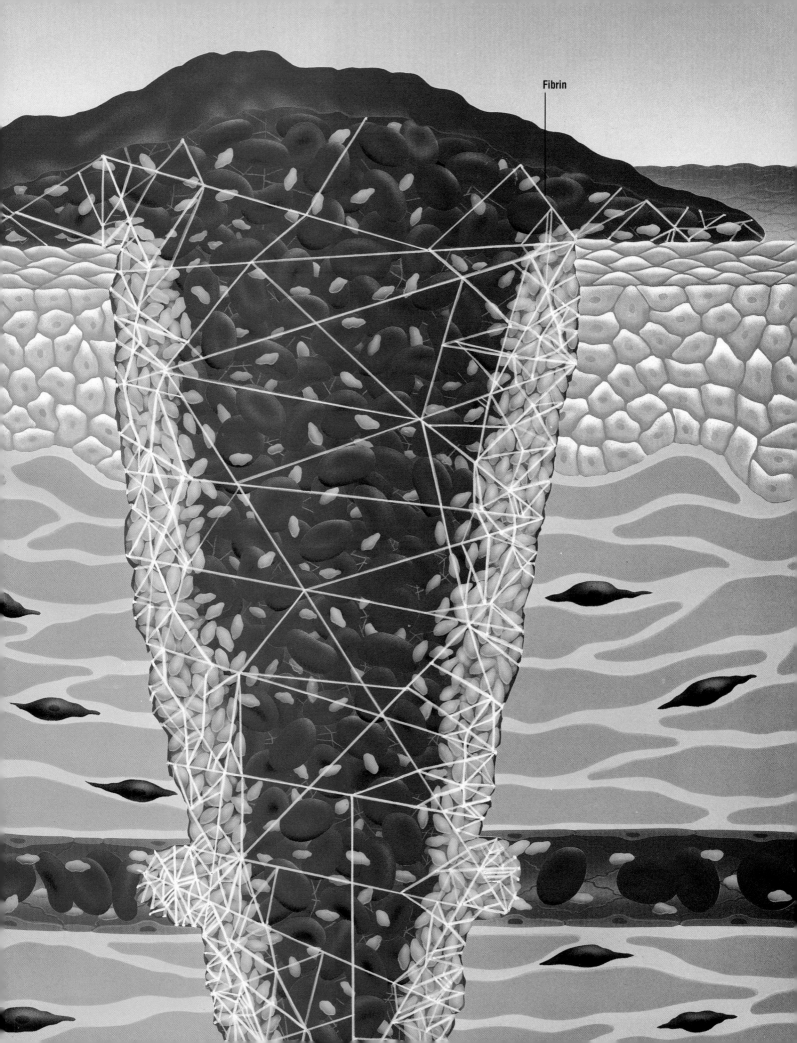

Fibrin

DEFENDING AGAINST INVADERS

Factors released during the clotting process cause blood vessels near the wound to swell in diameter. This dilation increases their permeability by spreading the endothelial cells apart, leaving gaps through which blood components escape into the adjacent tissue. Accumulating at the wound site, this mixture of fluid and white blood cells produces tissue swelling that marks the beginning of what is known as the inflammatory response (*reddish cast in illustration*).

Much of the activity in the wound involves phagocytes (literally, "devouring cells"), scavengers that destroy foreign cells and microbes. The first of this cleanup crew to arrive in great numbers are neutrophils, which initially adhere to endothelial cells and then migrate into surrounding tissue and the wound itself. With an appendage called a pseudopod, a neutrophil may grab a microbe, engulf it, and then digest it with chemicals; neutrophils can also dispatch foreign material by spraying these chemicals on it.

The number of short-lived neutrophils within the wound peaks about a day after the injury, then drops as more macrophages, a longer-lived phagocyte, arrive. Macrophages not only devour microbes but also clean up the edges of the wound by ingesting dead and injured cells—including neutrophils. Also, they set the stage for repair by releasing growth factors.

Reconstruction commences while the defensive battle continues. The upper portion of the blood clot, dried by contact with the air, hardens into a scab. Epithelial cells farthest from the surface begin dividing and migrating through the clot, bridging the gap.

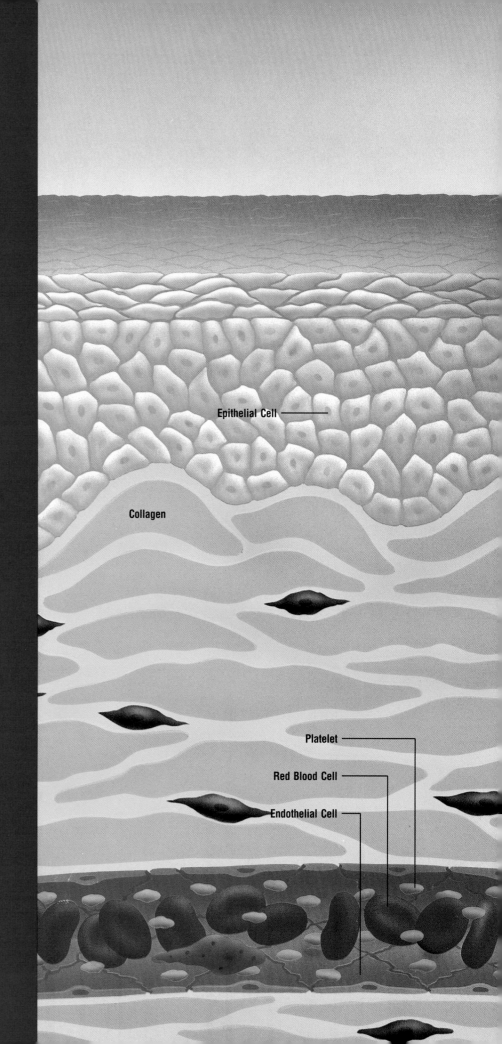

Epithelial Cell

Collagen

Platelet

Red Blood Cell

Endothelial Cell

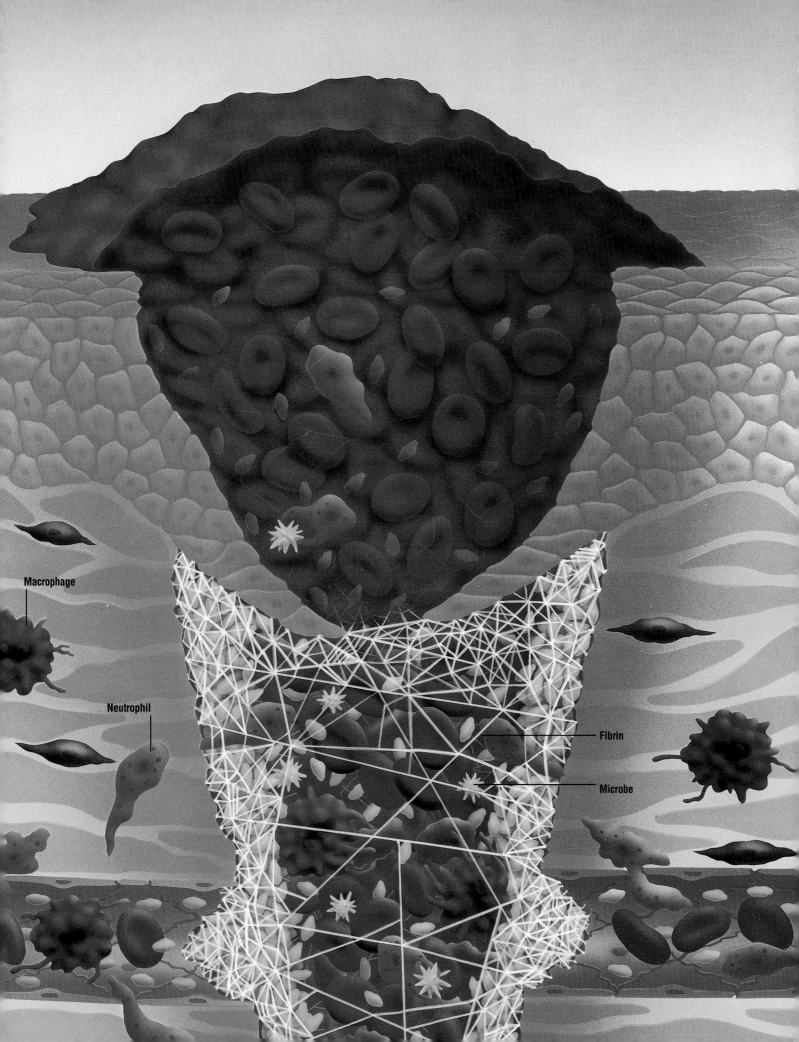

Macrophage

Neutrophil

Fibrin

Microbe

REBUILDING THE SYSTEMS

Restoration of the damaged area, which begins with expansion of the layer of epithelial cells, continues at deeper levels as connective tissue and blood vessels are repaired. At the same time, the clot breaks up, its component blood cells and fibrin degrading into their constituent proteins.

Through a process known as contact inhibition, in which epithelial cells moving toward the wound site encounter others of their type in the gap beneath the scab, the epithelial cells stop migrating and start to multiply, building up a new layer of epidermis. Cell division around the edges of the wound provides replacements for epithelial cells that migrated.

In the underlying connective tissue, fibroblasts proliferate and move to the wound. These cells ordinarily build connective tissue by secreting fibers of collagen and a material called ground substance. Penetrating the blood clot, they travel along the fibrin threads and synthesize connective tissue fibers—mainly collagen—as they go. These building blocks are randomly deposited, transforming the clot into so-called granulation tissue, an intermediary connective tissue that supports growing blood vessels.

Blood vessels regrow in a process known as angiogenesis (*page* 77). Factors released by cells involved in cleanup and repair trigger the proliferation of the blood vessels' endothelial cells. These lining cells rebuild damaged blood vessels and grow from existing small vessels into the region of the wound, where they establish new capillaries.

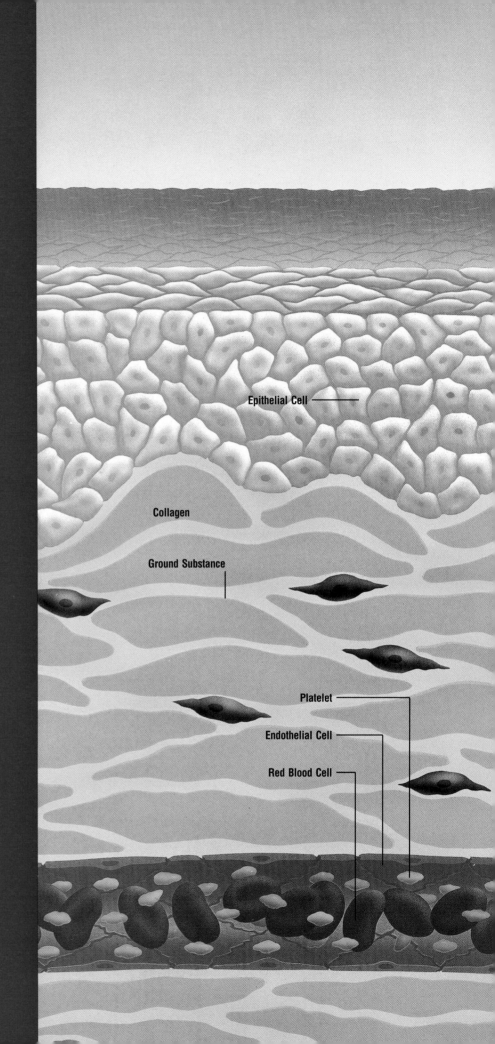

Epithelial Cell

Collagen

Ground Substance

Platelet

Endothelial Cell

Red Blood Cell

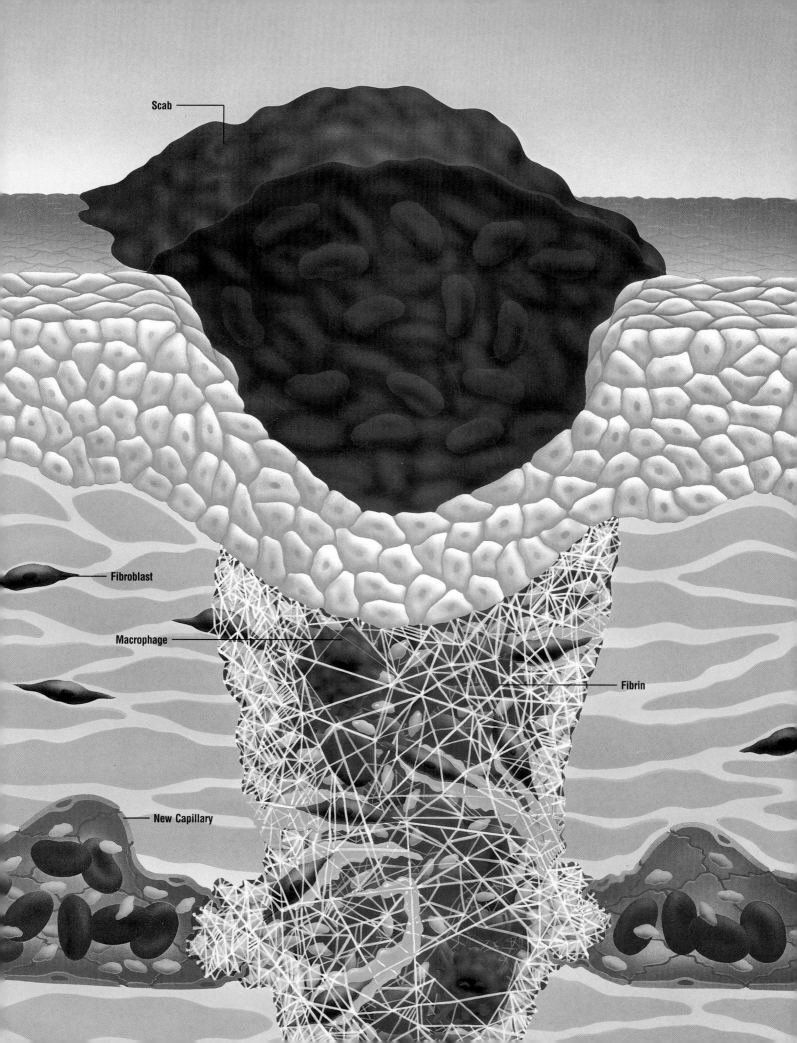

Scab

Fibroblast

Macrophage

Fibrin

New Capillary

RESTORATION COMPLETED

The final stage of wound healing continues at a slower pace than the emergency repairs. Specialized fibroblasts within the granulation tissue tug at the sides of the wound, causing it to contract. Proliferating epithelial cells restore the epidermis to its normal thickness, and the scab begins to loosen. Eventually the scab will slough off as the tissue below forms a raised, red scar (*not shown*), rich with new blood vessels and cells.

As the scar matures, new collagen gradually replaces fibers deposited earlier in the granulation tissue, in a process called remodeling. Over a period of weeks and months, the collagen itself matures and, as it does so, forms tighter bundles. These bundles are stronger than the fibers they replaced, but they never fully duplicate the organized pattern, and the consequent strength, of the original tissue.

The severed blood vessels complete their regeneration, not necessarily following the same paths as their damaged predecessors; in the illustration here, they form an arch. As healing continues, the stubs of the old blood vessels will be reabsorbed by macrophages. Meanwhile the increased blood supply to the wound site curtails the production of the factors that encouraged vessel growth, and new capillaries stop forming.

The increased density of collagen transforms the wound into a flat, white scar that differs from normal tissue in more than appearance. Although the skin is again whole, it may lack much of its original equipment, such as hair follicles, sweat glands, and sensory neurons.

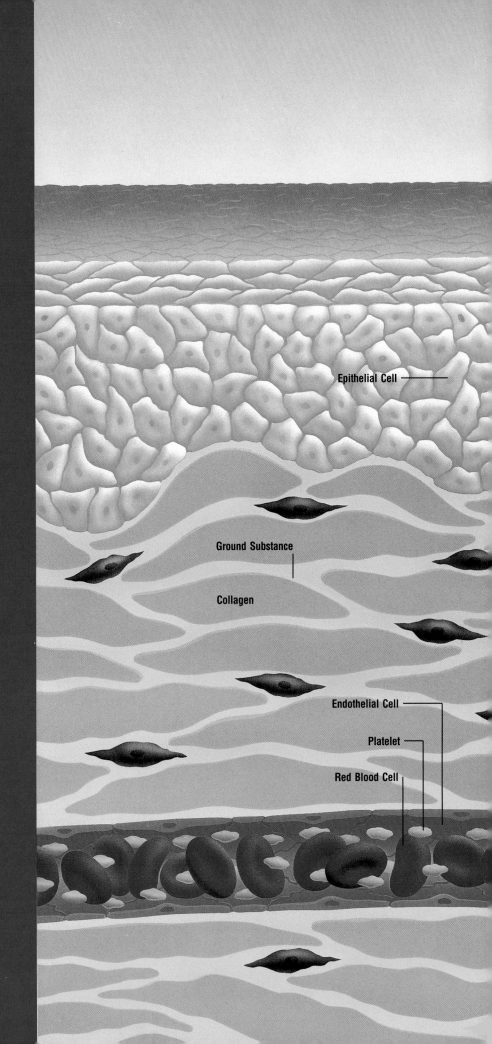

Epithelial Cell

Ground Substance

Collagen

Endothelial Cell

Platelet

Red Blood Cell

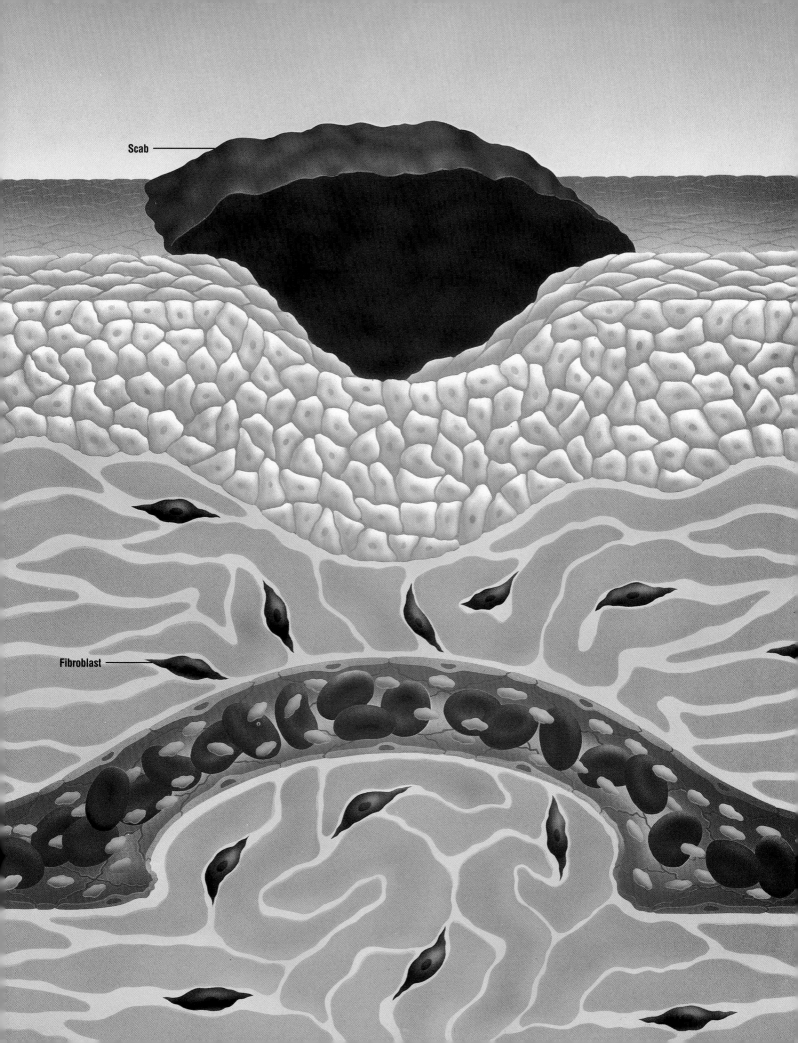

Scab

Fibroblast

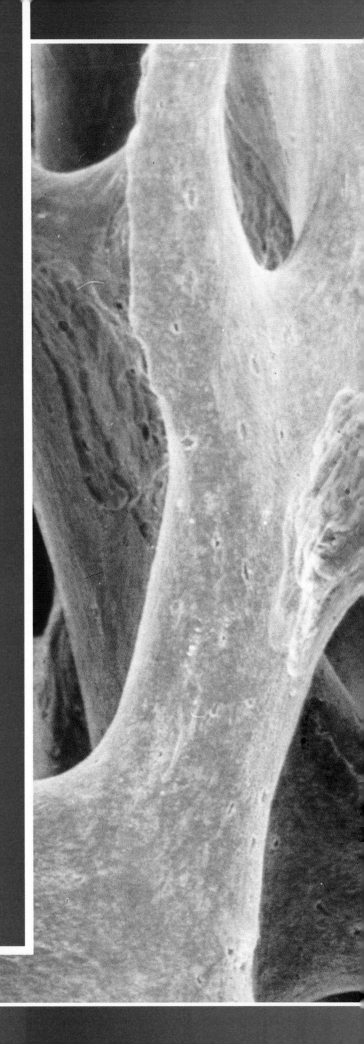

WHEN A BONE BREAKS

A broken bone is probably the most traumatic and painful of relatively common injuries. The body handles the damage through many of the same processes and stages—from inflammation to repair and remodeling—as in wound healing, but with a few added complications. Fractures usually call for the reconstruction of soft tissue around the bone, the marrow inside it, and vessels running through it. But the central task, of course, is the remaking of the bone itself.

Undifferentiated stem cells play a key role in bone regeneration. Like blood stem cells, they can become different types of cells as they proliferate. Through a mechanism that scientists understand only poorly, a class of proteins called morphogens apparently influence these stem cells to develop into chondroblasts, which produce a cartilage scaffolding around the break, or osteoblasts—the progenitors of new bone cells.

Because bone cells grow and divide slowly, and because of bone's complex architecture (including, as seen here, a thin web of bone that honeycombs the interior, where marrow resides), the repair and remodeling phases can take months. But in the end, healing can be so complete that the fracture line is not even visible on an x-ray.

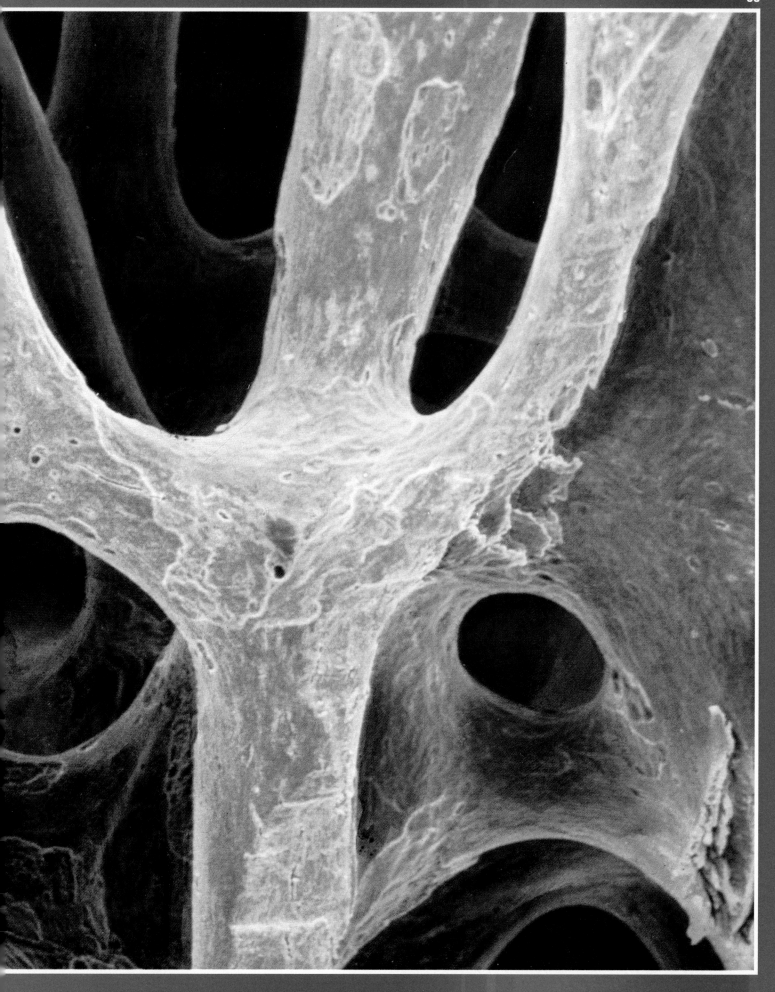

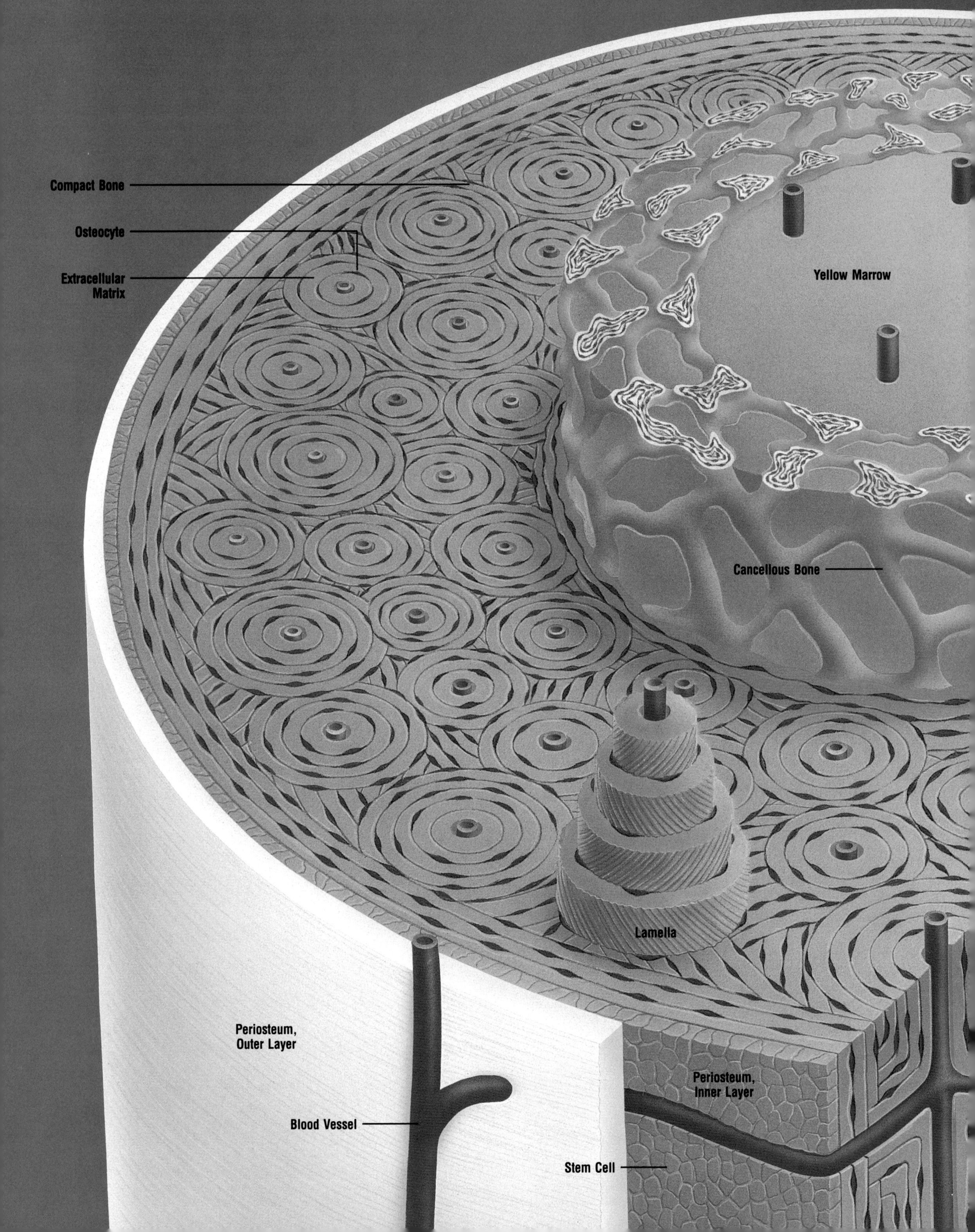

Compact Bone

Osteocyte

Extracellular
Matrix

Yellow Marrow

Cancellous Bone

Lamella

Periosteum,
Outer Layer

Periosteum,
Inner Layer

Blood Vessel

Stem Cell

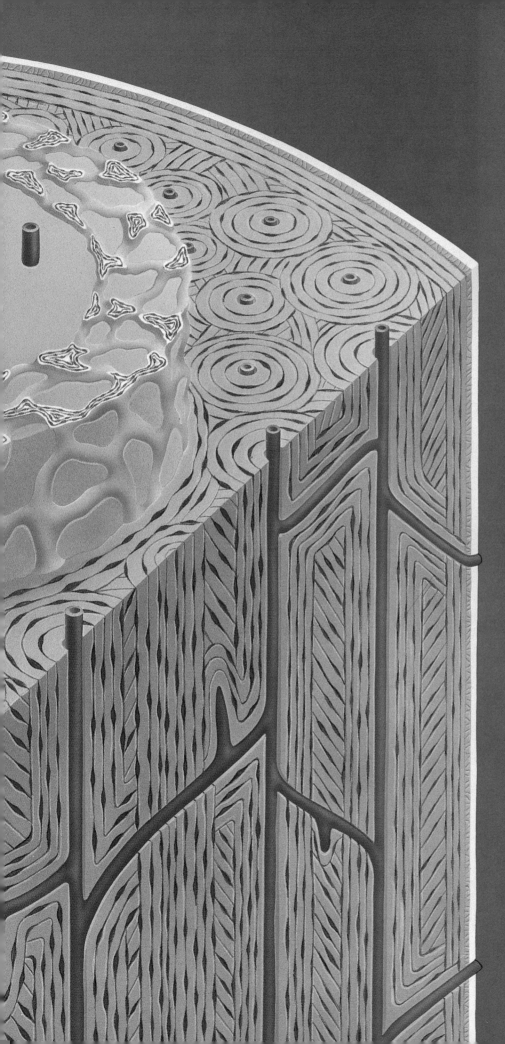

STRUCTURED FOR STRENGTH. Bone, which is actually a kind of connective tissue, consists primarily of a dense extracellular matrix *(pink)* and widely separated bone cells, or osteocytes *(blue).* In the broad region of what is known as compact bone, these cells and matrix are organized in groups of concentric rings, called lamellae; blood vessels supply nutrients and oxygen and also remove waste. The heart of the bone contains marrow—yellow marrow in this diagram of the shaft of a long bone—and the network of so-called cancellous bone. The exterior of the bone is encased in two layers: the tough and fibrous outer periosteum, and the inner periosteum, the repository of stem cells *(purple)* that are the source of new bone cells. Not shown are two other types of cells found in bone. Osteoblasts, which arise from stem cells, are the precursors of osteocytes, and they also secrete protein fibers and other compounds that make up the extracellular matrix. Osteoclasts are thought to derive from a type of white blood cell; they consume bone matrix as part of a process for forming new bone during both development and repair.

68

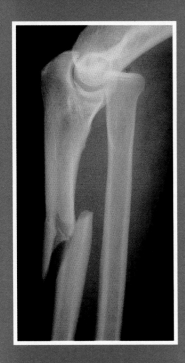

THE FIRST STAGES OF REPAIR. As part of the inflammatory response, which kicks in while the blood is clotting, stem cells in the area of the break are stimulated to proliferate and start differentiating. Some become chondroblasts, which create cartilage throughout the break *(below, blue)*, replacing the blood clot. The cartilage starts appearing about four days after the injury and can take up to a month to fully develop into what is called a soft callus. At the bone's outer edges—just within the layers of periosteum—the callus forms a bump on the bone's exterior that acts as a kind of splint to

A BLOOD CLOT IN BONE. Fractured bone, such as the broken ulna shown above in the x-ray of a forearm, typically causes bleeding, as blood vessels spanning the break are severed. As with skin, blood clotting to close the wound in the bone is the first order of business *(below)*. Platelets accumulate, and various transformations of substances in the blood give rise to fibrin, the filamentary protein that helps form clots by trapping red blood cells, platelets, and plasma. Usually within six to eight hours, clotting will have closed the fracture. Meanwhile, bone cells around the break have died and are being reabsorbed by osteoclasts; stem cells have also begun to migrate into the wound.

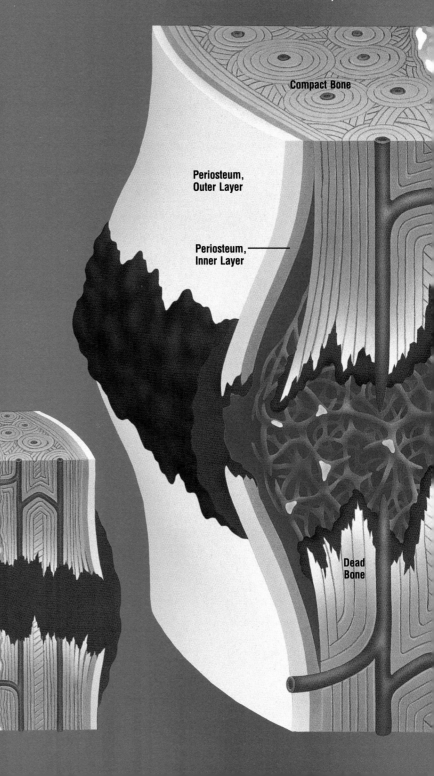

Compact Bone

Periosteum, Outer Layer

Periosteum, Inner Layer

Dead Bone

Blood Clot

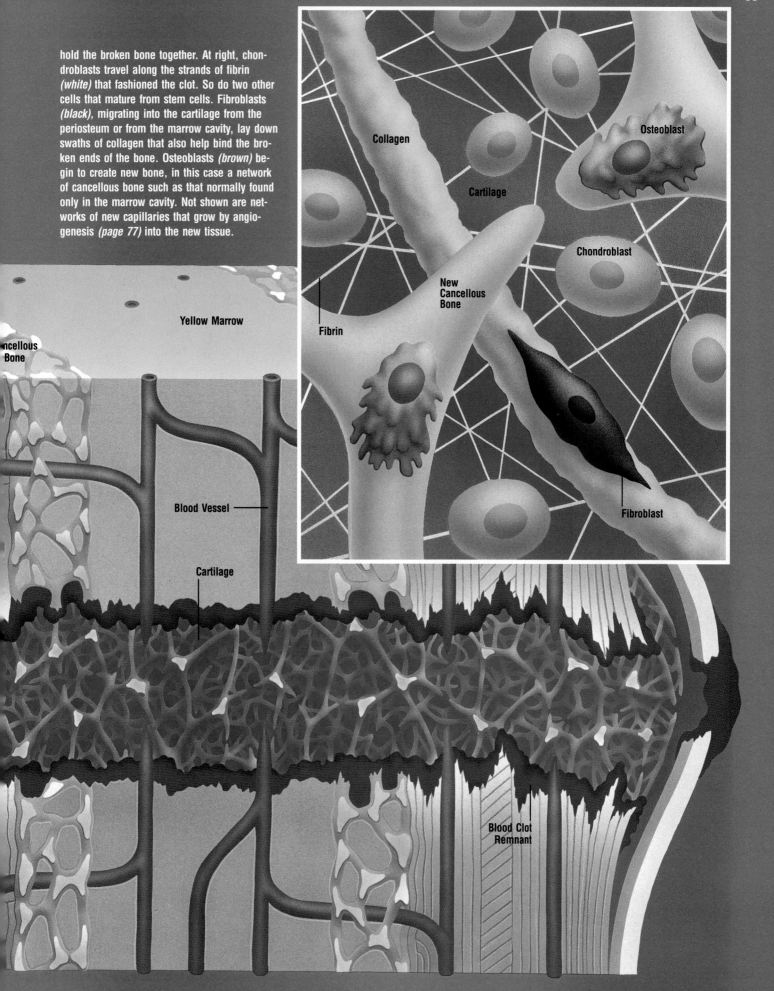

hold the broken bone together. At right, chondroblasts travel along the strands of fibrin *(white)* that fashioned the clot. So do two other cells that mature from stem cells. Fibroblasts *(black),* migrating into the cartilage from the periosteum or from the marrow cavity, lay down swaths of collagen that also help bind the broken ends of the bone. Osteoblasts *(brown)* begin to create new bone, in this case a network of cancellous bone such as that normally found only in the marrow cavity. Not shown are networks of new capillaries that grow by angiogenesis *(page 77)* into the new tissue.

Collagen

Osteoblast

Cartilage

Chondroblast

New Cancellous Bone

Fibrin

Fibroblast

Yellow Marrow

ncellous Bone

Blood Vessel

Cartilage

Blood Clot Remnant

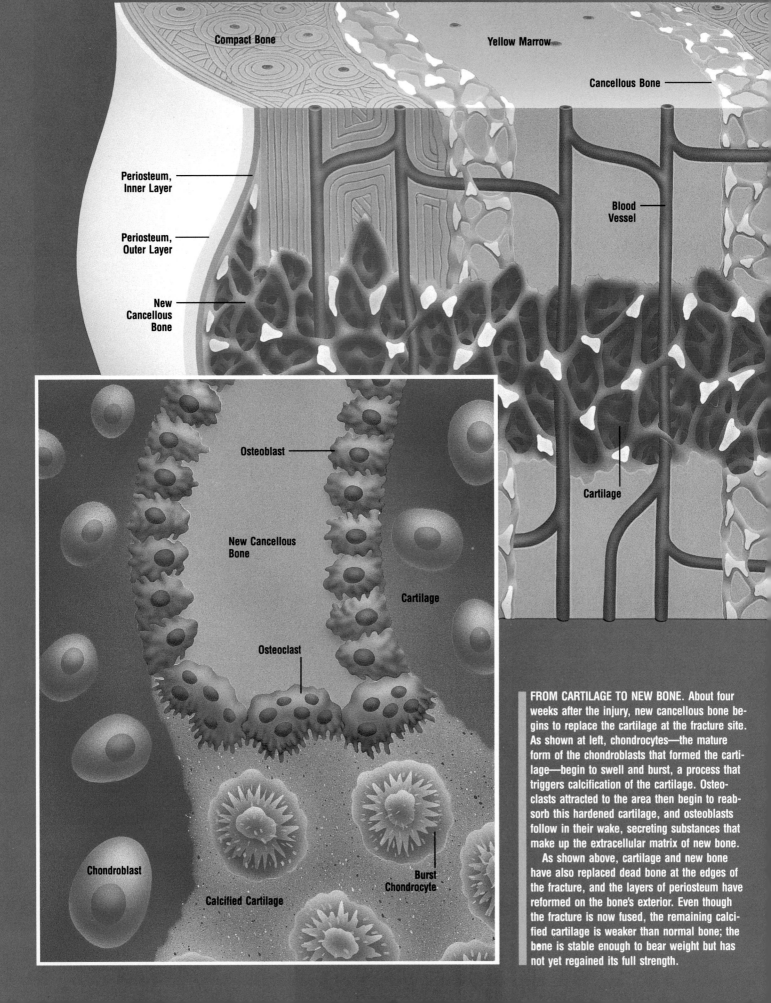

Compact Bone

Yellow Marrow

Cancellous Bone

Periosteum,
Inner Layer

Periosteum,
Outer Layer

Blood
Vessel

New
Cancellous
Bone

Cartilage

Osteoblast

New Cancellous
Bone

Cartilage

Osteoclast

Chondroblast

Calcified Cartilage

Burst
Chondrocyte

FROM CARTILAGE TO NEW BONE. About four weeks after the injury, new cancellous bone begins to replace the cartilage at the fracture site. As shown at left, chondrocytes—the mature form of the chondroblasts that formed the cartilage—begin to swell and burst, a process that triggers calcification of the cartilage. Osteoclasts attracted to the area then begin to reabsorb this hardened cartilage, and osteoblasts follow in their wake, secreting substances that make up the extracellular matrix of new bone.

As shown above, cartilage and new bone have also replaced dead bone at the edges of the fracture, and the layers of periosteum have reformed on the bone's exterior. Even though the fracture is now fused, the remaining calcified cartilage is weaker than normal bone; the bone is stable enough to bear weight but has not yet regained its full strength.

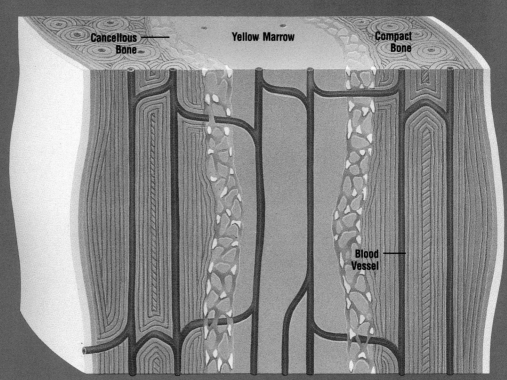

Cancellous Bone — Yellow Marrow — Compact Bone — Blood Vessel

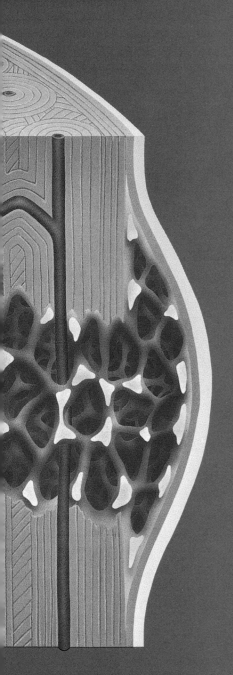

COMPLETING THE JOB. In remodeling, the final stage of fracture repair, one group of cells destroys old extracellular matrix while another class creates new matrix until compact bone has replaced cancellous bone along so-called force lines that bear the most weight. Osteoclasts continue to reabsorb dead parts of the original bone as well as unneeded callus, thus decreasing the size of the lump over the fracture site. Osteoclasts also burrow through the newly formed compact bone, creating tunnels into which new capillaries will grow. Osteoblasts follow along, gradually lining the tunnel walls and laying down concentric layers of new bone. The concentric layers gradually fill the tunnel, leaving only a narrow channel around the blood vessel. At the heart of the bone, yellow marrow moves in, returning the bone to its original architecture *(above)*. The entire remodeling process can continue for years after the fracture has fused.

A DANGEROUS CASE OF REPAIR

Normally, the body's cells repair and renew tissues and organs with speed, energy, and discretion—reproducing or dying off to make room for replacements. But sometimes, their reaction to damage can prove harmful.

In the circulatory system, the misguided response of some cells to injury can lead to atherosclerosis, the most common form of arteriosclerosis, or hardening of the arteries. Trouble seems to arise when cells that line the inner surface of blood vessels are damaged. Though these injuries may be minute, the body's normal response is to rush agents in to mend the breach. In this case, the repair team—like a road crew sent to fix a pothole on a busy highway at rush hour—may cause a major backup, or even an accident.

To sustain life, the heart must pump five quarts of oxygen- and nutrient-rich blood per minute into the aorta and up through a junction called the aortic arch (*right*), then on through the circulatory system. A backup can lead to a heart attack—a cardiovascular crisis, often brought on by atherosclerosis, that is the leading cause of death in the Western world.

As explained on the next pages, atherosclerosis begins at a microscopic level and can take years to become a threat. Doctors employ an arsenal of therapies for advanced cases, but the best approach is prevention.

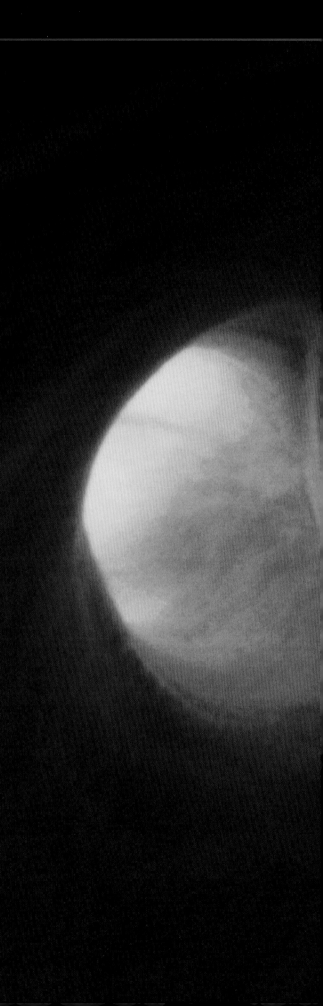

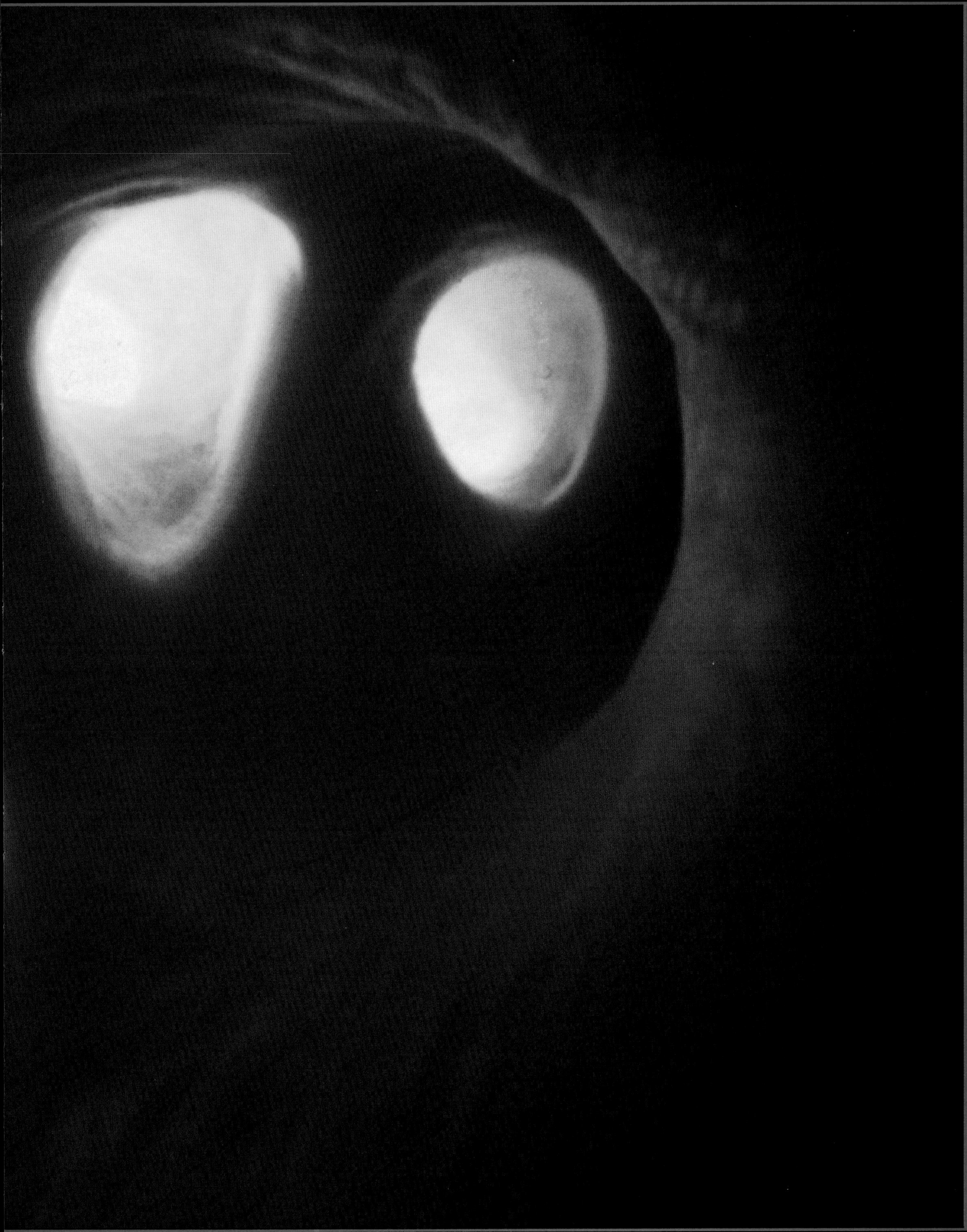

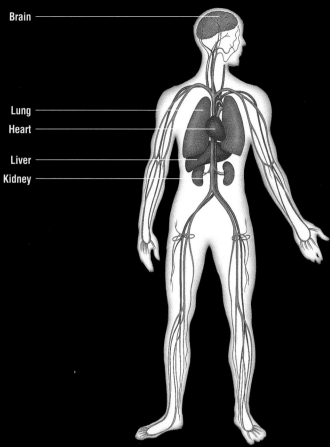

Brain

Lung

Heart

Liver

Kidney

A TIRELESS PUMP

The fist-size muscle that is the human heart beats 60 to 100 times a minute, or about 100,000 times a day—more than 2.5 billion times during a 75-year life span. Because the organ serves two separate circulatory systems, an impenetrable barrier called the septum divides the right side from the left. Each side is further partitioned into two sections: a thin-walled holding tank, or atrium, and a more powerful chamber called a ventricle that does the actual pumping.

Both sides of the heart beat at the same time. The right side sends blood a short distance to the lungs to get rid of carbon dioxide collected from throughout the body and to pick up fresh oxygen. Oxygenated blood from the lungs returns to the left side and from there is pumped to all of the body's other organs and tissues. The muscle wall of the heart's left ventricle thus works harder and is about four times thicker than that of the right ventricle.

A built-in electrical conducting system sets the pace, triggering the heart's chambers to fill and empty in a rhythmic cycle that lasts about a second. Valves open and close with each beat, guiding the flow of blood through the organ.

The heart supplies itself with oxygen and nutrients by way of small coronary arteries that tap the aorta and deliver blood deep into the muscle walls. If blood flow in a coronary artery is obstructed, sections of heart muscle downstream from the blockage will die within minutes, resulting in a heart attack.

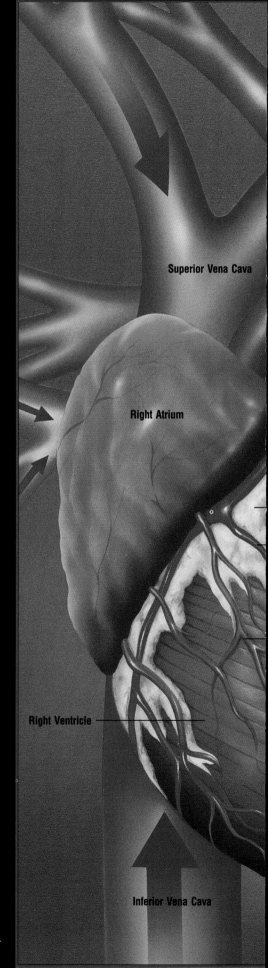

Superior Vena Cava

Right Atrium

Right Ventricle

Inferior Vena Cava

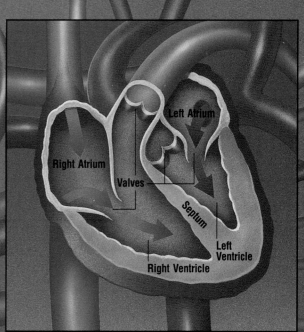

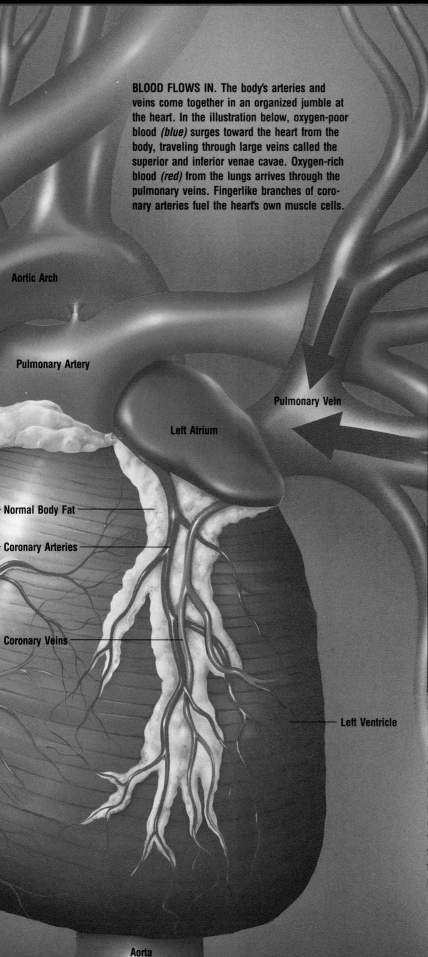

BLOOD FLOWS IN. The body's arteries and veins come together in an organized jumble at the heart. In the illustration below, oxygen-poor blood *(blue)* surges toward the heart from the body, traveling through large veins called the superior and inferior venae cavae. Oxygen-rich blood *(red)* from the lungs arrives through the pulmonary veins. Fingerlike branches of coronary arteries fuel the heart's own muscle cells.

Aortic Arch

Pulmonary Artery

Pulmonary Vein

Left Atrium

Normal Body Fat

Coronary Arteries

Coronary Veins

Left Ventricle

Aorta

Right Atrium

Left Atrium

Valves

Septum

Left Ventricle

Right Ventricle

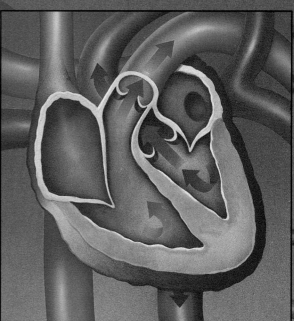

A HEARTBEAT. During the first phase of a heartbeat, called diastole *(top)*, blood flows into the right and left atria from the body and the lungs respectively. After the atria fill, specialized valves open and allow the collected blood to drain into the ventricles. In the pumping phase, known as systole *(above)*, these valves close to prevent backflow into the atria as the ventricles contract. Other valves open to allow the right ventricle to squeeze oxygen-depleted blood into the pulmonary artery (toward the lungs), while the left ventricle sends oxygenated blood to the rest of the body by way of the aorta.

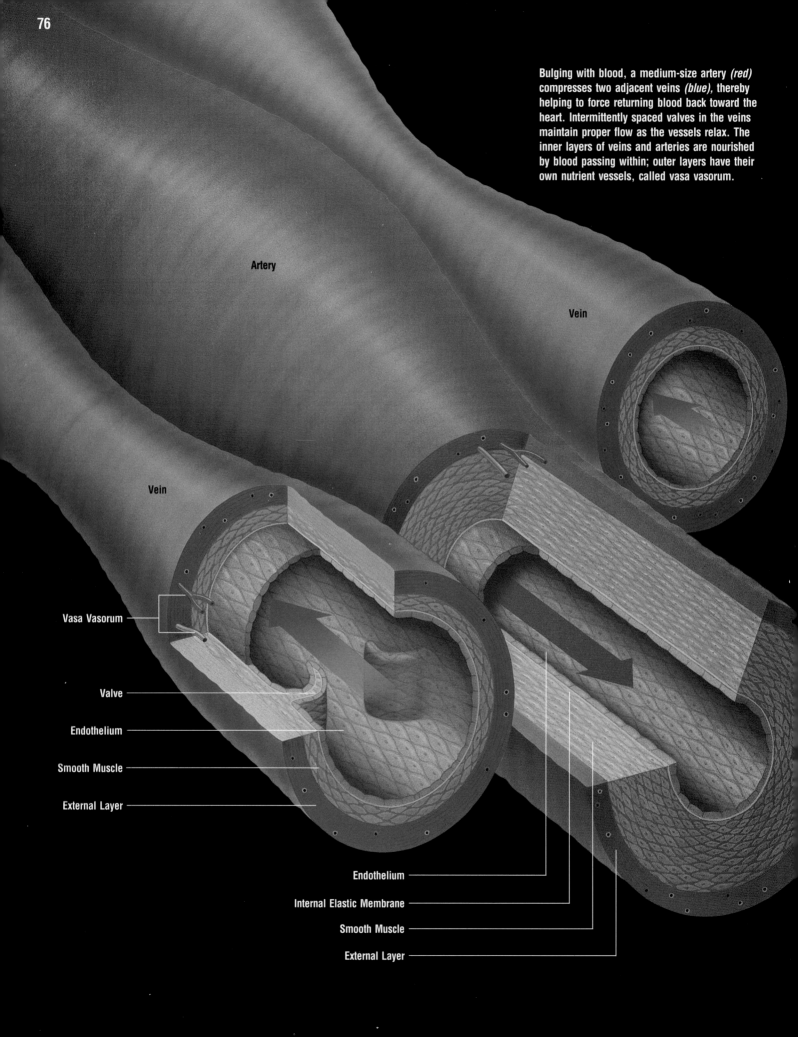

76

Bulging with blood, a medium-size artery *(red)* compresses two adjacent veins *(blue)*, thereby helping to force returning blood back toward the heart. Intermittently spaced valves in the veins maintain proper flow as the vessels relax. The inner layers of veins and arteries are nourished by blood passing within; outer layers have their own nutrient vessels, called vasa vasorum.

Artery

Vein

Vein

Vasa Vasorum

Valve

Endothelium

Smooth Muscle

External Layer

Endothelium

Internal Elastic Membrane

Smooth Muscle

External Layer

The heart's left ventricle pumps oxygenated blood into the aorta and other large arteries, which in turn branch into medium-size arteries and then into smaller vessels called arterioles. These supply tiny capillaries within the various body tissues.

Capillaries consist of a single layer of endothelial cells encased by a flexible basement membrane. As blood cells maneuver single file through these narrows, their oxygen cargo seeps through the thin capillary walls into surrounding tissue. Cell wastes and carbon dioxide, meanwhile, pass from the tissue through the capillary wall and into the bloodstream. Its oxygen spent, blood begins the return trip to the heart, entering small vessels called venules, which feed into progressively larger veins.

As shown at left, veins and arteries share a similar three-tiered structure: an inner layer, or endothelium, composed of endothelial cells, that keeps substances in the bloodstream from sticking to vessel walls and also helps regulate the interaction between blood and tissues; a middle layer of smooth muscle cells; and an external layer of fibrous collagen and elastic tissues. Arteries are stronger and more pliable than veins, because they contain extra sheets of elastic tissue and thicker layers of muscle. These traits allow arteries to withstand the pressure of blood being pumped from the heart, and to constrict or dilate as blood volume and heart rate change.

Pressure in the veins is generally low, approaching zero as returning blood nears the heart. Valves inside many veins open to let blood advance and close to prevent backflow. Muscle contraction, the pulsing of nearby arteries, and pressure changes from breathing also help squeeze the blood back toward the heart.

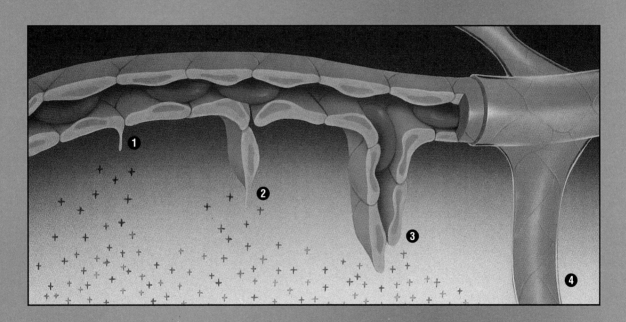

How Tissues Create Their Own Blood Supply

All blood vessels originate as capillaries, in a process known as angiogenesis. When tissues need oxygen—during growth, for example, or in response to injury—they emit chemicals called growth factors, which prompt endothelial cells to digest their way to the outside of the vessel. The cells extend sprouts called pseudopods (1), then grow toward the chemical lure (2) and reproduce by simply dividing (3). The resulting cells form the opening, or lumen, of a new capillary shoot. Red blood cells then begin to flow into the growing vessel, which remains somewhat leaky until it is completed (4). When the vessel joins others to become a working part of the circulatory system, the tissues shut down production of growth factors.

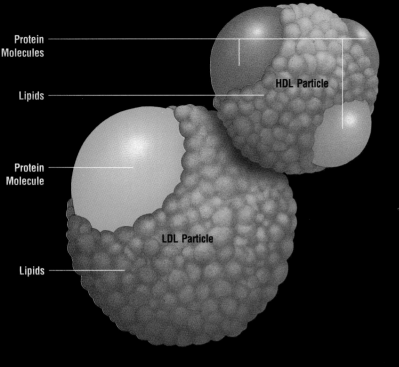

Protein Molecules

Lipids

HDL Particle

Protein Molecule

LDL Particle

Lipids

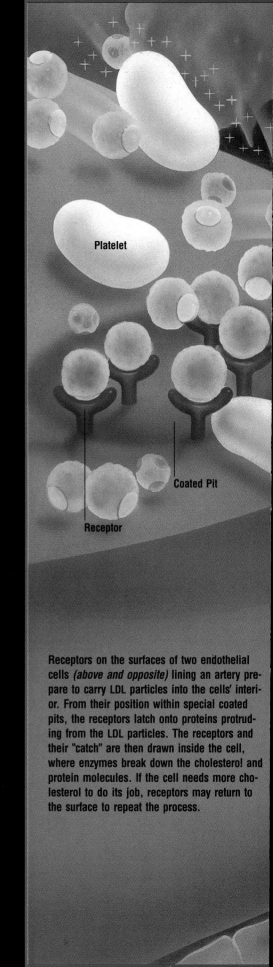

Platelet

Coated Pit

Receptor

Receptors on the surfaces of two endothelial cells *(above and opposite)* lining an artery prepare to carry LDL particles into the cells' interior. From their position within special coated pits, the receptors latch onto proteins protruding from the LDL particles. The receptors and their "catch" are then drawn inside the cell, where enzymes break down the cholesterol and protein molecules. If the cell needs more cholesterol to do its job, receptors may return to the surface to repeat the process.

A CELL NECESSITY TURNS DEADLY

As is often true in life, too much of a good thing can be bad for you. Such is the case with cholesterol, a fatty substance essential to all animal cell membranes and also used to create bile acids and steroid hormones. Some of the body's cholesterol is derived directly from food, but most is synthesized by the liver and dispatched to cells by way of the blood.

Because cholesterol is not water-soluble and thus cannot enter the bloodstream in its pure form, the liver combines waxy cholesterol molecules, or lipids, with dissolvable protein carriers, called apolipoproteins, to form microscopic particles called lipoproteins. These vary in size and density according to their content. A high ratio of low-density to high-density lipoproteins (LDLs and HDLs)—and not the overall concentration of cholesterol in the body—is a sign of susceptibility to disease.

Often referred to as "bad" cholesterol, LDLs are so called because they consist primarily of low-density cholesterol and have only one large protein molecule. Smaller HDLs—"good" cholesterol—are denser because they have multiple protein molecules.

LDLs are the primary carrier of the body's circulating cholesterol. They bind to receptors on cell membranes, enter the cells, and are broken down into free cholesterol and amino acids. Once cells have collected enough cholesterol for the body's various needs, they stop making receptors.

If, for dietary or other reasons, the ratio of LDLs to HDLs is too high—and in patients with atherosclerosis, LDLs can outnumber HDLs five to one—excess LDLs in the bloodstream can begin to penetrate the endothelial lining of blood vessels, as illustrated at right. The job of HDLs, meanwhile, is to remove excess LDLs from vessel walls and ferry them either to cells for their use or to the liver for disposal.

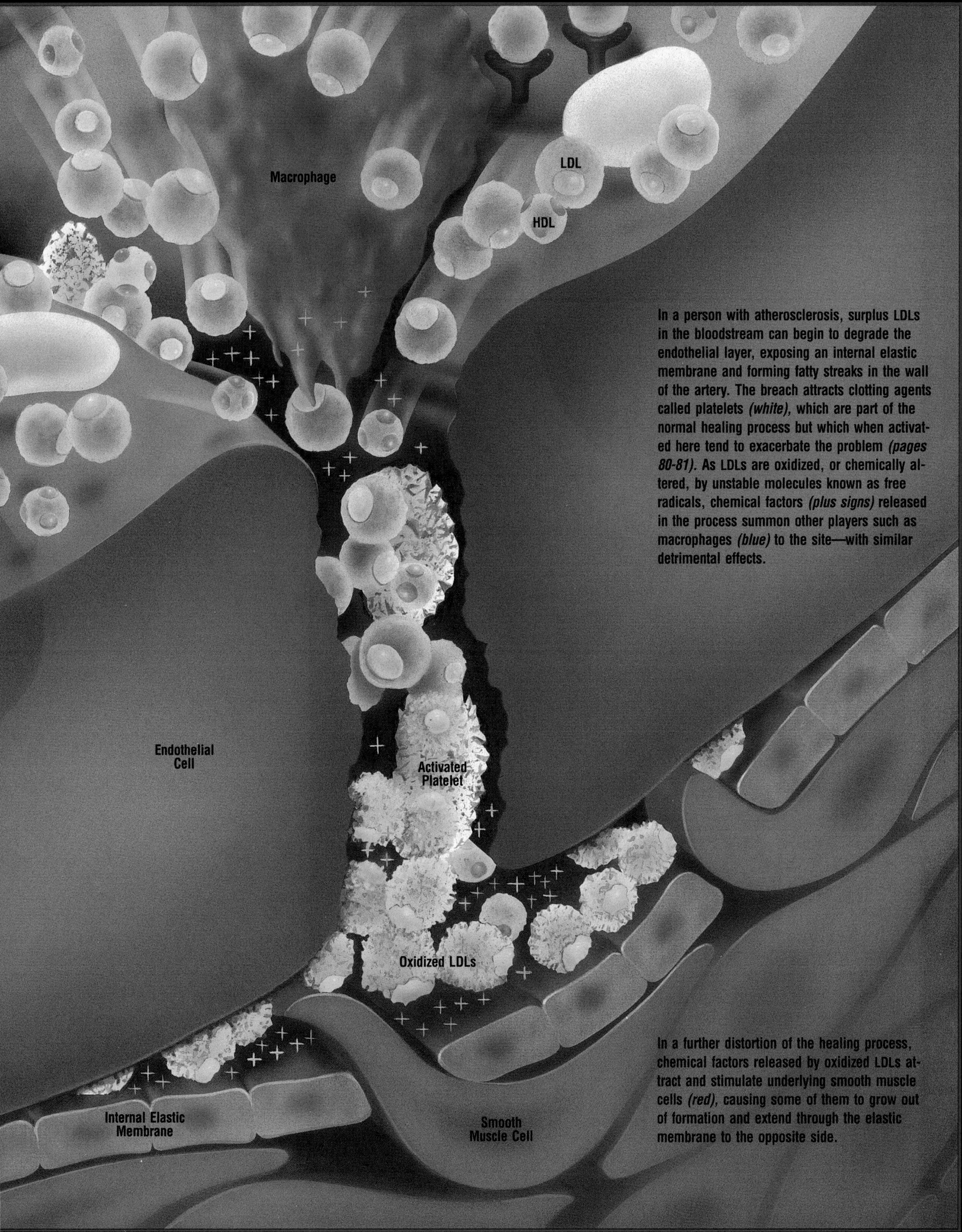

Macrophage

LDL

HDL

In a person with atherosclerosis, surplus LDLs in the bloodstream can begin to degrade the endothelial layer, exposing an internal elastic membrane and forming fatty streaks in the wall of the artery. The breach attracts clotting agents called platelets *(white)*, which are part of the normal healing process but which when activated here tend to exacerbate the problem *(pages 80-81)*. As LDLs are oxidized, or chemically altered, by unstable molecules known as free radicals, chemical factors *(plus signs)* released in the process summon other players such as macrophages *(blue)* to the site—with similar detrimental effects.

Endothelial
Cell

Activated
Platelet

Oxidized LDLs

In a further distortion of the healing process, chemical factors released by oxidized LDLs attract and stimulate underlying smooth muscle cells *(red)*, causing some of them to grow out of formation and extend through the elastic membrane to the opposite side.

Internal Elastic
Membrane

Smooth
Muscle Cell

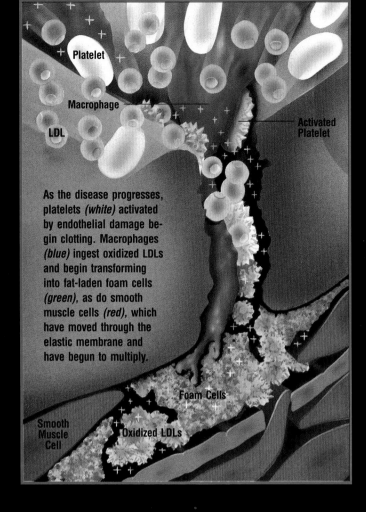

Platelet

Macrophage

LDL

Activated
Platelet

As the disease progresses,
platelets *(white)* activated
by endothelial damage be-
gin clotting. Macrophages
(blue) ingest oxidized LDLs
and begin transforming
into fat-laden foam cells
(green), as do smooth
muscle cells *(red)*, which
have moved through the
elastic membrane and
have begun to multiply.

Foam Cells

Smooth
Muscle
Cell

Oxidized LDLs

A DANGEROUS OBSTRUCTION

As the buildup of LDL cholesterol in arterial walls continues, it can trigger a chain of events leading to the formation of atherosclerotic lesions, or plaques. For example, when the endothelial layer is damaged, platelets that would normally be repelled by chemicals on the surface of endothelial cells instead stick to the cells and to the elastic membrane below them. The platelets aggregate and start a chemical chain reaction that will form a blood clot *(pages 56-57)* to prevent blood from leaking out of the vessel.

Meanwhile, scavenging macrophages, immobilized by the oxidized LDLs they have ingested, as well as by toxins emitted by the LDLs, are converted into stagnant, fat-filled foam cells. The same fate befalls some of the smooth muscle cells that have invaded the area, adding to the growing plaque, which is also fed by connective tissue and various bits of cell debris.

As the plaque expands, it intrudes into the artery, interrupting blood flow and creating turbulence. This can cause additional damage and attract yet more platelets. Eventually the plaque develops a fibrous cap, made primarily of foam cells, smooth muscle cells, immune cells, and connective tissue. The cap can repeatedly rupture, enlarging the protrusion and also leading to the formation of a thrombus, or clot. Atherosclerotic plaques may take 20 or 30 years to develop, often becoming calcified in the process, making the artery brittle and even more vulnerable to injury.

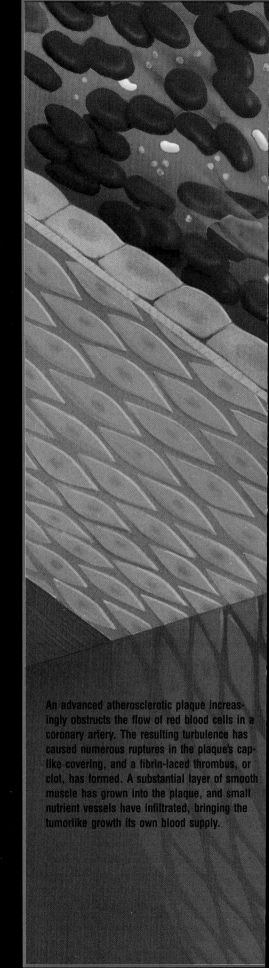

An advanced atherosclerotic plaque increasingly obstructs the flow of red blood cells in a coronary artery. The resulting turbulence has caused numerous ruptures in the plaque's cap-like covering, and a fibrin-laced thrombus, or clot, has formed. A substantial layer of smooth muscle has grown into the plaque, and small nutrient vessels have infiltrated, bringing the tumorlike growth its own blood supply.

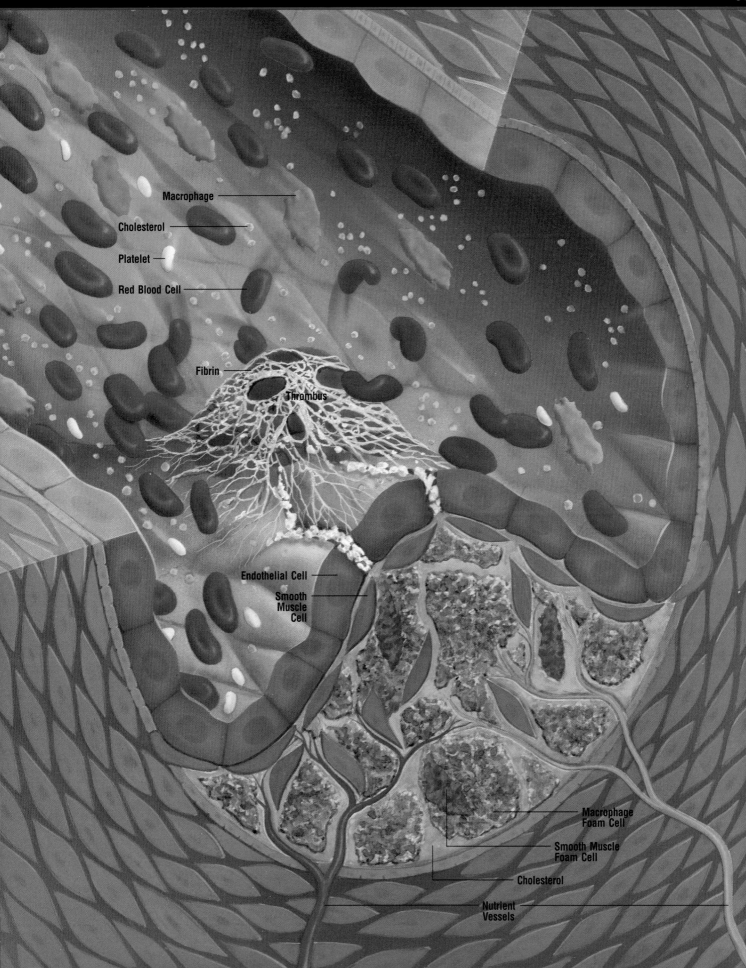

Macrophage

Cholesterol

Platelet

Red Blood Cell

Fibrin

Thrombus

Endothelial Cell

Smooth
Muscle
Cell

Macrophage
Foam Cell

Smooth Muscle
Foam Cell

Cholesterol

Nutrient
Vessels

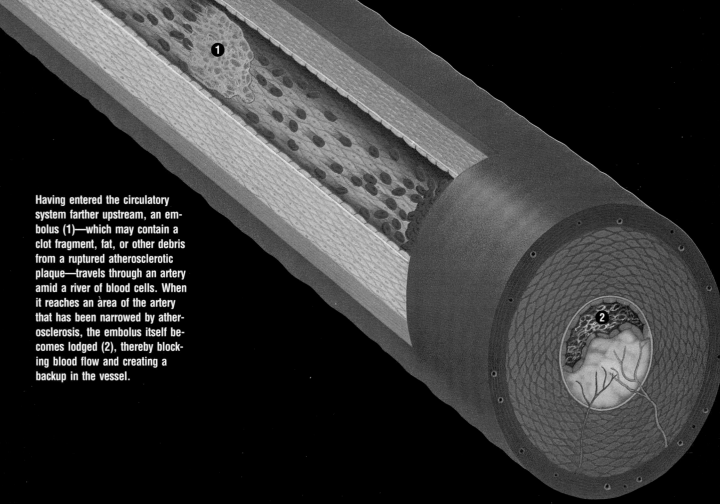

Having entered the circulatory system farther upstream, an embolus (1)—which may contain a clot fragment, fat, or other debris from a ruptured atherosclerotic plaque—travels through an artery amid a river of blood cells. When it reaches an area of the artery that has been narrowed by atherosclerosis, the embolus itself becomes lodged (2), thereby blocking blood flow and creating a backup in the vessel.

PRELUDE TO A HEART ATTACK

Although in advanced cases of atherosclerosis, a thrombus often forms directly over the plaque buildup—further narrowing the vessel—it is also common for a clot that has developed elsewhere in the body to break free and become what is known as an embolus. As it travels through the bloodstream, an embolus can lodge in an area constricted by a plaque, blocking the vessel even more. If an artery becomes so obstructed that blood flow is reduced to less than 30 percent of the normal rate, tissues beyond the bottleneck may no longer receive the oxygen and nutrients they need to survive.

Blockages in the arteries supplying blood to the heart muscle can have disastrous consequences. Temporary oxygen deprivation to cardiac muscle,

a condition known as ischemia, can be reversed if blood flow is restored within a few hours. Such a short-term oxygen deficit may cause chest pressure and discomfort called angina pectoris, which can arise when a person with blocked coronary arteries suddenly needs more oxygen because of increased physical activity or a heightened emotional state. Angina patients usually recover from an attack when they relax or take medications that dilate their arteries and allow increased blood flow.

If oxygen and nutrients are not restored soon enough, the affected area of the heart muscle will die, resulting in a myocardial infarction—a heart attack. The severity of the attack depends on the location and size of the affected region. Often, dam-

aged areas surrounding dead tissue can be saved if oxygen flow and nutrient delivery are restored in time, but the greater the muscle loss, the less effective will be the heart's pumping action. Death of cardiac muscle can also disrupt the heart's electrical system, causing the organ to beat erratically or to stop beating entirely.

Researchers have found that, as atherosclerosis develops, some blood vessels enlarge to compensate for the obstruction and maintain normal vessel capacity. Some atherosclerosis sufferers, particularly those who have survived a heart attack, grow secondary vessels, known as collaterals, that create a natural bypass around the blockage. Consequently, not all individuals with atherosclerosis will experience life-threatening symptoms.

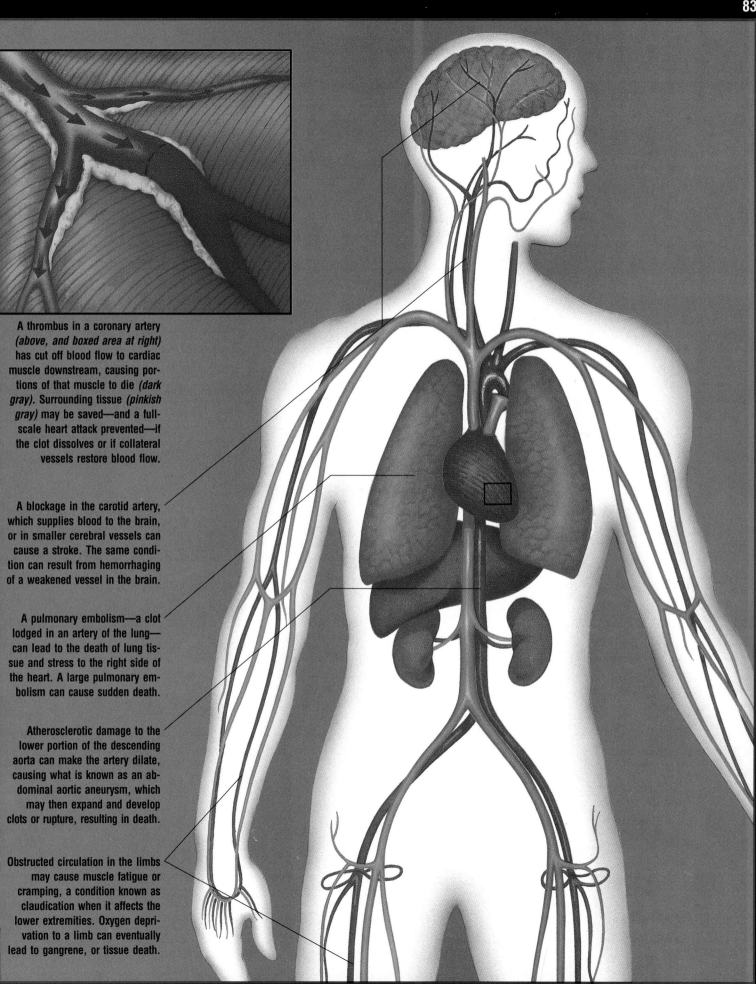

A thrombus in a coronary artery *(above, and boxed area at right)* has cut off blood flow to cardiac muscle downstream, causing portions of that muscle to die *(dark gray)*. Surrounding tissue *(pinkish gray)* may be saved—and a full-scale heart attack prevented—if the clot dissolves or if collateral vessels restore blood flow.

A blockage in the carotid artery, which supplies blood to the brain, or in smaller cerebral vessels can cause a stroke. The same condition can result from hemorrhaging of a weakened vessel in the brain.

A pulmonary embolism—a clot lodged in an artery of the lung—can lead to the death of lung tissue and stress to the right side of the heart. A large pulmonary embolism can cause sudden death.

Atherosclerotic damage to the lower portion of the descending aorta can make the artery dilate, causing what is known as an abdominal aortic aneurysm, which may then expand and develop clots or rupture, resulting in death.

Obstructed circulation in the limbs may cause muscle fatigue or cramping, a condition known as claudication when it affects the lower extremities. Oxygen deprivation to a limb can eventually lead to gangrene, or tissue death.

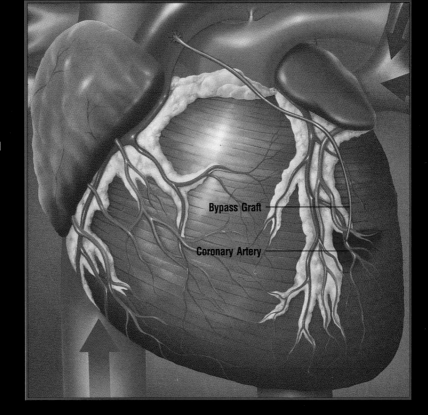

In this illustration, a clogged coronary artery *(red)* has been bypassed surgically by a vein graft *(blue)* that routes blood from the aorta above the obstructed area to a vessel in the heart muscle below it.

Bypass Graft

Coronary Artery

ARTIFICIAL REPAIR AND THERAPY

Most medical strategies to treat cardiovascular disease fall into three categories: treatment of symptoms, reversal of the disease process, and disease prevention.

One of the most frequently used forms of treatment involves coronary bypass surgery, once a risky procedure that in recent years has become fairly routine. An artery graft from the patient's chest or a vein graft from the leg is attached to the aorta at one end and then to an area of the vessel below the site of the obstruction. The graft acts as a conduit that bypasses the blocked area and restores blood flow to the deprived muscle. Multiple bypasses can be performed if more than one artery is clogged. But if the disease continues unchecked, eventually even these new vessels will narrow and need to be replaced.

In another technique, called balloon

angioplasty, a thin catheter is threaded through the femoral artery in the groin, up the aorta and into a coronary artery. A smaller catheter with a tiny, deflated balloon on its tip is then passed through the first catheter to the blockage. Doctors inflate the balloon, displacing the plaque and stretching the vessel wall to widen the artery. Catheters can also be used to deliver atherectomy devices—miniature drills, lasers, and suction tools—that can bore through, vaporize, or suck out a blockage.

In 30 to 40 percent of angioplasty and atherectomy patients, however, blockage recurs. Damage from the process itself may cause immediate formation of a thrombus or, over a period of months, trigger smooth muscle cells to proliferate, blocking the vessel even faster than would an atherosclerotic plaque. In some cases,

a small stainless-steel coil called a stent can be inserted at the site of an atherectomy or angioplasty to prop the vessel open.

As both a treatment and a preventive measure, certain medications can help curb the formation of dangerous blood clots. Common aspirin, for example, has been found to block one of the enzymes that cause platelets to cluster and blood vessels to constrict. Some drugs, known as thrombolytic agents, activate plasminogen, the body's own clot dissolver; often administered during a heart attack, they can eradicate a newly formed thrombus and prevent further clotting. Drugs called anticoagulants also prevent thrombi from forming.

The cornerstone of cholesterol management—effective in efforts both to reverse the course of the disease and to prevent its onset—is a low-fat diet.

BALLOON ANGIOPLASTY. A tiny balloon attached to a catheter reaches a plaque that has narrowed an artery.

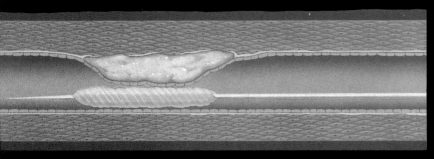

The balloon is inflated, compressing the plaque into the artery wall and dilating the vessel to allow greater blood flow.

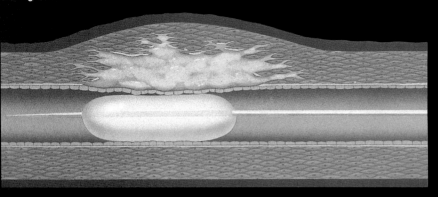

Although cholesterol is found only in animal products, foods derived from both animals and plants can contain fat, which, depending on the type, may increase the amount of cholesterol in the blood. Saturated fats—those that remain solid at room temperature, such as animal fats or coconut and palm oils—raise blood cholesterol levels more than other fats do, because they can reduce the number of LDL receptors on cells. Eating soluble fiber may help lower blood levels of "bad" LDLs, while exercise and weight loss have been found to raise levels of "good" HDLs.

Some patients with excessively high levels of LDLs (usually because of a genetic condition) can receive liver transplants or regularly undergo a process called LDL-pheresis, akin to dialysis, which removes excess LDLs from the blood. Medications can also improve blood serum cholesterol, in some cases by acting on the liver to inhibit production of LDLs. Other drugs work to raise HDL levels.

Some techniques used to treat atherosclerosis are still in the experimental stage. Many scientists, for example, think that specific doses of antioxidant vitamins such as A, C, and E may prevent oxidation of LDLs and thus inhibit plaque formation.

Researchers are also working on high-tech remedies for atherosclerosis, including gene therapy for people whose cells have a shortage of LDL receptors, and antibodies that may someday provide a vaccine against excess blood cholesterol. Other laboratory-engineered antibodies may eventually be used to deliver special clot-dissolving proteins to a deadly thrombus without disrupting the body's normal clotting ability.

Ingredients of a Disease

Experts cite a number of factors that increase the risk of atherosclerosis:

Endothelial injury. Pounding of the arterial wall caused by high blood pressure can injure the endothelium and accelerate LDL invasion of vessel walls. Excess stress hormones or toxins such as those found in cigarette smoke and city smog also seem to harm the endothelium.

Cholesterol levels. Heredity, age, and diet can affect serum cholesterol levels. One in 500 people inherits a gene that reduces the cells' ability to make LDL receptors and, thus, to absorb cholesterol. Receptor-making ability can also be reduced by age, obesity, and excess dietary fat or cholesterol, raising levels of "bad" cholesterol in the blood. Blood levels of "good" cholesterol are diminished by smoking and increased by aerobic exercise.

Demand on the heart. A heart that has been strengthened by regular exercise has a greater pumping capacity and works at a lower rate, saving wear and tear on vessel walls. Exercise also keeps vessels dilated, lowering blood pressure and further reducing the risk of disease. In the absence of regular exercise, higher heart rates can boost vulnerability to disease. Increases in the heart's work load will thus tax the whole circulatory system. Obesity and nicotine from cigarette smoke can drive up the heart rate, as can stress, anger, and fear.

Overactive clotting. Smoking, stress, and diabetes can make platelets more prone to harmful clotting. High blood levels of lipoprotein(a)—a substance structurally similar to LDL and to plasminogen—seem to increase the risk of clots, possibly by competing with the body's own clot dissolver and keeping it from doing its job.

MIND AND BODY: HEALING THE WHOLE

The human body is always healing, repairing flesh and bone damaged by injury, regenerating cells destroyed by infection, and renewing various systems after natural, everyday losses. For years these processes have been seen as nothing less than small miracles taking place beyond our conscious control. However, the possibility that the physical restoration of the body might be subject to the mind's powerful influences has surfaced time and again as our view of how we heal has evolved.

Ancient societies linked healing ability to a life in balance and to a respect for the interconnectedness of mind, body, and spirit. But as medicine became more science than art, the focus shifted to practical techniques for contending with illness or injury, and the patient was sometimes almost lost in the shuffle.

Today, however, there is a growing tendency to merge scientific and alternative practices, and to put the patient once more at the center of attention. As a result, healing has changed. It has become not just restoration but also a transforming experience that challenges longstanding attitudes and roles of both the patient and the healer as together they discover what it means to heal and be whole.

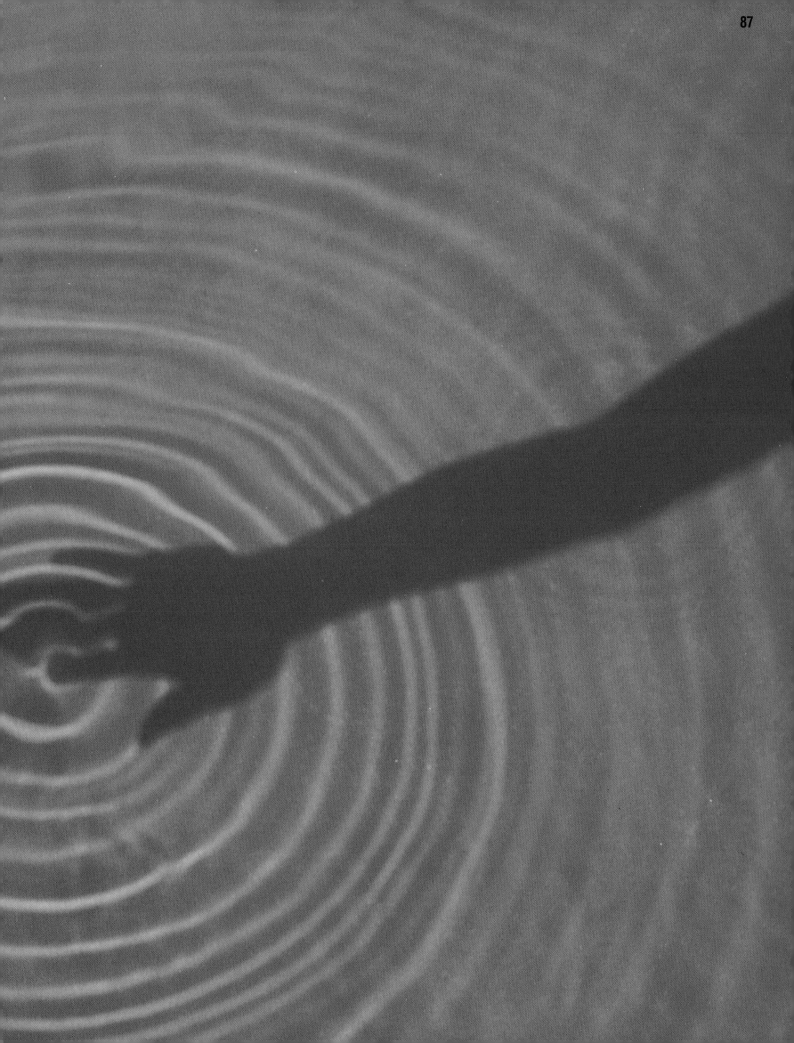

A NATURAL FLOW OF ENERGY

The primal force behind healing, say some healing experts, is a continuous stream of energy connecting the three levels of the self—body, mind, and spirit. An interruption in this vital flow, it is thought, can prevent the body's natural healing abilities from taking effect. According to this view, the culprit is often the mental trauma of the experience of illness or injury. As endocrinologist and author Deepak Chopra has noted, "You can say that the body is made out of molecules, but with equal justice you could say that it is made out of experiences."

Many healers throughout time have used the simple act of touch as a way of restoring energy flow and thereby enabling the body to cure itself. One particular technique, developed in 1986 by Steven Vazquez of The Health Institute of North Texas, combines a form of therapeutic touch—where the healer places his or her hands on or near areas of the patient's body—

with psychotherapy. Vazquez asserts that the difference in how fast someone heals depends on the emotional reaction associated with the experience of the injury. By reliving the event mentally, he says, the patient is able to "reprocess" any negative emotions and induce positive physiological changes. Through touch therapy, the healer is thought to help guide the energy flow within the body.

In one case in 1988, Vazquez used his approach with an eighth-grade girl who had suffered a hairline fracture to her ankle during a track meet. In two 20-minute sessions, Vazquez used what he calls hands-near intervention on the girl's ankle while discussing with her the fear she still felt from seeing her badly scraped and bleeding leg at the time of the injury. A week and a half later, the young runner placed fifth in a race despite her original doctor's claim that she would be on crutches for at least six weeks.

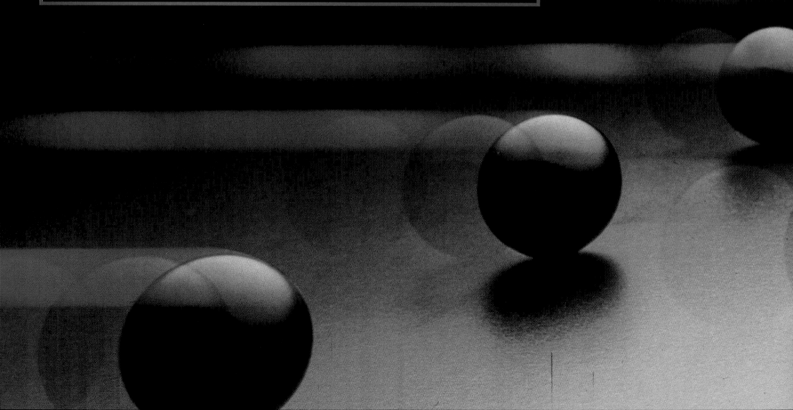

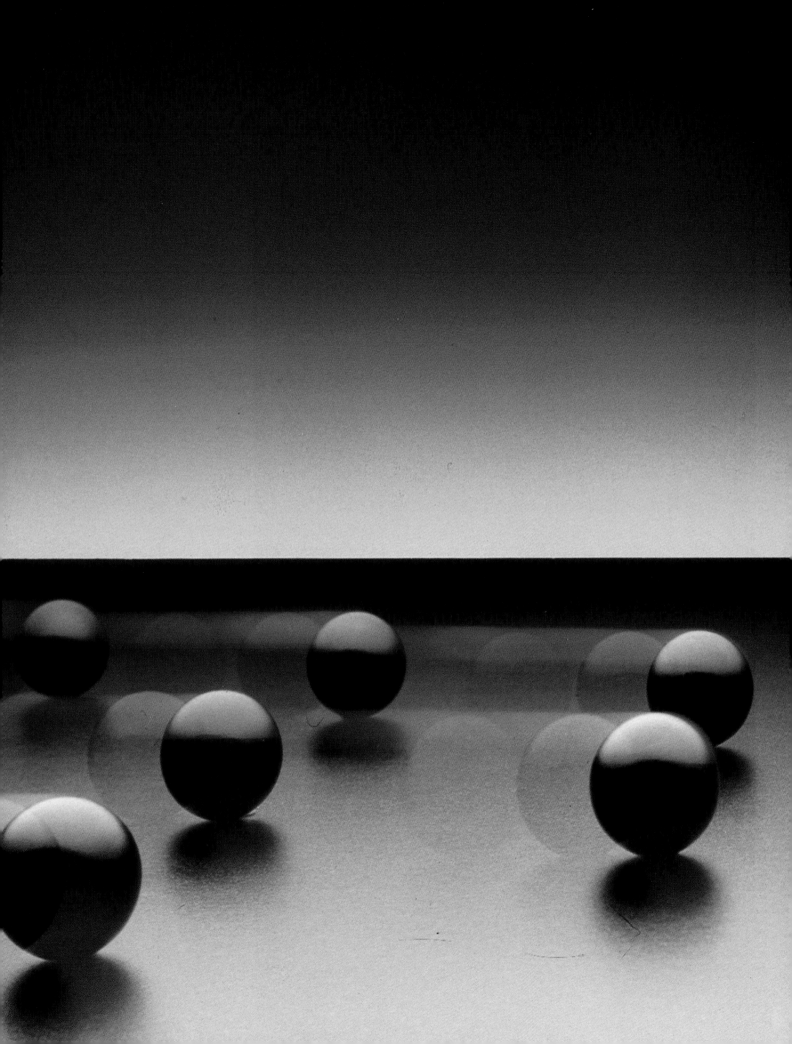

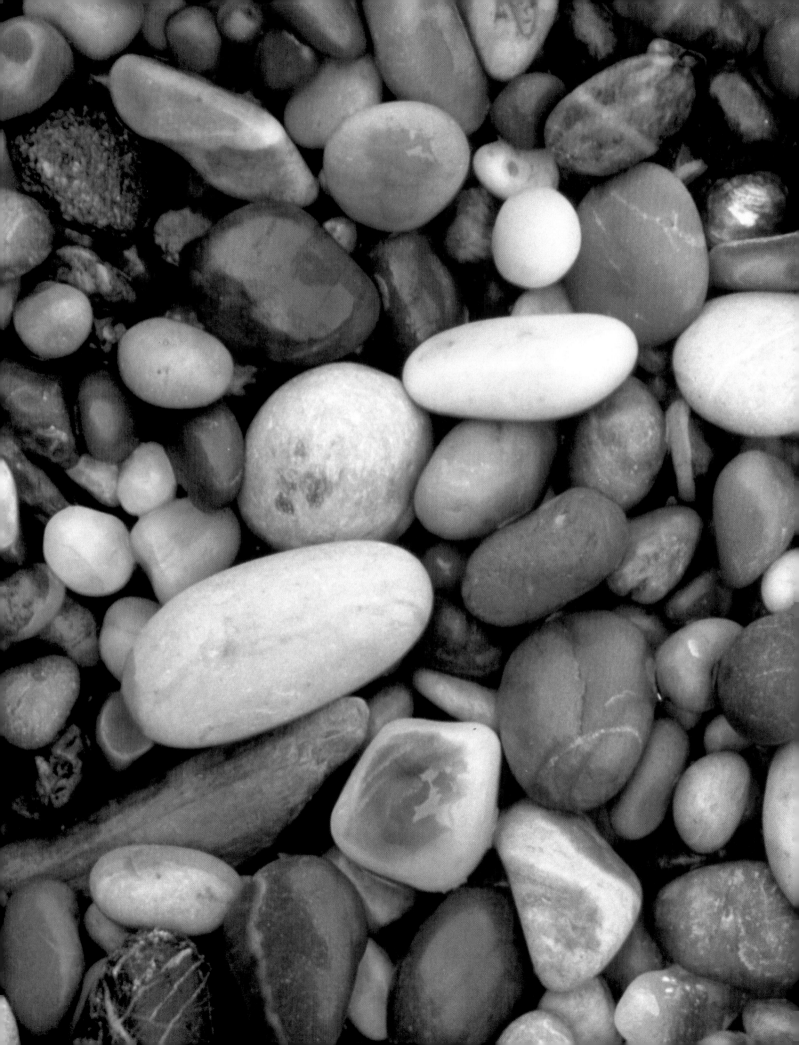

EACH INDIVIDUAL A SPECIAL CASE

Standard present-day medicine often relies on statistical averages and diagnostic categories in the evaluation of patients. In reality, however, numbers and labels say very little about the unique characteristics that set each patient apart and that can play an important role in the healing process. Indeed, many circumstances of life—from educational background to social status and financial resources—can influence a person's response to sickness or injury and thus the ability to heal.

Sometimes circumstances affect patients' attitudes and motivations in clear-cut ways. For example, a patient who has recently become unemployed and has a child to support may be reluctant to undergo lab tests that are considered optional, whereas a patient with a well-paying job and health insurance may actually ask for the tests. In other cases, the influence of circumstance may be more difficult for the healer to gauge. A patient who is caring for an elderly parent at home, for instance, may attempt to hide the increased anxiety she feels upon learning that she must remain in the hospital for several nights— anxiety that could prove detrimental to her recovery.

In Dallas, Texas, healers at Parkland Hospital—a public institution serving people from all socioeconomic backgrounds, regardless of their ability to pay—are attempting to create a caring environment that focuses on treating the patient and not simply the ailment. As Ron Anderson, chief executive officer of Parkland, has commented, "We can be very competent in dealing with the trauma, or the disease, but until we deal with the illness and the wholeness of that individual, we are not good doctors."

Anderson looks at each patient "as a mosaic," taking due note of the myriad fragments of personal history that he or she brings to the experience of illness. By understanding the patient's background, needs, and desired outcome, the healer is equipped with the knowledge it takes to facilitate the healing process.

MAKING USE OF THE TIES THAT HEAL

For many patients, the words of a disturbing diagnosis pose a threat all their own. According to Deepak Chopra, a diagnosis that receives too much focus can acquire a "kind of magic" that darkens the patient's outlook regardless of the reality of the situation. Above all, Chopra advises, healers must work to "break the spell of this magic, which can be uncannily powerful." Among the most potent weapons that can be brought to bear are the various personal relationships in the patient's life.

Of prime importance is the relationship between the healer and the patient. Ideally, both of them should foster an uninhibited two-way flow of ideas, concerns, emotions, expectations, and information—about everything from the illness or injury itself to possible coping methods and applicable healing techniques. Such communication not only helps the patient feel more in control but also enables the healer to better guide the patient on the healing path.

Thomas Delbanco, a Boston physician working to enhance the healer-patient relationship, believes it is also important to get to know a patient's family. "I have trouble seeing patients in isolation," he has noted. "We learn more from people when we see them in context." He often arranges to meet patient and family together, and by involving the family members—whose lives have also likely been affected by the patient's ills—he helps strengthen the patient's support network.

At Stanford University School of Medicine in California, David Spiegel also uses the idea of a support network to assist patients in the healing process. In a landmark study published in 1989, he showed that participation in a support group for women undergoing standard medical care for breast cancer may increase their life expectancy. Women who attended a 90-minute group session each week lived an average of 18 months longer than women in the study who did not attend the sessions. The results may owe to an improved quality of life achieved through the release of anxieties, fears, and emotional pain in a supportive, nurturing environment.

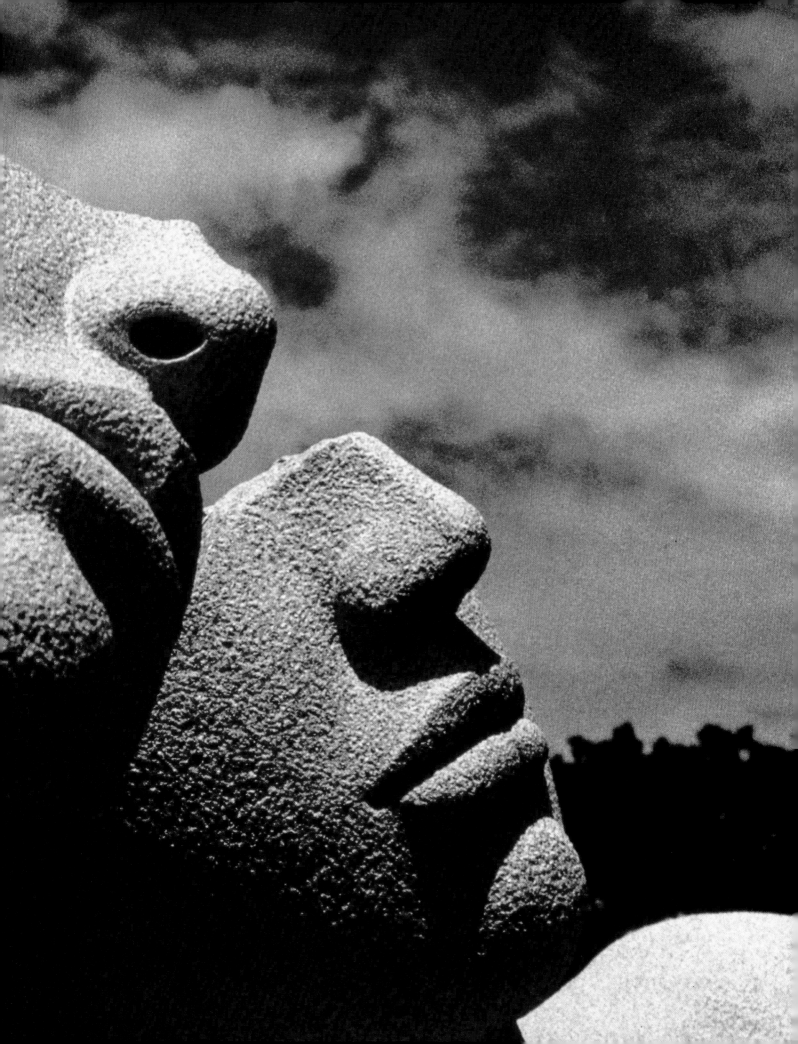

LEADING THE WAY TO SELF-HEALING

The Nobel Prize-winning physician Albert Schweitzer once said, "We doctors do nothing but aid and encourage the doctor within. All healing is self-healing." His words have been taken to heart by growing numbers of healers and patients who work together to move beyond their traditional roles.

Combining personal experience and the knowledge acquired through years of practice, healers today are doing more than simply treating patients: They are teaching patients ways to treat themselves. Part of the goal is to instill in patients a greater sense of responsibility for their own care by making clear that healing is a process that takes place before, during, and after office visits.

Self-healing techniques vary from biofeedback and meditation to regimens of healthful eating and exercise.

The common element in almost every such method is that the patient plays an active role in the treatment course.

Through his work with heart disease sufferers, Dean Ornish of the University of California at San Francisco has discovered the invaluable contribution patients can make to their own healing abilities. His ongoing study of arterial blockage and lifestyle has shown that cholesterol and other deposits in the arteries may actually begin to disappear within a year when patients replace harmful habits with better ones, such as a strict low-fat diet, regular exercise, and stress reduction techniques such as yoga. In short, Ornish teaches a new way of living that, he believes, can be more successful than a bypass (*page* 84). He calls it "emotional open-heart surgery."

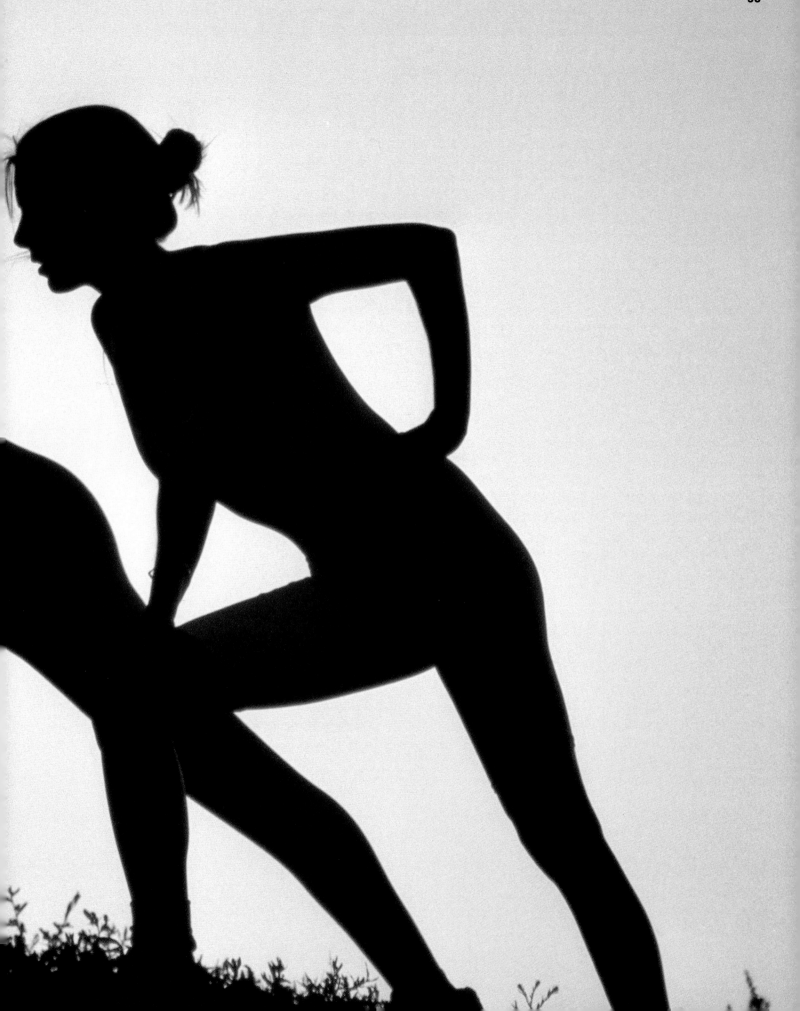

CROSSING A THRESHOLD THAT TRANSFORMS

The negative aspects of illness and injury are all too apparent, from the actual physical pain and debilitation to the feelings of hopelessness and despair that may also occur. Finding the positive side—particularly when the situation is dire—can seem next to impossible, and yet some people do indeed manage to transform affliction into an opportunity. The effort is often life changing and in some cases can even be lifesaving.

According to some healers, the experience of physical distress is the body's way of saying "Slow down, pay attention, enjoy this life." Research suggests that viewing illness or injury as a learning experience not only fosters optimism and a sense of control but also provides an effective vehicle for self-examination and psychological growth. For some patients, healing may involve looking within and changing old habits; for others, it may mean considering the future for the very first time and making a conscious effort to choose the sometimes tortuous path of survival.

A Dutch woman named Geertje Braakel made such a choice in the late 1970s. Throughout her early adult years, Braakel saw little reason to embrace life. "I didn't like the real world. I didn't want to see all the terrible things. I knew my life was falling through my hands but I couldn't do anything about it." But a diagnosis of ovarian cancer at the age of 28 forced her to make some decisions: "All my life I had been afraid but on this moment I was only thinking, 'I want to become better. I want to stay alive.' "

Despite her refusal of conventional treatment, Braakel's tumor went into remission. However, seven years after her first bout with the disease, cancer struck again. Braakel appeared to face this second battle with even greater resolve, her defeatist perspective on life seemingly transformed—by circumstance and by choice—to that of a survivor.

"There are some people who haven't really made the choice to be here," says Marco De Vries, a Dutch pathologist who studied Braakel's case. For Braakel and others like her, De Vries suggests, the trigger is "the real facing of a life-threatening crisis. These people suddenly become awake."

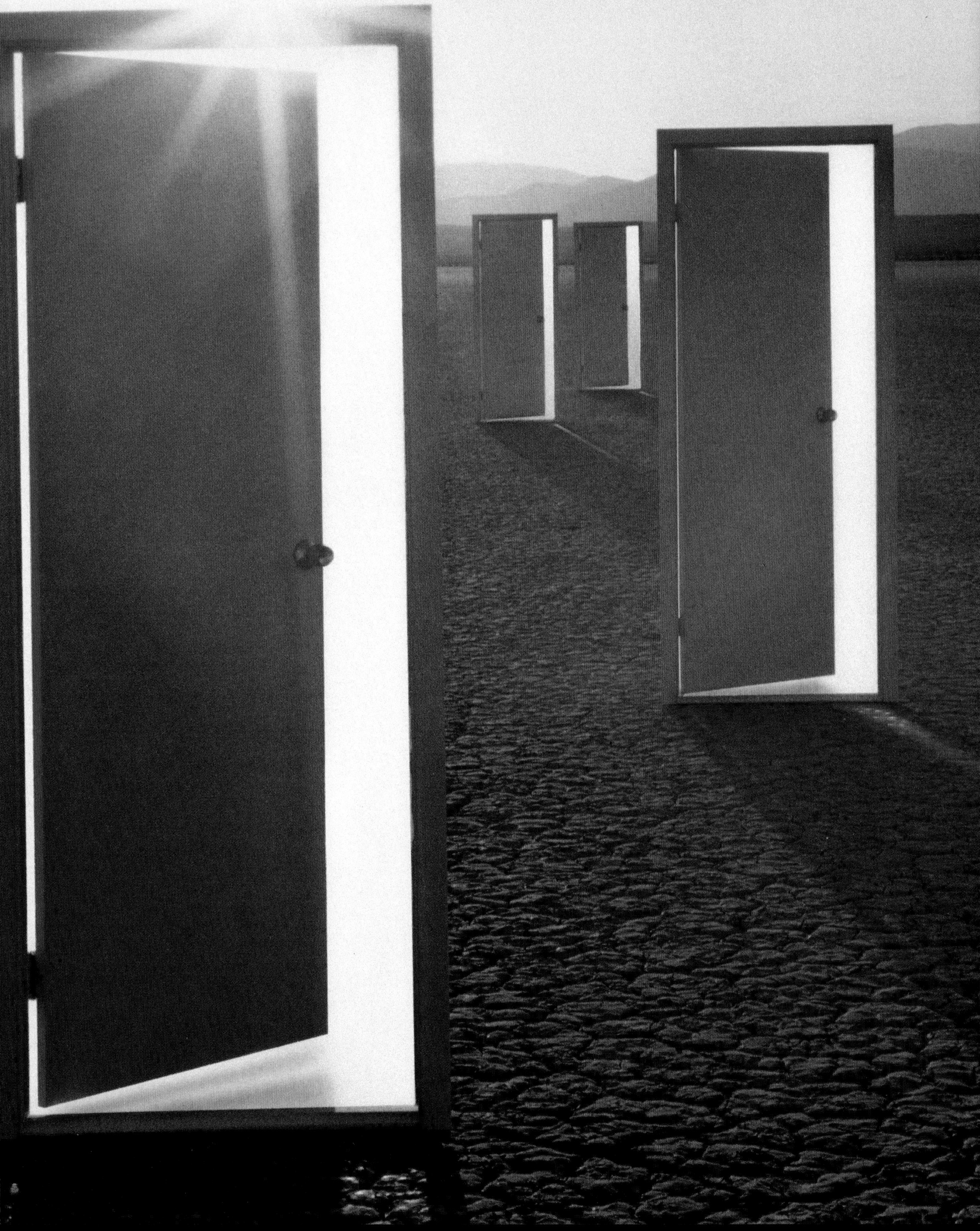

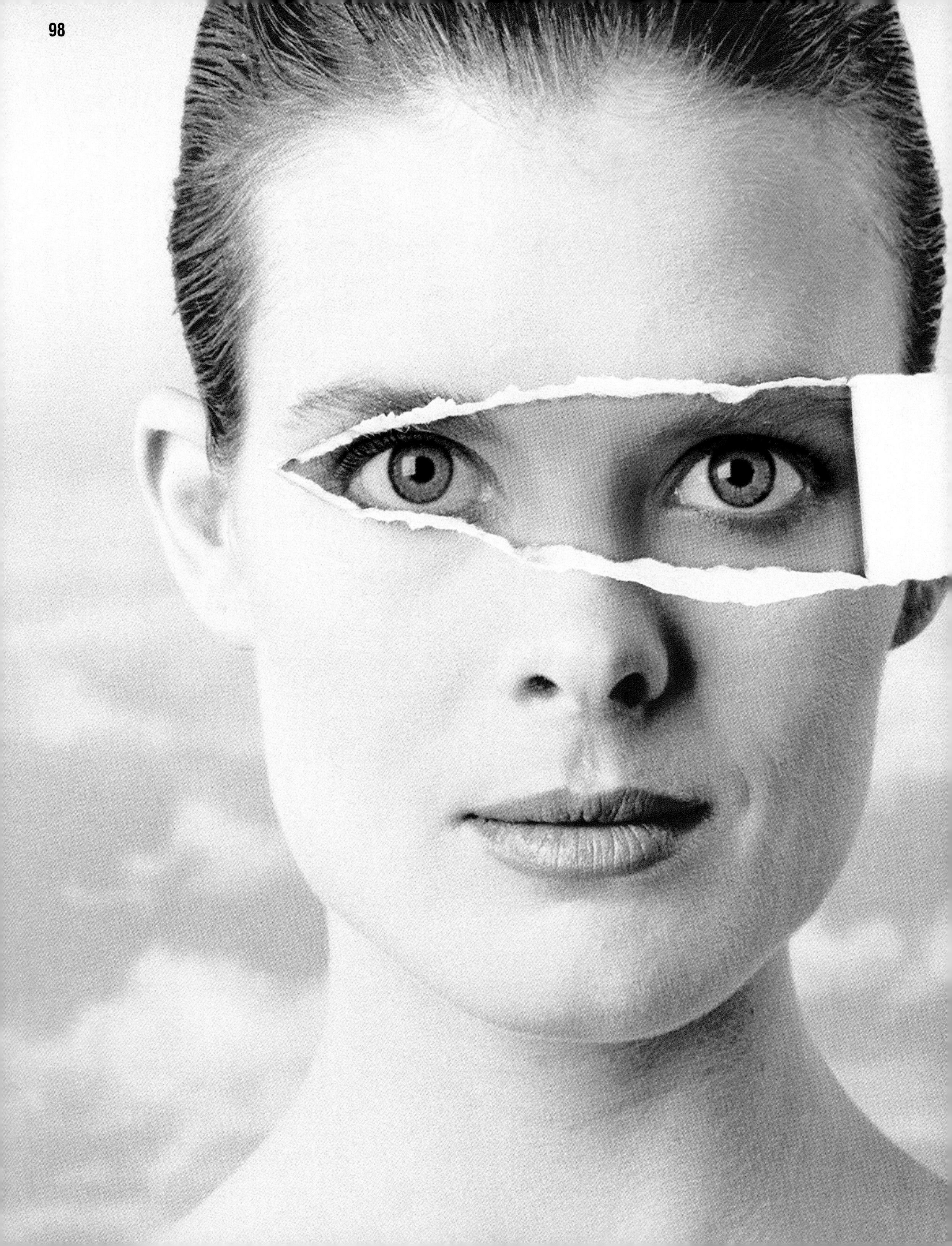

A NEW VISION OF BODY AND MIND

There is no longer much doubt that healing is not simply a function of the body but a function of the mind as well. Many healers today recognize that beliefs and expectations, attitudes and emotions all may contribute to the messages the mind sends to the physical self. Although the specifics of how the mind and body interact are still difficult to observe, techniques based on the existence of such a connection have been tailored to a variety of purposes—from wart removal to anesthesia. For example, studies show that patients who receive preoperative information that addresses their fears and other matters of personal concern often have a more positive recovery following surgery.

While some mind-body approaches employ the powers of the conscious mind to facilitate healing, others reach into the depths of the subconscious. Dabney Ewin, clinical professor of surgery and psychiatry at Tulane University in New Orleans, is among those who believe that patients have the ability to play an unconscious role in their own healing.

Ewin focuses on the period immediately following a traumatic accident and employs the psychological technique of suggestion. One of Ewin's patients was a man named Jerry Baggett, who suffered second-degree burns to his arms, face, and neck in a boiler room explosion. Within two hours after the accident, before hormones were released that would cause the second-degree burns to progress to the more severe condition of third degree, Ewin says he talked to the unconscious Baggett, telling him that his thoughts and attitude would affect his healing and to let his body feel "cool and comfortable." These early messages, Ewin claims, helped to block inflammation, which delays the body's natural healing process and contributes to the pain, swelling, scarring, and skin rejection that burn victims commonly suffer.

Although most severe burns take a minimum of six weeks and an average of three months to heal, according to Ewin his patient experienced no pain or swelling a mere 36 hours after treatment. Eleven days after the accident, Baggett returned home, and he was back to work three days later. "Even to this day, it's hard to understand," reflects Baggett, "but we haven't even started to tap what's in the subconscious mind."

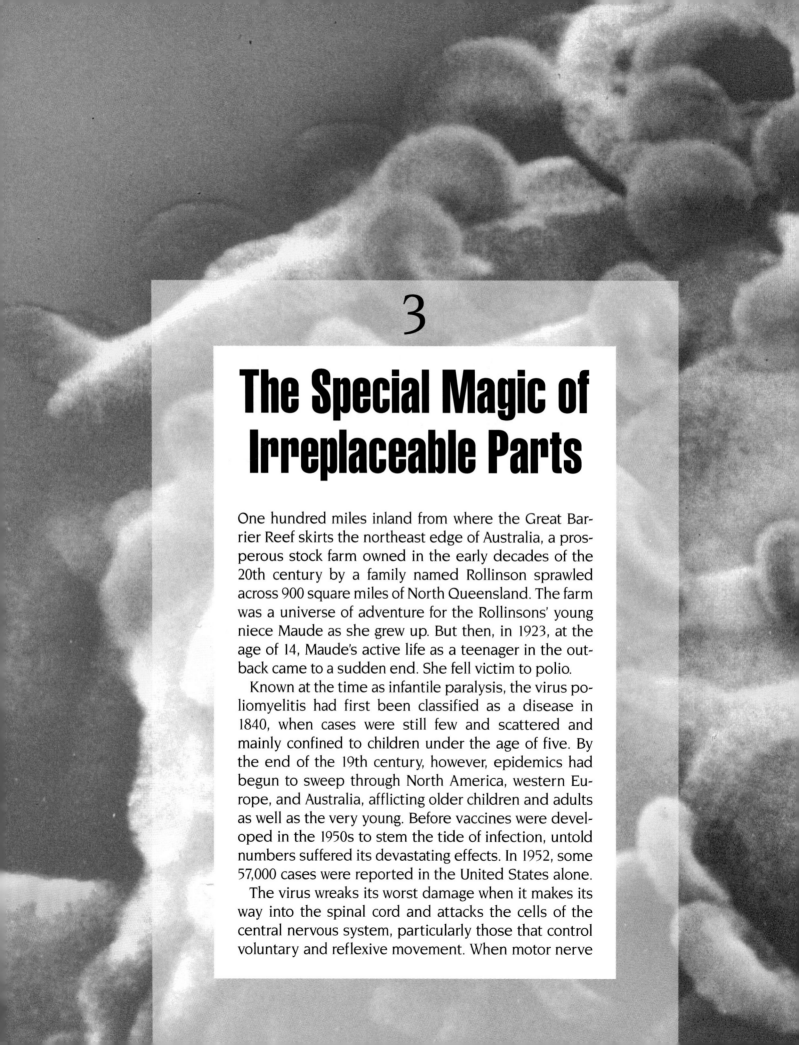

3

The Special Magic of Irreplaceable Parts

One hundred miles inland from where the Great Barrier Reef skirts the northeast edge of Australia, a prosperous stock farm owned in the early decades of the 20th century by a family named Rollinson sprawled across 900 square miles of North Queensland. The farm was a universe of adventure for the Rollinsons' young niece Maude as she grew up. But then, in 1923, at the age of 14, Maude's active life as a teenager in the outback came to a sudden end. She fell victim to polio.

Known at the time as infantile paralysis, the virus poliomyelitis had first been classified as a disease in 1840, when cases were still few and scattered and mainly confined to children under the age of five. By the end of the 19th century, however, epidemics had begun to sweep through North America, western Europe, and Australia, afflicting older children and adults as well as the very young. Before vaccines were developed in the 1950s to stem the tide of infection, untold numbers suffered its devastating effects. In 1952, some 57,000 cases were reported in the United States alone.

The virus wreaks its worst damage when it makes its way into the spinal cord and attacks the cells of the central nervous system, particularly those that control voluntary and reflexive movement. When motor nerve

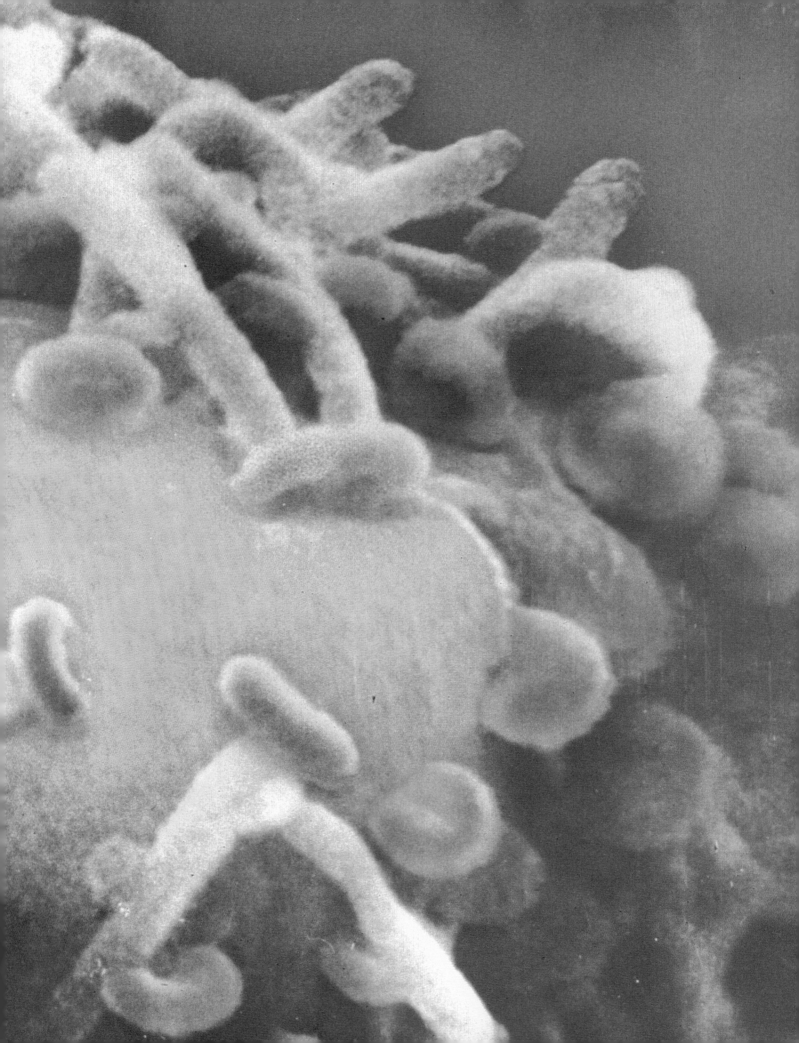

PRECEDING PAGE: Arriving from all areas of the brain and body, nerve fibers (yellow) establish contact with the cell body of a neuron (green) through knoblike features called synaptic buttons (orange) in this false-color image. The ability of healthy nerve cells to form such connections makes possible learning, sensing, movement—and healing when the nervous system suffers damage.

cells—which are permanent and irreplaceable—are invaded, they swell up and then shrivel and die, while uninfected cells, partially crushed by the pressure of their swollen neighbors, stop functioning properly. As a result, any muscle ordinarily activated by these nerves is paralyzed; almost immediately it begins to weaken from disuse, and eventually to waste away. If none of the nerves recover, the paralysis is permanent.

Despite the best medical treatment Maude's well-to-do family could arrange, both of her legs were left paralyzed by the disease. She was confined to the house and could only move around arduously with the aid of heavy crutches. By 1931, eight years after contracting polio, she had resigned herself to a lifetime of severe constraints. But that year her prospects changed dramatically through the ministrations of Elizabeth Kenny, a strong-willed Australian nurse who would change Maude's life—and eventually the lives of many polio victims—forever.

Kenny arrived to treat Maude at the behest of two Rollinson relatives who had met the nurse while traveling in Europe in 1929. At 50 years of age, the bluff, outspoken Kenny was a self-made practitioner, having parlayed a few years of outback schooling and lessons from her mother into a career that included a stint with the Aus-

tralian army during World War I. She treated her first polio victim in a simple hut under a gum tree in the Australian bush in 1911, before she even knew the name of the disease. Kenny's formal knowledge of polio was only slightly more advanced by 1931, but she had seen enough of its crippled victims to conclude that the standard medical treatment was little short of disastrous.

When Maude met Elizabeth Kenny on the veranda of the Rollinson home in 1931, the shy young woman managed just a few clumsy steps in the nurse's presence, dragging her useless legs behind her; exhausted by the effort, she had to be carried back into the house. Her condition was typical of many polio survivors of the time. In the early 1930s, most doctors believed that all paralysis from the disease was permanent and that lifelong disability was the inevitable outcome.

Specialists had concluded that deformities—twisted spines, skewed joints, wizened limbs—resulted from the distorting effects of strong, undamaged muscles pulling against paralyzed or weakened ones. If nothing could be done to reverse the paralysis, then the only way to prevent deformities was to hold the affected

parts of the body in normal alignment while the patient rested to help beat the virus itself. To protect weak muscles and enforce rest, doctors routinely applied wooden splints or plaster casts to paralyzed limbs, or even strapped the patient into a rigid whole-body frame. This treatment lasted through the acute phase of the disease—about two weeks—before brief periods of exercise were added to the regimen. The immobilization might continue for months or even a year with only these fleeting snatches of relief from confinement. In some cases even this respite was denied in the belief that the muscles needed protection more than exercise.

This was the sort of treatment Maude had received in 1923, but Kenny had another approach in mind. Drawing on her own experience with wartime meningitis patients, she decided to try a rigorous program of physical and mental exercise to rehabilitate Maude's long-neglected muscles. She began by placing her patient in a bathtub filled with hot salt water and trying to "reach Maude's brain," as one of the Rollinson kin put it. Moving Maude's legs back and forth in the bath, Kenny told her to think of the muscles being manipulated. Then she urged her to try to use those muscles to touch the end of the tub with her feet. After an hour of this exercise first thing in the morning, Kenny

Encouraged by Australian nurse Elizabeth Kenny, a five-year-old New Jersey girl stands on her own for the first time since she was stricken with polio months earlier in 1943. Sister Kenny, as everyone called the self-taught innovator in physical rehabilitation, believed in—and demonstrated—the effectiveness of touch, heat, and exercise for restoring activity to once-paralyzed muscles.

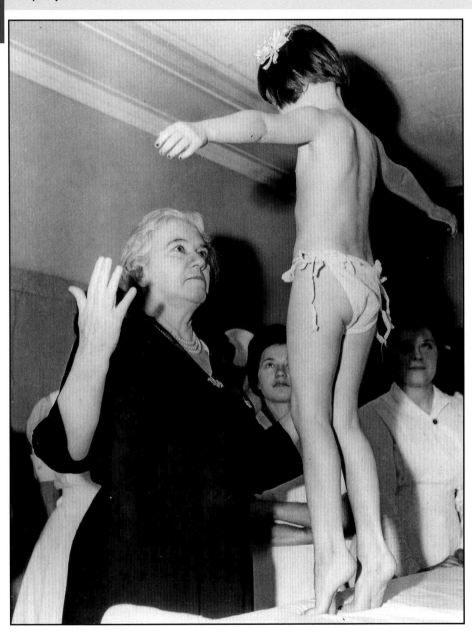

brought Maude down to a table on the veranda where she worked the paralyzed legs back and forth with her strong, sensitive hands. "Some of your cells are dead," she told Maude, "but some are dormant. We have to make you aware of the dormant cells. We have to reeducate them."

As this routine went on day after day, all of Maude's concentrated effort seemed unavailing: The legs still flopped lifelessly when Kenny released them. But the nurse's fierce will bolstered her patient's resolve, and one morning, after two months of treatment, Kenny detected a faint flicker of movement in one of the legs. It was the moment she had been waiting for. Kenny declared to the family that soon Maude would start to move the leg herself.

Indeed, in the months that followed, Maude began to move both of her legs, a little more each day, and her wasted limbs gained bulk as their muscle tone improved. Finally the day came to put the reactivated legs to the test. Chalking a set of footsteps on the porch, which wrapped around the house, Kenny positioned Maude before them and told her to walk. Maude tottered uncertainly, then asked for her crutches. Kenny gave her a light walking stick instead, and Maude took her first unsteady steps. Three months later, Maude got herself halfway around the house, a trip that

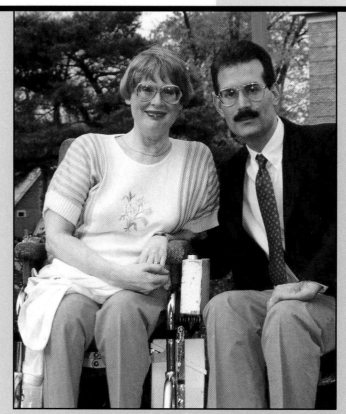

Richard Bruno and Nancy Frick, pictured here in 1993, collaborate in their research on post-polio sequelae. Bruno also treats polio survivors at the Kessler Institute in New Jersey, and Frick conducts educational programs worldwide.

Returning Symptoms of a Virus Once Defeated

During the late 1980s, one president of a prominent Wall Street insurance brokerage firm began to experience difficulty concentrating and an inexplicable, overwhelming fatigue. By 1992 the 45-year-old executive had to be in bed at 3:00 in the afternoon in order to function the next morning; soon afterward he retired on disability. Little did he realize when his symptoms first appeared that they would be traced to the polio infection he suffered during infancy—and thought he had vanquished.

Hearing of such cases, in 1982 Richard Bruno, a clinical psychophysiologist at Columbia University, assembled a team to investigate what would come to be called post-polio sequelae, or PPS. The group has found that nearly half of the 1.63 million living Americans who were afflicted with poliomyelitis decades ago are now experiencing symptoms of muscular weakness and mental fatigue.

Bruno and his colleagues have concluded that part of the problem has to do with motor nerve cells in the spinal

took an hour but so buoyed her spirits that she laughed most of the way. Her confidence and strength continued to grow, and in another few months she was walking daily with Kenny to a lagoon near the house. Rambling along the bank, Maude listened to the nurse's tales of war, polio, and the possibilities of a life no longer limited by physical disability.

Maude Rollinson regained her legs, and Elizabeth Kenny gained a following. By the next year Kenny was operating an open-air rehabilitation clinic in the small port city of Townsville. As she treated more patients she honed

her methods, but the fundamentals never changed. First she used heat to relieve the pains and sores of unused arms and legs, which would start taking on the pink flush of healthy blood circulation. Then she began to manipulate the limbs, talking to the patients all the while, pointing out the muscles involved, urging her listeners to think hard about moving them. When telltale flickers of movement occurred, she pressed her patients to redouble

their efforts while nurturing their optimism about recovery. Not every case ended in success, but enough did to provide a legacy of discarded crutches—and a model of treatment that Kenny eventually carried to the United States, where its broad acceptance radically altered the standards of polio therapy in the 1940s.

The success of Kenny's methods came at a time when doctors and researchers were questioning longstanding assumptions about damage and recovery in the nervous system. Nerve cells, or neurons, are the most essen-

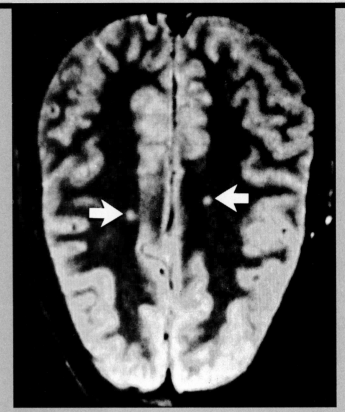

cord that, among other things, control a person's ability to walk. After the virus destroyed some of the cells, those that remained increased their work load as much as a thousandfold by, in effect, adopting the orphaned muscles—allowing the person to continue functioning. Years later, though, as these cells began to fail through normal aging as well as overuse, the deficit started to affect performance. A second source of PPS lies in the brainstem, which governs alertness. Here, too, if neurons were killed by the virus long ago, problems with concentration may beset polio survivors once normal attrition claims a certain number of the remaining cells.

These symptoms are "very treatable," according to Bruno. Part of the solution may be drug therapy, but most important is the need for polio survivors to conserve their body's resources—ironically, the opposite of the "use it or lose it" strategy that helped them overcome the debilitating effects of the disease the first time around.

An MRI taken in 1992 of a 45-year-old man who battled polio in 1948 reveals two lesions in the area where the brainstem links to the cerebral cortex. Such lesions appear in brain scans of polio survivors suffering from mental fatigue.

tial of the body's permanent tissues, which also include certain internal organs—such as the heart—and the lens of the eye. Because the cells that make up these tissues do not reproduce, the effects of damage would seem to be particularly dire. If each cell has a job to do, then every one that dies must lead to some reduced capacity. The greater the destruction, it would appear, the greater the loss.

In some cases this direct link between cell death and lost ability holds true. The lens of the eye, for example, cannot adapt to the destruction of its cells. If a person with a severe cataract—a clouding of the lens—is ever to see normally again, he or she must have the lens surgically removed and then be fitted with a lens implant, eyeglasses, or a contact lens. Other permanent body tissues, however, show a remarkable resiliency. Surviving nerve fibers around the site of an injury sometimes sprout new shoots that retrace the intricate paths of devastated neural networks. And some of the body's inner organs, al-

though constructed of irreplaceable tissues, can maintain at least some of their functionality by substituting a tougher, if less efficient, type of cell for the original.

In the inner lining of the lungs, for example, delicate ciliated epithelial cells die when they are continually exposed to the harmful ingredients of tobacco smoke. These special cells ordinarily help keep the lungs clean by producing a sticky mucus that traps

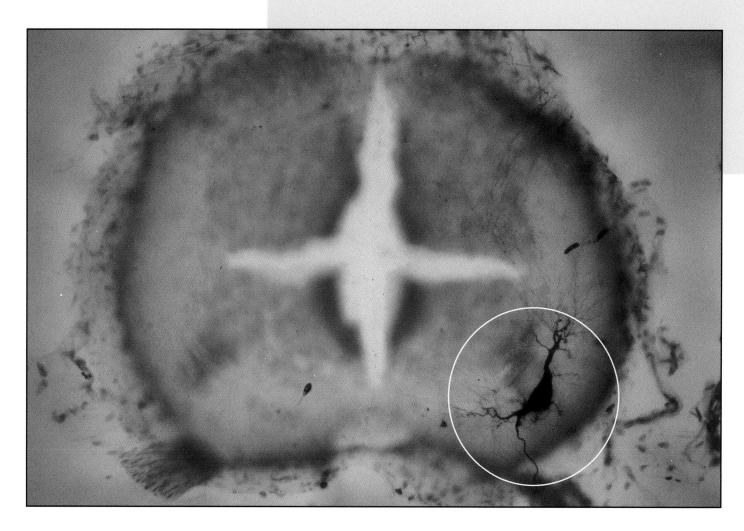

foreign particles; the cells' hairlike cilia, always in motion, transport the captured alien matter up the respiratory tract to be expelled by coughing or sneezing. When ciliated epithelial cells die, they are replaced by more rugged but less specialized cells that form what is called the stratified squamous epithelium. Cousin to skin cells, the squamous cells maintain the integrity of the lung lining, but they cannot cleanse the organs of potentially damaging substances. Similar replacements—of squamous cells for more easily damaged epithelia—may also occur in the salivary glands, the pancreas, and bile ducts of the gallbladder when stones injure its lining.

Although these substitutes keep the organs intact after they have been injured, the organs themselves usually cannot perform as well.

There is no substitute for the cells of cardiac muscles, which power the beating of the heart. But like skeletal-muscle cells, cardiac cells are highly responsive to the demands placed on them, and they enlarge to meet the needs of a greater work load—an adaptive mechanism that unfortunately does not always work to the good. For example, when the heart is forced

to pump against excessive pressure in the aorta, as when a person has high blood pressure, so much strength is required of the cardiac muscles that the heart can actually double in size as a result. This response works in the short run by keeping the blood circulating, but eventually it leads to muscle-cell injury—and heart failure.

The nervous system has its own method of adapting to loss. All of a person's neurons are present at birth, and the human body has no way to produce any sort of replacement once the neurons are destroyed. Instead, most repairs depend on the ability of existing neurons to put out new extensions through tissues that have

been burned, cut, withered by disease, or otherwise damaged. When this kind of reconstruction is impossible, the nervous system sometimes falls back on another strategy, one that works like a telephone operator searching for an intact line into a disaster area: The brain simply finds alternate pathways for sending and receiving neural impulses.

Every neuron has a cell body with a single nucleus and a number of thin appendages, known as processes. These typically include one long strand called an axon, which carries signals away from the cell body, and several shorter fibers—the dendrites—that accept signals across so-called synaptic gaps from the axons of other neurons. The cell body itself can also receive nerve impulses. The axon, which in humans may be up to a yard long in nerves running to the foot, can branch profusely at its far end in order to reach numerous target cells. Dendrites also split into many branches, creating a dense fringe of endings that accept as many as 100,000 inputs. Weaving through the organs and limbs of the body, these processes form the connections of the peripheral nervous system, which conducts signals into and out of the central nervous system—the spinal cord and the brain.

The meaning of the signals transmitted by a neuron varies according to the role the cell plays in the nervous system. In a motor neuron, an impulse is a command that causes a particular muscle to contract. A sensory neuron, on the other hand, carries reports of various stimuli, such as light, sound, heat, and pressure, to the brain from a specific part of the body—the eye, the ear, the fingertips.

The nervous system makes new neural connections throughout a person's life. Under everyday conditions, processes lengthen and retract slowly and to a limited degree, adapting to changes in the body and to constantly shifting stimuli. But the ability is called into play on a grand scale when connections are suddenly disrupted as a result of injury to the peripheral nerves or to their target tissues. Neurons that survive the damage quickly set about rebuilding the neural infrastructure by reestablishing links, sometimes over relatively long distances. With the added help of skilled surgeons, such reconnections often verge on the miraculous.

One of the most remarkable instances of surgical neural repair involved a 22-year-old man known in the medical literature as M. M., who lost his left arm during an accident in 1982 when his out-of-control automobile collided with a guardrail. Part of the guardrail pierced the car, roughly cutting through M. M.'s upper arm a few inches above the elbow. A search of the chaotic accident scene finally turned up the severed limb some 400 yards from the vehicle; attendants carefully sealed it in a refrigerated bag and sent it on to the hospital where M. M. had been taken. Three hours later, the arm had been x-rayed, cleaned, and reattached, the bone ends—shortened by two inches in surgery—held

Why Humans Don't Regenerate Limbs

Some simple organisms—such as flatworms, starfish, and salamanders—can perform a feat beyond the talents of more sophisticated creatures, including humans: They can regenerate amputated limbs or body parts. The process, illustrated at right, is remarkable, but no less intriguing to some investigators is why supposedly more advanced organisms lack this apparently useful ability.

Many researchers believe that evolution selected against regenerative powers in certain species, and that warm-bloodedness may have been a determining factor. Warm-blooded organisms such as humans have higher nutritional demands than cold-blooded ones, so presumably they would have a harder time keeping their energy fires stoked—and thus keeping themselves alive—through the lengthy period of incapacity when a limb was regrowing. Naturally enough, then, the ability would have died out in those creatures unable to survive the process.

Furthermore, warm-blooded species are more prone to infection, which some researchers speculate may have led to the development of rapid and efficient wound healing. A wound that seals quickly and forms scar tissue, however, creates precisely the wrong environment for regeneration. Research has shown that slow healing at the point of severing allows for the crucial cellular activity that eventually produces a new limb.

In the 1970s, doctors demonstrated this in dramatic fashion. Working with young children who had lost fingertips, they found that when they did not follow the common practice of stitching a flap of skin over the wound but instead left it open (though carefully dressed), a new fingertip—complete with fingerprint and fingernail—would grow. The study seemed to confirm that to some extent humans do retain the evolutionary traces of this lost talent, but that wound healing itself ultimately proved more important to our species' survival.

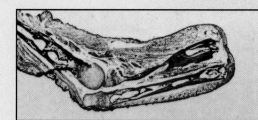

Regeneration begins with wound healing.

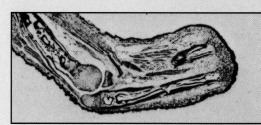

A blastema *(right)* forms beneath the surface.

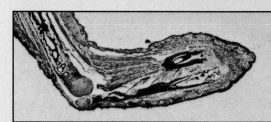

The blastema grows and cells redifferentiate.

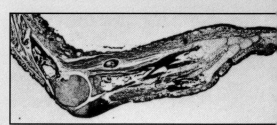

A new limb takes shape.

Mechanisms of Regeneration

During limb regeneration, a functional replica of an amputated appendage develops at its severed cross section, provided an adequate nerve supply is present and some part of the appendage is left behind to serve as a blueprint for its replacement. The regenerating newt limb shown in the images at left highlights the various stages of this intricate process.

When the skin's wounded epidermal layer begins to heal across the injured stump, researchers believe it induces changes within the remaining tissues, causing their cells to lose their definitive traits and collect in an undifferentiated clump, or blastema. With the potential to become any part of the new appendage, these cells rapidly divide, extending the blastema outward. Presumably regulated by unknown growth factors, proliferation continues in the far end of the appendage, while cells closest to the body begin to redifferentiate into the specialized structures that will form an often flawless copy of the original.

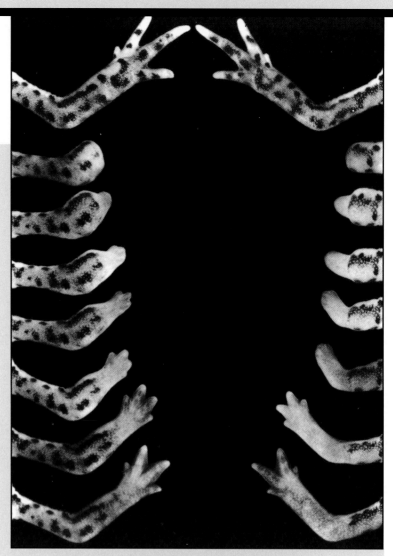

STAGES OF REGROWTH. The composite image above shows two newt limbs in their original condition *(top)* and then at seven stages in their regrowth over a period of 70 days. Cells in the limb on the left, which was severed below the elbow joint, redifferentiated more quickly.

A NEAR MATCH. A five-lined skink pauses on a leaf, displaying its regenerated tail *(purple)*. For reasons unknown, new appendages do not retain original coloring.

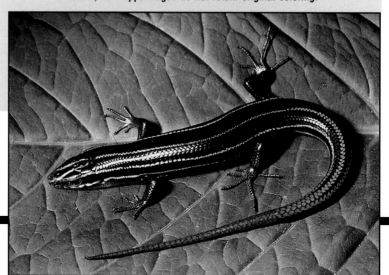

together by a metal plate. Working with an operating microscope and suturing thread only 15 millionths of a meter in diameter—thinner than the finest human hair—the surgeons stitched arteries and veins back together, returning circulation to the arm within five hours of the accident. During the surgery doctors also repaired M. M.'s torn muscles.

The following day saw the first of a series of additional operations to reconnect the three main nerves running the length of the arm. The surgeons first tackled the ulnar nerve, a cable of nerve fibers up to a quarter-inch thick whose thousands of individual axons control muscles in the forearm and hand. The team trimmed back the frayed stumps of the nerve so that individual bundles of nerve fibers, called fascicles, could be distinguished clearly. Then they matched up the severed fascicles from each stump and sutured them back together one by one.

Seven months later, with the healing of the earlier repairs well under way, the surgeons began to reconstruct the median nerve. The largest and most important of the three nerves, the median controls the flexor muscles of the forearm, hand, and thumb, directs the fist to close in a tight grip, and also relays sensation from much of the surface of the palm. At the same time, M. M.'s doctors also worked on the ra-

dial nerve, which governs the triceps and the back of the forearm and receives sensory nerve branches from the skin. Because portions were missing between the stumps of the median and radial nerves, end-to-end reconnections were impossible. Instead, the surgeons took nerves from the calf of M. M.'s leg and used them as grafts. Before the patient was put under anesthesia for the joining of the nerves, the doctors stimulated each fascicle above the point where the arm had been severed while asking M. M. what he felt. By comparing his responses with the known map of the nervous system, they were able to identify the function of most of the nerve bundles as they prepared to splice them to the graft.

M. M. began to regain movement in his arm about nine months after the accident. The first signs of sensation in the hand and arm appeared a few months later. During the next few years, both motion and sensation continued to return. He could move his arm and all of his fingers, although he never regained the strength he had possessed before the accident. He also reported high levels of sensitivity to light touching, pinpricks, and temperature. Curiously, however, his abili-

ty to feel vibration did not return.

Other peculiarities marked M. M.'s recovery. He could identify the sensation of touch, for example, but had a hard time telling just where a touch was occurring. When the tip of his middle finger was stimulated with a light brush, he described feeling the stroke simultaneously on the outside of his little finger and near the base of the index finger. Another time he believed that he was being touched on the wrist when in fact the brush was stroking the end of his thumb.

The outcome of M. M.'s case reflects both the possibilities and the problems involved in attempting to repair nerves. The fact that surgically joined nerve fibers could eventually function again confirms that the nervous system does have certain regenerative abilities. But the vagaries of M. M.'s recovery demonstrate that there is still much to be learned about the way the human body is wired. Even the most informed investigators continue to be challenged by the complexities of this system.

The study of the nervous system's secrets has been very much a 20th-century science. Many experts trace the roots of neurological investigations to a book published in 1899 by Spanish researcher Santiago Ramón y Cajal. A paragon of medical scholarship, Ramón y Cajal brought an artist's

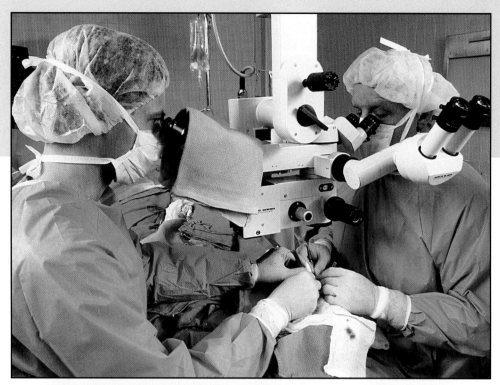

sensibility to his work. His authoritarian father, a barber-surgeon, had discouraged the son's youthful interest in art and apprenticed the rebellious lad first to another barber and then to a shoemaker. Ramón y Cajal finally yielded to his father's greatest wish that he follow directly in the paternal footsteps and attended medical school, graduating in 1873. The actual practice of medicine held no appeal for Ramón y Cajal, however; he turned instead to the laboratory research that would consume most of his long career—and eventually, in 1906, win him a Nobel Prize in medicine. He focused on the nervous system, drawn to it by his own belief that its intricate structure provided the material basis of thought. Throwing light on that structure, he concluded, could provide answers to many questions in physiology and psychology alike.

Ramón y Cajal's seminal book, His-tology of the Nervous System of Man and the Vertebrates, described in detail every part of the brain and the peripheral nervous system. Building on the existing—albeit slim—body of neurological knowledge, he added a wealth of meticulous observations, which he supplemented with beautifully drawn illustrations. Primarily

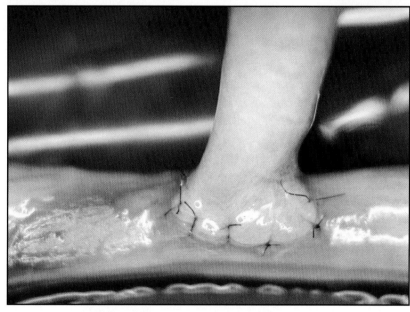

MICROSURGERY. With the aid of powerful microscopes, surgeons reattach a severed thumb (top), using nylon thread and needles finer than human hair to repair tiny blood vessels and nerves. Although the blood vessel (bottom) is only the diameter of a narrow string, the surgeon must suture it so securely that no fluid leaks and yet leave a hollow interior through which blood can flow.

In 1899 the Spanish neuroscientist Santiago Ramón y Cajal *(below)* published nearly 600 illustrations that revealed the structure of neurons in unprecedented detail. Among them was the drawing at bottom of a human brain cell, showing an axon *(a)* descending from the cell body and branching out *(b)*; all other fibers are dendrites surrounding spaces filled by capillaries *(c)* and other cells *(d).*

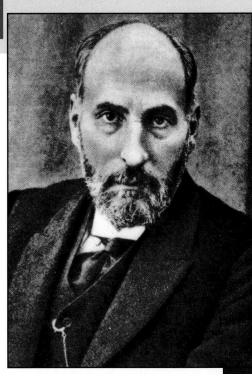

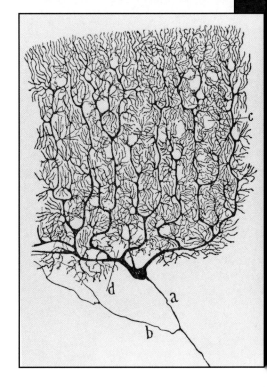

through the use of recently developed staining techniques, he was able to examine individual nerve-cell processes in unprecedented detail. His ability to focus on a single axon or dendrite led to several important new findings, including the first conclusive demonstration of the existence of synaptic gaps between neurons. Fifteen years in the making, Ramón y Cajal's work is still considered a classic of medical science.

Not satisfied with describing the nervous system in stasis, Ramón y Cajal went on to study its development, and particularly the problems of damage and regeneration in certain nerve structures. Here again he took a body of existing knowledge, added the results of his own research, and produced superb pictures of his experimental preparations. The expense of publishing his work in 1913 was borne by expatriate Spanish physicians living in Argentina, who wished to honor Ramón y Cajal's Nobel Prize. The book, *Degeneration and Regeneration of the Nervous System*, prefigured by nearly half a century some of the most important discoveries made about the nervous system.

Neurologists of Ramón y Cajal's time knew that a severed axon could regenerate across the site of an injury, as long as the cell body of the neuron had escaped damage. But precisely how this happened was unclear. All human nerve tissue contains two main kinds of cells. Neurons play the most important role in a healthy nervous system by receiving, conducting, and transmitting signals throughout the body. However, they are greatly outnumbered by their supporting cast, the various types of glial cells, which surround neurons and fill up the spaces between them. One of the tasks of glial cells is to produce a fatty substance known as myelin that encases the elongated neurons and serves as electrical insulation. Unlike neurons, most glial cells remain capable of division throughout life—a feat that allows them to play a significant role in the rebuilding of damaged networks of nerves.

In the early 20th century, one school of thought held that regenerated fibers arose from glial cells called Schwann cells (named for Theodor Schwann, the 19th-century German physiologist who discovered them) that had been wrapped around the original axons, forming a kind of tube. When a cut axon degenerated, these theorists guessed, its Schwann cells underwent some kind of transformation and grew back toward the body of the damaged cell. Eventually the changed Schwann cells would meet

A modern false-color micrograph of an axon terminal *(yellow)* and a muscle fiber *(red)* attests to the accuracy of Ramón y Cajal's research. Tiny vesicles *(brown)* in the axon produce chemicals that diffuse across the narrow synapses between the cells—a form of noncontact communication whose discovery was made possible by the early neuroscientist's work.

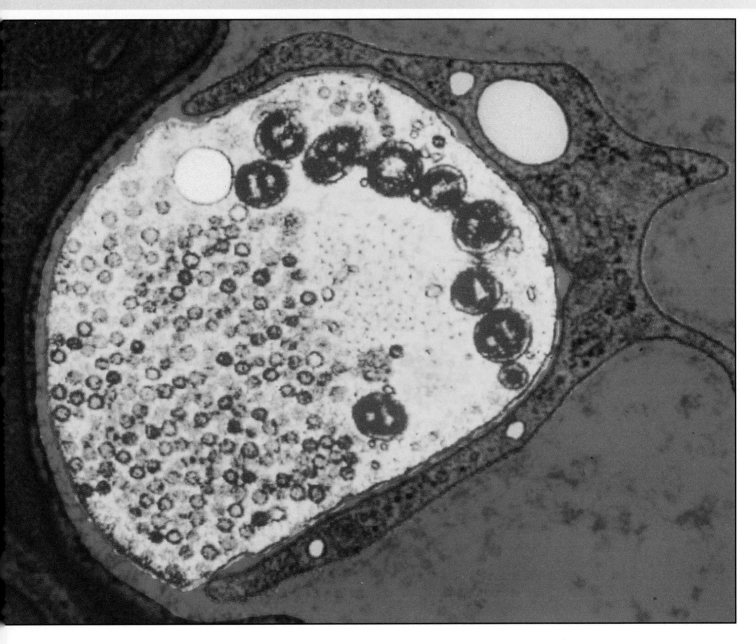

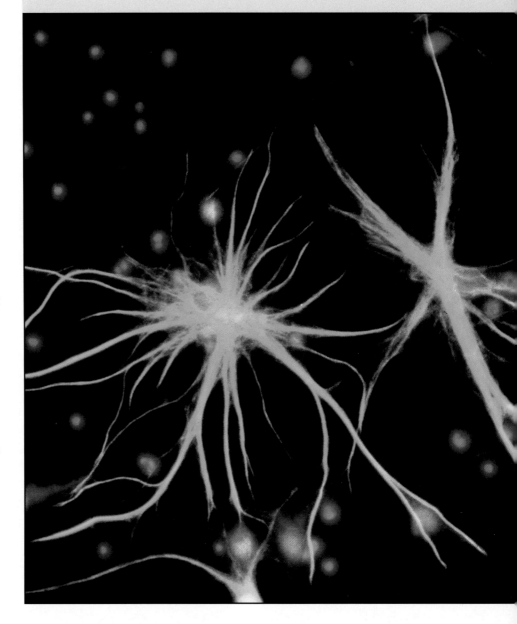

up with and fuse to their related nerve cells, filling the place and function of the severed axon and reestablishing the neural link. This was, however, a theory more of speculation than of observation and fact.

Ramón y Cajal cleared up some of the mystery, showing conclusively that another mechanism was responsible for the repairs. Observing the stumps of cut axons, he found that soon after an injury, spiky enlargements began to form at their tips. These structures, named growth cones for their distinctive shape, appeared to crawl through the surrounding tissue, heading in the direction of their former connection sites. An injury to one neuron also signaled intact neurons nearby to sprout growth cones.

Cones on the intact cells grew from the gaps between the individual Schwann cells sheathing their axons. The sprouts appeared to seek out synaptic sites on target tissues that showed no sign of activity; those that succeeded in connecting to muscles survived. In most cases unsuccessful sprouts disappeared, but where no connection was even possible, as in the stump of an amputated limb, they might continue to grow in wild profusion, developing into clumpy masses of tissue called neuromas.

Building on these findings, other researchers discovered that growth cones serve as mobile workshops

where new components are assembled to extend the axons. Materials for the expansion are synthesized within the cell body and then transported along minuscule tubes to the growth cone, where they are combined to form new nerve tissue. Serviced in this manner, the grow-

ing axon progresses at the rate of about one millimeter per day. Santiago Ramón y Cajal was not familiar with these internal workings, but he recognized that the growth cone was the engine that drove expansion. He also believed that in the growth cone he had discovered the trailblazer of regeneration, a steering apparatus that directed the axon's course. Ramón y Cajal theorized that growth cones sprouted and navigated in

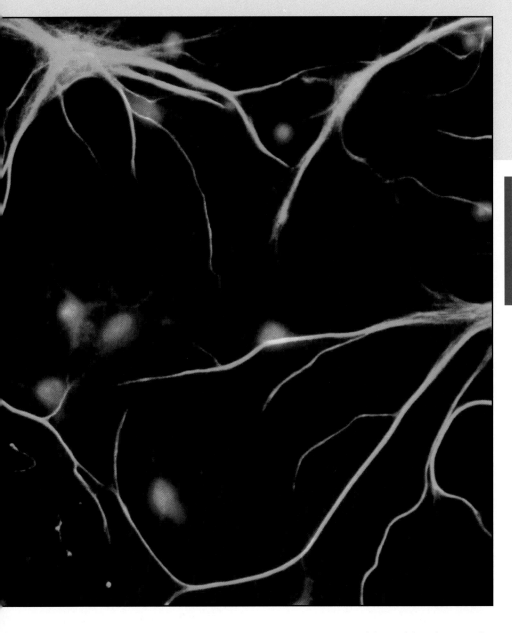

Neurons *(red)* and glial cells *(green, blue)* resemble fireworks in a night sky in this false-color stained micrograph of mammalian spinal cord tissue. Glia provide nourishment and other support for the neurons and—unlike neurons—remain capable of dividing throughout life.

response to chemicals released by both the structures they were trying to reach and the Schwann cells that had insulated the severed processes. These attractants—or neurotropic agents, as Ramón y Cajal called them —must somehow be produced in response to damage to the nerve cells.

Ramón y Cajal based his theory of neurotropism on the observation that growth cones often follow the paths of degenerated axons through the surrounding tissue. They make their way down tunnels of what is known as basal lamina—continuous thin mats of extracellular matrix secreted by the Schwann cells that sheathed the now-absent axons. In effect, the basal lamina preserves the original tissue architecture, providing a scaffolding along

which regenerating nerve processes can maneuver.

Despite his rigorous experimental approach, Ramón y Cajal was unable to produce more than circumstantial evidence of the existence of the neurotropic agents that governed such events. Later research by others was no more successful, and the theory of neurotropism gradually fell into disfavor. By the 1930s, experiments with neurons kept alive outside the body showed that growing axons would follow artificially constructed pathways. This research supported what are known as mechanical theories of axon regeneration, which rejected the notion of chemical agents and proposed instead that the tunnels of the basal lamina were the only necessary guides for nerve regeneration.

Mechanical theories, however, failed to account for the way that specific neurons usually found their way to the right target cells. This difficulty gave rise to yet another hypothesis, also contrary to Ramón y Cajal's: that each neuron and its processes had a specific chemical affinity for particular pathways and connections, a predilection that allowed nerve fibers to retrace the proper course during regeneration. But this notion in turn left no room for the occasional erroneous connections sometimes formed by regenerating nerves, as in the case of some of the nerves in M. M.'s reattached arm. Growth cones sometimes become confused about their destinations, taking wrong turns as they progress along old pathways. If they fall in with other nerve fibers, they can end up growing down foreign routes. Sensory fibers can even go so far astray as to regenerate along motor pathways, although when they reach a muscle they are unable to form synaptic connections and so fail to function.

The understanding of nerve regeneration was still sketchy in the 1950s when the work of Rita Levi-Montalcini and Stanley Cohen began to build evidence in support of Ramón y Cajal's original ideas. Further studies indicated that the nerve growth factor

isolated by Cohen does far more than simply instigate the sprouting of nerve fibers. A 1963 experiment demonstrated that a regular supply of the growth factor is essential to the survival of neurons in a culture dish. Subsequent work indicated that neurons in the body also require a steady supply of growth factor. Target cells that connect with neurons produce nerve growth factor and other similar growth enhancers, which are transferred to the axons of the associated neurons. Microtubules in the axons carry the proteins back to the nerve cell bodies. When growth factors are absent, neurons contract their processes or degenerate altogether. And when a synaptic connection is broken because of some other damage to a neuron, the target cell begins to broadcast its growth factors—increasing the amount of the proteins available to initiate regeneration in surviving nerve cells.

The discovery of nerve growth factor also provided scientists with an opportunity to reconsider Ramón y Cajal's long-neglected theory of neurotropism. In an elegant experiment conducted at Harvard Medical School in the mid-1970s, neurobiologist Robert Campenot created a cell-

culture system with three chambers separated by impermeable barriers. In the center chamber Campenot seeded neurons with nerve growth factor, allowing the resulting sprouts to grow under the barriers through scratches in the bottom of the culture dish. He then filled the chamber on one side with a solution containing nutrients and nerve growth factor; he filled the other side with the same solution minus the growth factor. The nerve fibers sprouting from the central chamber grew only into the side containing the growth factor. When Campenot removed the solution from that side, the nerve fibers that had worked their way over began to degenerate, even though their cell bodies in the central chamber remained in good condition.

The results of Campenot's and other experiments indicated that Ramón y Cajal had been largely correct in his hypothesis, posited a half-century earlier, that regenerating neurons need chemical guidance. Target cells such as muscles do indeed produce nerve growth factor and other neurotropic agents that have the same attractant effect. In addition, subtle chemical differences among motor neurons help them find the specific muscles that they activate; the neurons' growth cones have specialized receptors that cause them to follow the trail of the proteins generated by

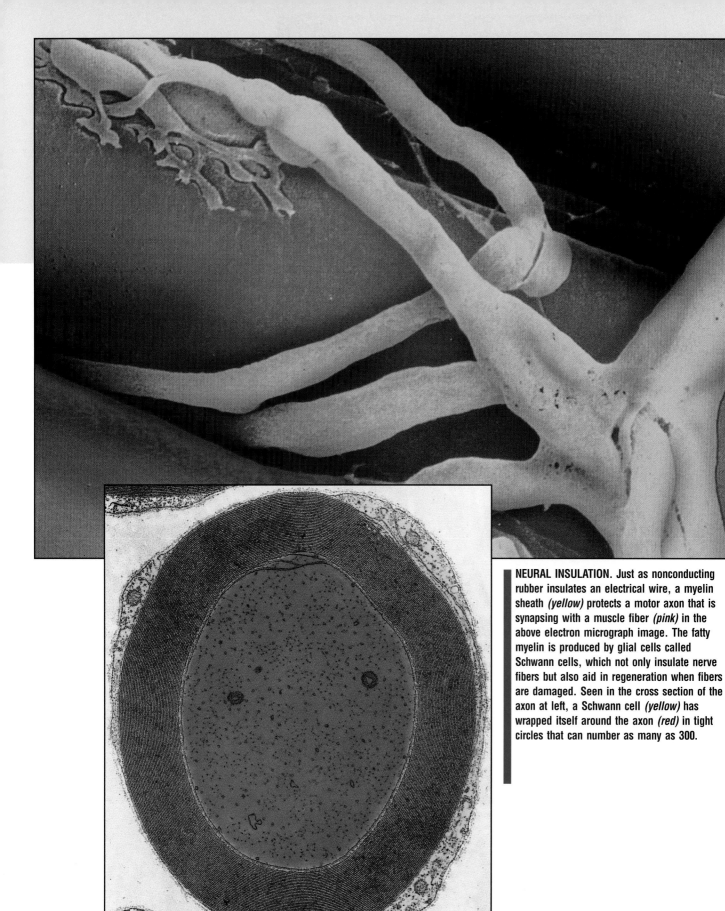

NEURAL INSULATION. Just as nonconducting rubber insulates an electrical wire, a myelin sheath *(yellow)* protects a motor axon that is synapsing with a muscle fiber *(pink)* in the above electron micrograph image. The fatty myelin is produced by glial cells called Schwann cells, which not only insulate nerve fibers but also aid in regeneration when fibers are damaged. Seen in the cross section of the axon at left, a Schwann cell *(yellow)* has wrapped itself around the axon *(red)* in tight circles that can number as many as 300.

their particular target tissues. When growing axons reach their goal and connect with target cells, the renewed electrical activation causes changes within the targets—the most significant being that the production of growth factors then drops to the level required only to maintain the synaptic connection. The reduced supply no longer supports the sprouting and migration of new nerve processes, and hence the regenerative activity draws to a close.

Target cells are not the only sources of the chemical factors that guide the process of nerve regeneration. In the event of an injury to nerve fibers, the Schwann cells that house the fibers begin to divide. Soon these proliferating glial cells start to produce growth factor and other nerve-growth proteins; they then gather the nerve growth factor they have manufactured and pass it along to the regenerating axons. Proteins in the basal lamina play a slightly different role. Acting as neural signposts, they bind to specialized receptors on the advancing growth cones to signal that the cones are on course.

As research has revealed more about both the physical and the chemical bases of regeneration, surgeons have become more successful with damaged peripheral nerves in the operating room. One relatively new technique, called entubulation

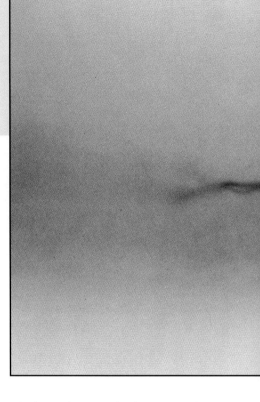

A pair of growth cones at the head of an axon make their way from the brainstem of a frog embryo to motor neurons in the lower spinal cord. The leading cone *(far right)* has a bulkier and more complex shape than the elongated cone behind it, because, in the role of pioneer, the leading cone must survey and route through unfamiliar territory. In humans, axons sprout similar growth cones during periods of development and regeneration.

repair, uses artificial tubes or conduits to reconnect nerves that have been severed. The tubes, made out of natural or synthetic materials, are attached to each end of the injured nerve when the gap between them is too wide to simply suture the ends back together.

Once in place, the tubes establish a friendly wound-healing environment, and the body's own systems quickly fill them from both ends with a variety of internal tissue cells, including Schwann cells. Nerve processes then grow into the tube and create a cable of fibers. Growth factors often concentrate there as well, assisting regeneration, and the tube also limits the growth of cells that create scar tissue,

which might impede the regrowth of nerve fibers. When surgeons add nerve-growth proteins to the whole mix, the rate of regeneration picks up, with axons making new connections within a few weeks.

By the early 1990s, entubulation repairs over short gaps were often proving more successful in restoring nerve function than grafts—such as those used in M. M.'s arm—and almost as effective as directly reconnecting severed nerve endings. In some cases, tube repairs have helped patients almost completely recover the sensations and abilities they lost through nerve injury.

Repairs to the brain and spinal cord are far more complex than those in the peripheral nervous system, and seldom as successful. Neurons of the human central nervous system (CNS) do not regenerate spontaneously. At-

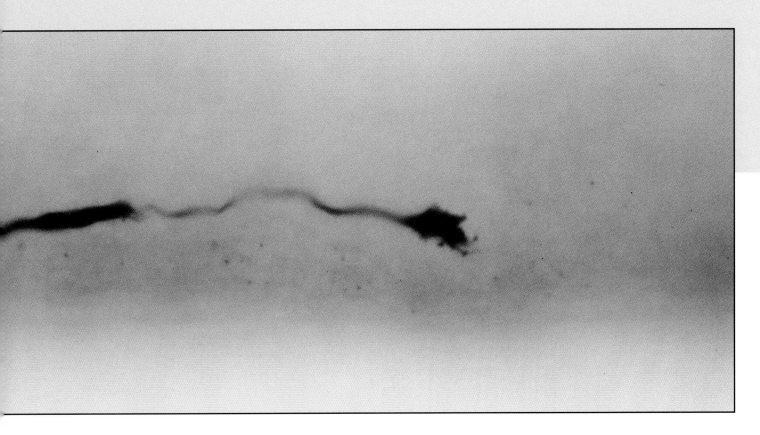

tempts to explain this inability generally point either to deficiencies in the neurons themselves or to an unfavorable environment for nerve fiber growth. Whatever the reason, the failure of CNS neurons to regenerate means that victims of head and spinal cord injuries—up to half a million people each year in the United States alone—often suffer permanent paralysis and brain damage.

Paradoxically, though, humans tend to benefit from the recalcitrant nature of CNS neurons. In the complex web of axons and dendrites in the brain and spinal cord, making and retaining just the right connections with billions of other cells is essential to survival. If neurons in the human brain or spinal

cord could divide, the chance of disrupting these links—and impairing any number of essential functions—might be unacceptably high.

Interestingly, not all creatures are incapable of regrowing brain and spinal cord cells. In newly hatched fish, whose nervous systems are far simpler than humans', damage to the spinal cord is repaired in a matter of days. Adult fish can also recover fully from spinal cord injury, but they usually need more time. Cells from the lining of the fish's spinal canal can multiply profusely and migrate down the length of the spinal cord, then transform themselves into new neurons. Replacement and repair take place in a similar fashion in some parts of the brains of fish and amphibians. Indeed, scientists have discovered that when entire cerebral hemispheres are removed from em-

bryos and larval forms, they grow back. And even though adult fish cannot replace a missing part of their brain in its entirety, the nerve fibers of the CNS can regrow and restore original synaptic links. Scientists speculate that some fish have retained the ability to develop new brain cells and connections because their bodies continue to grow throughout their lives and need ever larger brains to manage them.

Although the human CNS has almost no natural ability to make physical repairs, its cells share an important characteristic with regenerating peripheral nerve cells: Severed nerve fibers in the CNS commonly sprout new processes. Such processes tend to stop growing before they make it all the way across a damaged site, meaning that no functional connections can be established, but the phenomenon is a tempting beacon for researchers seeking new medical treatments for CNS injuries.

Santiago Ramón y Cajal was one of the first scientists to suggest that the problem with CNS regeneration lies not in the neurons themselves but in their less-than-hospitable surroundings. The first signs that his theory was in fact true began to emerge in the early 1980s during a series of experiments replicating Ramón y Cajal's methods and directed by neuroscientist Albert Aguayo at McGill University in Montreal. Aguayo's technique, which he called an "environment transplant," involved repairing injuries to the central nervous system using peripheral nerve tissue.

In a typical experiment, Aguayo used a portion of the sciatic nerve from the leg of a rat to bridge the site of an injury in the animal's brain. The peripheral nerve processes quickly degenerated, but their Schwann cells stayed healthy, dividing and retaining their tubelike alignment. Unlike the glial cells that ordinarily bracket central nervous system cells, Schwann cells produce basal lamina and growth factors, which proved to contribute the same regenerative capacity to the CNS that they do in the peripheral

system. Amazingly, some of the damaged nerve cells in the rat brain sprouted new axons, which readily grew into the grafted "environment."

Aguayo discovered that the axons entering the grafted tissue sometimes covered far greater distances than their ordinary span in the brain. In his experimental rats, severed axons from the retina, for example, sometimes grew as long as three centimeters— twice the length of a normal optic nerve cell. He also discovered encouraging signs of electrical activity in the neurons: When a light was directed at the rat's retina, electrical activity within the regenerated axons was indistinguishable from the response seen in axons of an undamaged optic nerve cell. In a further study, Aguayo entirely replaced a rat's optic nerve with a peripheral nerve graft linking the retina to the brain. Axons sprouted through the graft and spread out radially as they emerged at target areas in the brain.

Growth factors from peripheral nerve tissues played an important role in these studies. Since then, research has confirmed the existence of growth factor receptors in the retina, and has demonstrated that injections of specific growth factors can prevent

the degeneration of injured neurons in the eye. But in spite of the convincing proof that damaged central nervous system cells can be preserved and even persuaded to initiate regrowth, evidence that specific functions—such as vision in Aguayo's rats—have been successfully restored is harder to come by. Electrical impulses along the nerves in the rats clearly indicated some form of activity, but Aguayo could not be certain that the rats were actually perceiving visual images. The difficulty in restoring vision or any particular function may be due in part to the difficulty of controlling exactly where regenerating axons terminate in the brain.

Regeneration of the central nervous system may be further hindered by substances found in the CNS environment that actually stifle growth. These inhibitory factors probably serve in an uninjured system to prevent new neural connections that could jumble the exquisitely complex circuits of the brain. When the brain or spinal cord is damaged, however, successful repairs depend on somehow suppressing those restraining chemicals themselves. Approaching CNS regeneration from that angle has shown promising results in laboratory tests, such as those performed in 1993 by a team led by Martin Schwab, a University of Zurich neurochemist. Schwab's group partially severed the spinal cords of

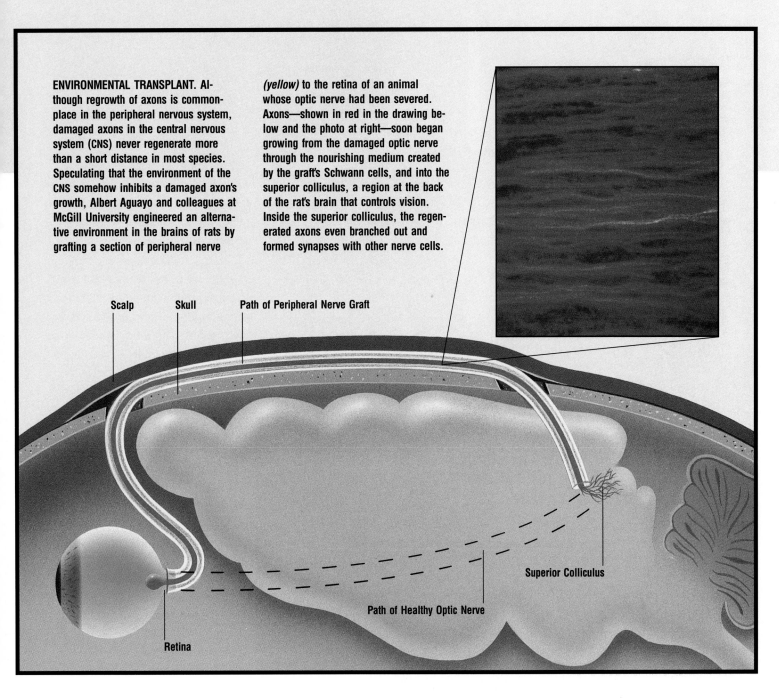

ENVIRONMENTAL TRANSPLANT. Although regrowth of axons is commonplace in the peripheral nervous system, damaged axons in the central nervous system (CNS) never regenerate more than a short distance in most species. Speculating that the environment of the CNS somehow inhibits a damaged axon's growth, Albert Aguayo and colleagues at McGill University engineered an alternative environment in the brains of rats by grafting a section of peripheral nerve *(yellow)* to the retina of an animal whose optic nerve had been severed. Axons—shown in red in the drawing below and the photo at right—soon began growing from the damaged optic nerve through the nourishing medium created by the graft's Schwann cells, and into the superior colliculus, a region at the back of the rat's brain that controls vision. Inside the superior colliculus, the regenerated axons even branched out and formed synapses with other nerve cells.

Scalp   Skull   Path of Peripheral Nerve Graft

Superior Colliculus

Path of Healthy Optic Nerve

Retina

rats, then applied a combination of a growth factor called NT-3 and antibodies that suppressed the growth-inhibiting proteins of the rats. The result was a prolific sprouting in the spinal neurons, with some fibers growing as much as two centimeters.

Other chemical and biological interventions also show promise for the repair of spinal cord damage. In an experiment at Kyoto University in Japan, a team led by neurosurgeon Yasushi Iwashita used grafts to repair severed spinal cords in newborn rats. The researchers bridged the injured regions with spinal tissue from rat embryos, in which developing neurons multiply and grow vigorously. The procedure was performed on 32 rats; of the 22

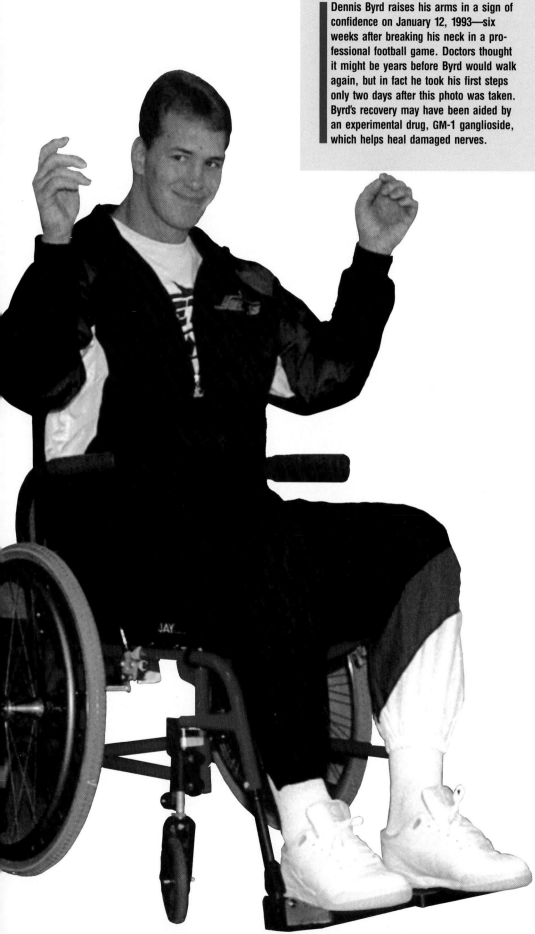

Dennis Byrd raises his arms in a sign of confidence on January 12, 1993—six weeks after breaking his neck in a professional football game. Doctors thought it might be years before Byrd would walk again, but in fact he took his first steps only two days after this photo was taken. Byrd's recovery may have been aided by an experimental drug, GM-1 ganglioside, which helps heal damaged nerves.

who survived, 14 showed almost complete recovery. They behaved just as normal rats do—walking, running, climbing, and even landing on their feet when dropped upside down. However, when Iwashita's team tried the experiment with adult rats, they were unable to duplicate the success they had had with the newborns, suggesting that the results of the earlier study were possible only because the nervous systems of newborn rats are extremely resilient.

Despite the mixed results of experiments in spinal cord repairs, particular types of damage have shown response to treatment. Some paralyzing injuries to the spine, for example, occur when spinal neurons are merely compressed rather than severed. Once crushed, the cells often degenerate, making the damage permanent, but in a few cases, prompt treatment has helped victims regain a substantial amount of nerve function.

A chemical that seems especially promising is a steroid known as methylprednisolone, which has restored an average of 20 percent of lost motor and sensory functions when administered within a few hours of injury. Another involves a complex molecule called GM-1 ganglioside, that is found in abundance in the membranes of neurons in humans and other mammals. Animal studies have demonstrated that this substance is essential to supporting life, although its specific function is unknown. In one study, human patients who received injections of GM-1 ganglioside during the first months after spinal cord damage recovered a measure of movement in paralyzed limbs, but other studies have not been able to duplicate the results with assurance. Nevertheless, in one highly publicized case, GM-1 ganglioside may have played a critical role in recovery from what could have been a permanently disabling injury.

On a cold Sunday afternoon in late November 1992—the height of the football season—New York Jets defensive end Dennis Byrd collided head-first with one of his own teammates during a game against the Kansas City Chiefs, hitting with such force that he broke his neck. Surgeons at Lenox Hill Hospital in Manhattan spent seven hours removing shattered bone, adding bone grafts taken from Byrd's pelvis, and stabilizing his spine with three permanent metal plates. In spite of their efforts, the prognosis was not good: The spinal cord was severely compressed, leaving the 26-year-old athlete paralyzed from the waist down. Byrd was told that it might be as long as two years before anyone could determine whether he would ever be able to walk again.

At the time, doctors also began administering GM-1 ganglioside—and to their astonishment, only a week passed before their determined patient began moving muscles in his lower legs. Four months later he was walking with a cane, and less than a year after the injury, Byrd strode proudly and unaided into training camp to greet his former teammates.

Unfortunately, successes such as Dennis Byrd's are not yet the usual outcome of spinal injuries, and even rarer is recovery from harm to the brain itself, where proper function relies on the interconnected operations of 100 billion nonrenewable neurons. As a consequence, brain-injury researchers have concentrated on promoting the survival of intact neurons endangered by disease, and on strategies that help the brain work around the loss of abilities caused by damage. In the 1980s, many investigators began turning their attention to a class of proteins called neurotrophic factors. Confusingly similar to *neurotropic*, the word is derived from the Greek words for "nerve" and "nourish." Neurotrophic molecules, which include nerve growth factor, appear to have three basic functions: setting up the embryonic nervous system; repairing damaged neurons; and promoting growth and connection between neurons as part of the process of learning and remembering.

One of the first of these important chemicals to be isolated was discovered in 1987 after a decade of searching by Hans Thoenen at the Max Planck Institute in Munich. Known as brain-derived neurotrophic factor, or BDNF, it can protect brain cells against damage, and it helps ensure the survival of some of the brain cells that commonly degenerate in the course of Parkinson's and Alzheimer's diseases. Another brain-oriented chemical, glial cell line-derived neurotrophic factor (GDNF), was discovered in 1993 by Frank Collins, a researcher with a Colorado biotechnology company. Glial cells constitute a full 90 percent of the brain's cells, and they were once thought to be little more than a gluelike (hence *glial*) medium that holds the neurons in place. As it turns out, though, they are the most significant producers of neurotrophic factors in the brain—playing an integral part in the organ's survival and communications.

In a petri dish, GDNF caused brain cells to live longer and develop dense thickets of sprouts. It also caused embryonic neurons to mature much faster than normal, and it proved to protect certain nerve cells, promoting the survival of neurons that produce the neurotransmitter dopamine. This ability makes GDNF a promising treatment for Parkinson's disease, a degenerative brain disease that causes severe motor disturbances, including tremors of the fingers and hands, rigid muscles, a shuffling gait, and halting speech. Affecting more than a million people in the United States, Parkinson's is believed to result from a reduced supply of dopamine in the brain. Recent studies indicate that not all of the dopamine deficiency in the brains of Parkinson's victims is the result of cell death; some nerve cells apparently become dormant, unable to function. Researchers hope that these cells can be protected and eventually switched back on with neurotrophic factors such as GDNF.

Scientists have also found that the brain possesses a surprising ability to accommodate implanted cells and to incorporate them into its established circuitry—pointing the way toward another possible treatment for Parkinson's disease. The most successful such transplants are fetal neurons, which survive in the laboratory longer than more mature cells and make new connections more easily, because

they have not yet formed extensive axonal links. In experiments using rats with brain damage paralleling parkinsonism, small pieces of fetal brain tissue were implanted into spaces between folds of the brain. The new cells formed normal synaptic contacts with previously disconnected neurons and produced an incomplete but nonetheless significant recovery of motor functions that had been lost to the brain damage.

Similar procedures, using tissue from unintentionally aborted human fetuses, have been carried out on humans suffering from parkinsonism. Although the technique is highly controversial, the results have been remarkable. In one of several studies reported in 1992, the effects of the surgery were still evident a year and a half later: The subjects moved more freely than they did before treatment, and they resumed some of the activities of normal daily life that had been lost to them, such as dressing and eating without assistance.

While tissue implants offer much-needed hope to the victims of degenerative brain diseases, many other kinds of brain damage do not respond to such treatments. Indeed, recovering mental functions after injury or disease often depends on the brain's own ability to adapt to its diminished resources. Surprisingly, that ability is considerable, particularly in

young children, as demonstrated by the near-miraculous success of a surgical procedure called hemispherectomy. In this operation half of the brain is removed in an attempt to quell epileptic seizures that cannot be tamed by drugs.

In 1985 the landmark case of four-year-old Maranda Francisco of Denver helped win acceptance for this drastic measure in children. At the time, the little girl was suffering 120 seizures a day. With little hope that Maranda could lead a normal life, her parents consulted Benjamin Carson, a neurosurgeon at Johns Hopkins Hospital in Baltimore, who proposed stopping the seizures by entirely removing the left hemisphere of Maranda's brain. The possibility of negative side effects was of course substantial: The left hemisphere contains the brain centers that ordinarily process speech and control movement on the right side of the body.

The first hurdle, the operation itself, went off without a hitch. Almost immediately afterward, Carson could see evidence that Maranda's brain was adapting to its reduced state: She never lost her ability to talk, probably because the healthy right hemisphere had already assumed this function

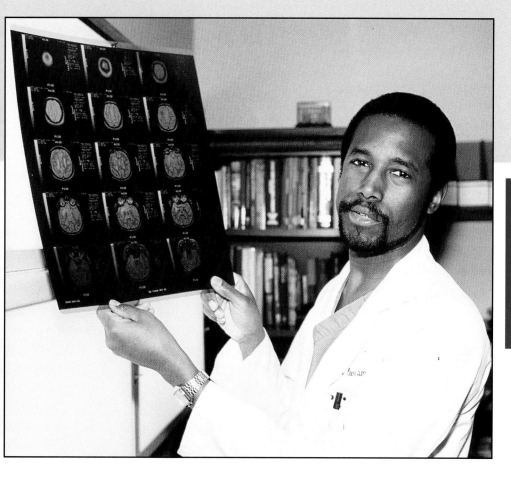

In 1985 Johns Hopkins pediatric neurosurgeon Benjamin Carson, shown here in 1993, made medical history when he successfully removed half of a young girl's brain in an attempt to control her near-constant seizures. The girl went on to lead a normal life, demonstrating the tremendous resilience of very young brain cells. Since then, dozens of children have benefited from the highly dramatic treatment.

from its damaged mate. The remainder of the missing left hemisphere's functions were taken over during the next few months, as physical therapy restored movement to her paralyzed right side. Freed of the seizures, Maranda recovered fully. In 1993 she was 12 years old, healthy—and taking tap-dancing lessons.

Neurobiologists use the term *plasticity* to describe this marvel of adaptation. Plasticity manifests itself in less dramatic circumstances as well. For example, blind people usually develop extraordinarily acute senses of smell, hearing, and touch to compensate for their lack of vision; similarly, the elderly can demonstrate high mental functioning in spite of the natural loss of brain cells through aging.

In both of these instances, the brain actually reorganizes some of the trillions of connections between its neurons. This kind of architectural change, once believed to happen only during periods of intensive development in infancy and childhood, has been shown to be a common phenomenon in the adult brain as well.

Sometimes reorganization of the brain's functional maps can lead to rather unusual results—as in the case of phantom limbs. Scientists once believed that a person who lost a part of the body continued to perceive sensation as if it were still present be-

cause of nerve stimulation around the area of amputation. But such an explanation could not account for reports from amputees that, for example, cold water on the face felt as though it were running down a phantom arm. In fact, recent studies show that when brain cells that process sensory information are cut off from their original source—a finger, for example, or a leg—the untethered nerve cells do not die but instead make new connections with other targets. The phantom limb thus stays alive in the mind long after it is gone from the body, because the brain apparently continues to process sensory information coming in from new targets as if it came from the original, and now missing, source. Understanding this remapping can help an amputee deal with its consequences—relieving an itch in phantom fingers, for instance, by scratching a spot on the cheek.

The brain's plasticity is called into play not only for repairing damage. Remapping occurs throughout life, as the brain reconfigures connections in response to what is typically a constantly changing external environment. This capacity is most pronounced in young, developing brains, which are predisposed to learn as much as they can, rearranging their circuitry as needed for mastering new skills. Rats raised in an environment rich with learning opportunities—plenty of cage mates and play equipment—show greater brain development than others raised isolated in small cages. The animals in the richer environment have many more neural connections in the cerebral cortex, the part of the brain associated with learning and memory.

Similarly, children who spend their time in invigorating spaces surrounded by playmates, interesting toys, and learning opportunities show marked differences in mental development. Surveys show that when youngsters from impoverished circumstances are placed in such an environment at an early age, they score significantly higher on IQ tests than do children from the same background who have not had the exposure. Scientists

Reproducing Neurons

One of the axioms in neuroscience is that neurons in the adult brains of nearly every species do not reproduce. But in 1991, two researchers from the University of Calgary put this notion to the test—with stunning results. Brent A. Reynolds and Samuel Weiss added one of three growth factors to each of several glass culture dishes. For each factor, they also treated some of the dishes with a sticky substance that mimics the normal environment of developing nerve cells. Then they placed 1,000 cells from the brains of adult mice in each container—and sat back and waited.

Two days later, most of the cells had died. But in nonsticky dishes that contained a hormone called epidermal growth factor, 15 of the original 1,000 cells not only had survived but had divided and later differentiated into neurons and glial cells (*right*). By inducing adult neurons to reproduce, Reynolds and Weiss had achieved the near-miraculous. The next challenge is to determine whether—and how—the same environment that assists developing nerve cells instead inhibits growth in adult nerve cells.

attribute this outcome to the same activity-related increase of synaptic connections observed in rats.

Learning has important effects on adult brains as well. People who read Braille, for example, develop a larger than normal brain map—a neuronal region devoted to a particular function—for their index finger. Monkeys trained to pick up pellets show expansion in the brain areas that control the finger muscles used to pick up small objects. Less-specific mental stimulation also changes the architecture of

Two days after they are placed in the bottom of a treated glass culture dish, a pair of nerve cells from an adult mouse brain begin to divide *(below, left)*. By the next day, they have developed into two growing clusters *(middle)*. Three to five days later, the clusters are much larger and have become buoyant, rising off the floor of the dish and floating in suspension *(right)*.

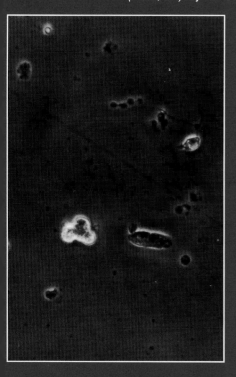
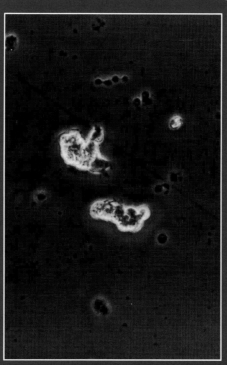
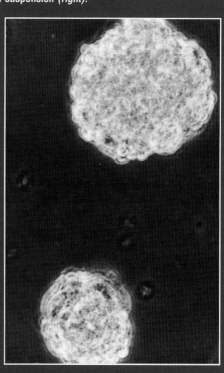

the brain. Autopsies of university graduates who remained mentally active all their lives showed that their brains had formed up to 40 percent more connections than the brains of high-school dropouts. The level of education, however, may be less important than continued use of the brain's circuits throughout life: More connections have been found in the brains of university graduates who throughout their lives continued to challenge themselves intellectually than in graduates who did not.

This continual adaptation allows the brain to maintain its level of functioning even as it suffers the inevitable organic losses of the aging process. After about 30 years of life, the human brain begins to lose neurons to cell death or atrophy at a rate of about 18 million each year. But neuron loss is not necessarily accompanied by loss of memory and mental function. A brain cell can grow new branches of dendrites at any time, if properly stimulated. Processing and storage of information is based on the connections established by the new dendrites—not on the number of cells remaining in the brain. Tests of mental acuity comparing 70-year-olds and 20-year-olds showed that the older people had better long-term memory—the ability to remember past events. The younger subjects scored better on tests of short-term memory—used to retain new information—but with a few minutes of practice every day, their elders nearly matched them in this category too.

With practice and repetition gaining acceptance as tools for redrawing mental maps, new possibilities have opened up for overcoming damage to the nervous system. One of the most promising is the technique of biofeedback, which allows people to exert conscious control over physiological processes that ordinarily take place in the realm of the unconscious. Biofeedback grew out of research in

the 1940s by Yale psychologist Neal Miller, who found that rats could learn to control their heart rate and blood pressure to obtain rewards of food. In the 1960s Miller extended his research to human subjects, using electronic equipment to monitor their heartbeats and brain waves.

Focusing on a dial that recorded heart rate, for example, a person could see when concentration produced a change. As it does in learning any new behavior, the brain takes a shotgun approach, firing neurons until it finds the right ones to do the job. In biofeedback, the brain is made conscious of the tricks that work. With repetition, the chance of activating the wrong cells drops; the right cells fire more reliably, and the new behavior becomes part of the subject's standard repertory.

Early biofeedback studies received little serious attention from health professionals, who considered the technique a fad of the thrill-seeking culture of the 1960s. The research continued, however, and the technique acquired more credibility as sophisticated electronics systems and computers made it possible to monitor almost any body function with ever finer distinctions. Thus it became possible for patients to see data about their skin temperature, muscle activity, heart rate, and brain waves, and to compare the information with

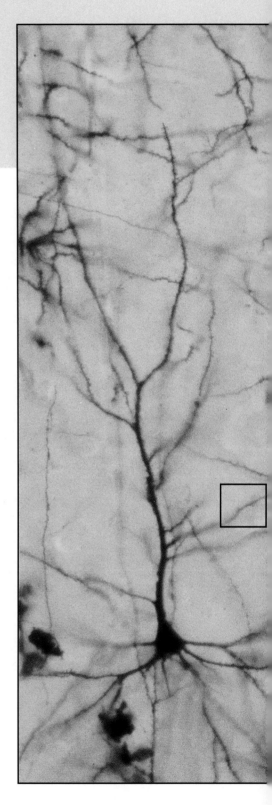

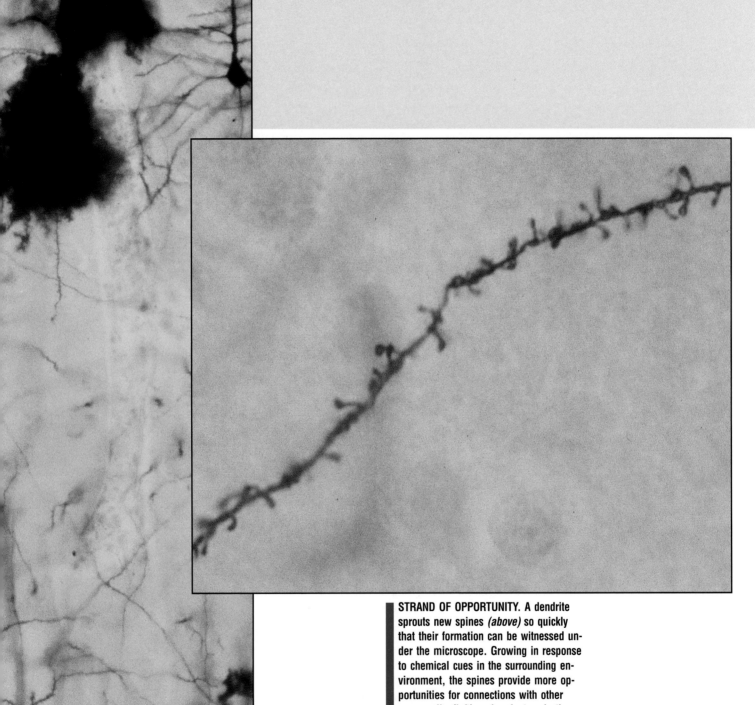

STRAND OF OPPORTUNITY. A dendrite sprouts new spines *(above)* so quickly that their formation can be witnessed under the microscope. Growing in response to chemical cues in the surrounding environment, the spines provide more opportunities for connections with other nerve cells *(left)*—a key feature in the regeneration of injured nerve tissue.

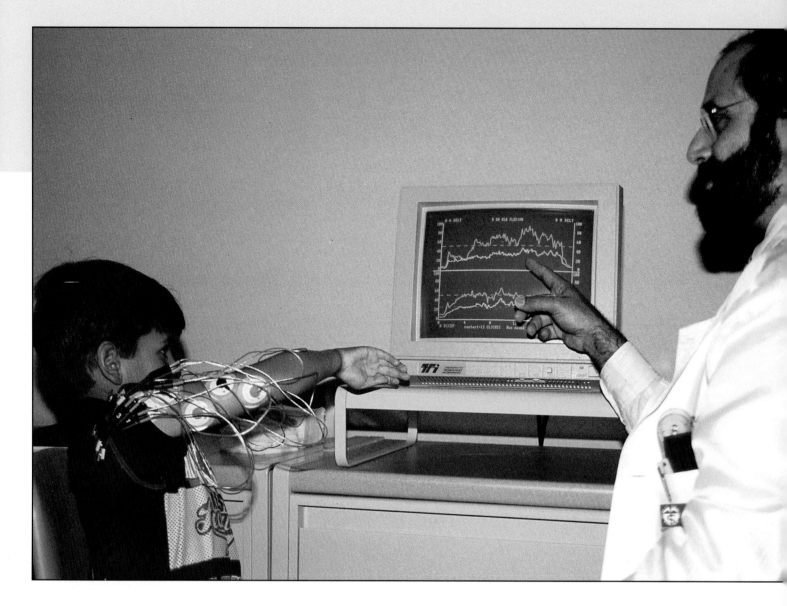

previous results and general standards. In fact, biofeedback tools became so precise that they could measure electrical activity as small as 10 millionths of a volt—the level of a single neuron firing.

By the 1980s, biofeedback research had advanced to the point that it was routinely used to teach muscle relaxation, or to help athletes build strength in specific muscle groups. Its most far-reaching application, however, was in efforts to restore function to paralyzed muscles. Psychologist

Bernard Brucker began treating paralysis and other motor disabilities in 1981 at a biofeedback laboratory associated with the Jackson Memorial Medical Center at the University of Miami. Throughout the next decade more than 2,000 people entered Brucker's program, with 90 percent experiencing improved functioning. More than a dozen were quadriple-

gics, with no movement in their arms and legs, and supposedly with no hope of recovery.

One of these patients was Tammy DeMichael, who suffered a broken neck and a crushed spinal column in 1985 when her fiancé fell asleep while driving and their car slammed into a guardrail and flipped. DeMichael entered Brucker's program after a year of extensive medical treatment that had failed to win back any function or feeling in her limbs. Her doctors told her that the crucial nerves in her

Through biofeedback therapy a boy with cerebral palsy has learned how to raise his arm and extend the elbow. By manipulating the lines on the screen into a pattern described by Bernard Brucker of the Jackson Memorial Medical Center at the University of Miami, the boy—whose condition resulted from a shortage of oxygen during his birth that killed a critical number of brain cells—has begun to use his remaining cells more efficiently.

spine were crushed and that she would be unable to move from the neck down for the rest of her life.

Brucker tested DeMichael with an electromyograph (EMG), an instrument that measures electrical activity in specific muscles. When he asked DeMichael to try raising her arm, she could not move, but the EMG showed that some nerve impulses were reaching the muscles—about 14 percent of the normal level. Even though the impulses were not nearly enough to trigger motion, Brucker told DeMichael, they offered a basis for hope. At least some motor nerves were still alive, he believed, and could regenerate fully if the brain could be retrained to send a strong enough signal to activate them.

To begin that process, Brucker asked DeMichael to watch a blue line running horizontally across the EMG monitor, which represented the impulses from the brain to the arm muscles, measured at intervals of one-tenth of a second. He then told DeMichael to try moving her arm again, which made the line slope upward. The arm never moved, but by the end of the session the line was approaching the vertical. DeMichael could not explain exactly what she was doing: "I just concentrated on watching the screen," she said, "and the line kept going higher." It took her only eight more sessions to improve her performance to 80 percent of normal capacity. Without knowing quite how, DeMichael was finding a way to fire more neurons.

However, there was still no movement, a fact that Brucker attributed to muscle atrophy after a year of paralysis. The muscle-to-nerve connection was reestablished, he told DeMichael, and now it was time to work on regaining strength. Brucker formulated a program that mixed biofeedback training with passive rehabilitation exercises such as massage and electrical stimulation. The progress was slow, but a year after the treatment began, DeMichael succeeded in moving her arm. Her recovery accelerated from this point, with biofeedback sessions focusing on other muscles—particu-

larly those of the legs—as DeMichael learned to move her arms without guidance from the equipment. Soon feeling was restored to all of her limbs, and she was launched on an exercise regimen to improve her strength and mobility.

Five years after entering the biofeedback program, DeMichael had better than normal arm strength, walked 60 feet with a cane, and with crutches could go nearly anywhere she wanted to. Like Maude Rollinson, who lived in a lower-technology time a half-century earlier, DeMichael was reconfiguring her nervous system to win back her lost mobility. She looked forward to the day when she would discard all supports to walk freely.

And Brucker looked ahead to what he considers the almost limitless possibilities in his chosen field. "Biofeedback offers us intimate evidence of what the brain can accomplish," he said in 1991. "In effect, we are looking into our own brains, and watching them encode new information into a few cells, based on what we think and do. It's opening up a whole new era in human learning." That era will doubtless bring ever greater understanding of the ways the human body heals—and the ways that the mind can help.

GLOSSARY

Alzheimer's disease: an affliction that destroys areas of the limbic system and other parts of the brain, resulting in gradual loss of memory and the ability to think rationally; named for German neurologist Alois Alzheimer, who identified it in 1907.

Antibody: a protein, produced by B lymphocytes, whose primary job is to neutralize invading pathogens such as bacteria and viruses.

Arteriole: a minute artery surrounded by smooth muscle.

Artery: a vessel that conveys blood away from the heart.

Atherosclerosis: a disease characterized by thickening of artery walls caused by cholesterol deposits and abnormal cell growth. Atherosclerosis is a leading cause of heart attacks and strokes.

Axon: the long fiber of a neuron, extending as much as three feet from the cell body in humans, that transmits electrochemical impulses. Axons generally branch only near their tips.

Bacteria: one-celled organisms, some of which can cause infection.

Basal lamina: also called the basement membrane, an extracellular layer underlying epithelial tissue. It is thought to have structural and filtering functions.

Biofeedback: a technique with which an individual learns to control a normally involuntary function such as blood pressure by responding to information, or feedback, about that function supplied by a monitoring device. Biofeedback can be used as a self-healing method.

B lymphocyte: also called a B cell, one of a class of white blood cells that mature into antibody-producing plasma cells.

Bone marrow: soft tissue at the center of bones. Red bone marrow is the fundamental production site for all blood cells;

yellow marrow stores fat cells.

Cancer: a disease characterized by the uncontrolled proliferation of cells; it has been linked to mutations in the cells' DNA.

Capillary: the smallest type of blood vessel.

Cartilage: dense, pliable connective tissue found in the joints, nose, and ears, and at the ends of some bones.

Catalyst: a substance capable of accelerating chemical reactions without undergoing chemical change itself.

Cell: the basic structural unit of virtually all living creatures.

Central nervous system: the part of the nervous system consisting of the brain and the spinal cord.

Cholesterol: a fatty substance that is essential to certain bodily processes. Made in the liver as well as consumed in foods from animal sources, cholesterol is thought to contribute to heart disease when present in large amounts over time.

Chromosome: a structure within a cell nucleus that consists of genes. In humans, 23 pairs of chromosomes carry the entire genetic code; each pair consists of one chromosome inherited from each parent.

Cirrhosis: a disease of the liver involving a buildup of connective tissue that interferes with the production of new, healthy tissue and causes extensive functional damage to the organ.

Clot: coagulated blood; the end result of a series of chemical reactions that changes blood plasma into a gelatinous substance composed mostly of fibrin.

Collagen: fibrous protein in connective tissue.

Cytokine: any of several types of chemicals, produced by various cells, that serve as messengers to facilitate cellular responses.

Cytoplasm: the fluid between a cell's outer membrane and its nucleus that contains a variety of cell components.

Dendrites: filaments that branch out from the body of a neuron to receive information transmitted by the axons of other neurons.

Dermis: the layer of skin just under the epidermis.

DNA (deoxyribonucleic acid): the complex molecule that, along with structural proteins, makes up chromosomes.

Elastin: a highly elastic protein in connective tissues and structures such as blood vessels and skin.

Endocrine system: the body's network of glands, organs, and other tissues that secrete hormones.

Endothelium: a thin layer of flat cells that lines blood and lymphatic vessels and heart cavities.

Enzyme: a type of protein that serves as a catalyst for a specific reaction such as breaking down molecules or repairing DNA.

Epidermis: the outermost layer of skin.

Epithelium: the layer of cells covering surfaces or lining cavities.

Fascicle: a small bundle of nerve fibers or muscle fibers.

Fibrin: the protein that is the primary constituent of blood clots.

Fibroblast: a cell that is capable of producing collagen fibers and other elements of connective tissue.

Free radical: an atom or a molecule bearing an unpaired electron. Free radicals destabilize other molecules in chain reactions that are thought to be potentially harmful to the body. Free radicals are neutralized in the body by antioxidants.

Ganglion: a bundle or mass of nerve cells outside the brain or spinal cord. In the autonomic nervous system, ganglia serve as relay points for impulses traveling from the central nervous system to various target organs in the body.

Gene: the basic unit of heredity, a length of DNA that codes for the production of a specific protein.

Glial cells: nonneuronal cells that support and possibly help to regulate the central and peripheral nervous systems.

Growth cone: an enlargement at the tip of a growing neuronal process that has special receptors for nerve growth factors.

Growth factors: substances that stimulate or inhibit cell division or cell differentiation in certain tissues.

Hormones: chemicals, secreted by specialized glands and other organs, that travel through the bloodstream and regulate the activities of specific tissues, organs, and other glands, thereby regulating such functions as growth, reproduction, and digestion.

Hypertension: chronic high blood pressure.

Hypertrophy: an increase in bulk of a tissue or organ caused by increased cell size rather than cell division.

Hypothalamus: a structure in the brain that controls many autonomic functions, such as body-temperature regulation, and also produces hormones and neurotransmitters.

Immune system: a network of tissues, cells, and cell products that mobilizes against foreign substances and organisms and removes debris from the body. The immune system includes the spleen, the thymus, lymph tissue and nodes, white blood cells, and antibodies.

Infection: invasion of the body by organisms that cause disease or injury to tissue.

Inflammation: a reaction of tissues to injury or infection, usually characterized by redness, pain, swelling, heat, and im-paired function. Inflammation may be a by-product of the immune system's response.

Liver: the largest internal organ, important to many metabolic functions.

Macrophage: a large immune cell that can ingest and destroy invading microbes, foreign particles, cancerous or diseased cells, and cellular debris. Macrophages need no direction from the immune system to act.

Malignant: tending to become worse; generally associated with cancer and implying invasion into surrounding tissue and the ability to spread to distant tissues via the blood or lymphatic system.

Membrane: a structural barrier of pliable tissue, serving as covering, lining, partition, or connection.

Microbe: a microscopic organism, such as a bacterium or virus.

Nerve cell: *See* Neuron.

Nervous system: the entire system of nerves and nerve centers in the body, including the brain, spinal cord, nerve processes, and ganglia.

Neuron: a nerve cell, consisting of a central body from which extend a number of branches called dendrites for receiving signals, and a single fiber called an axon for transmitting signals; the human brain contains up to 100 billion neurons.

Neurotransmitter: a chemical, synthesized by neurons, that carries information across the synaptic gap between two neurons or between a neuron and a muscle or a gland.

Neurotrophic factors: proteins that promote neuronal growth and connection in the embryo. These factors also nourish, guide, and repair neurons in adults.

Nucleus: a specialized component of almost all cells that contains, among other structures, the cell's chromosomes; it is encased in a membrane and often is located at or near the cell's center.

Oncogene: a gene that normally regulates cell growth and development but, if mutated or improperly activated, can give rise to cancer.

Parkinson's disease: an affliction in which a part of the midbrain called the substantia nigra stops producing the neurotransmitter dopamine; symptoms include muscle weakness, tremors, and difficulty speaking. It is named for English physician James Parkinson, who first described the disease early in the 19th century.

Peripheral nervous system: the nerves that extend from the spinal cord throughout the rest of the body. It has two subdivisions: the autonomic nervous system, made up of the nerves that regulate normally involuntary functions such as heart rate; and the somatic nervous system, made up of the nerves that control voluntary functions, such as walking.

Phagocyte: a white blood cell that can engulf and destroy pathogens, foreign particles, and cellular debris.

Pituitary gland: a structure, located in the brain near the hypothalamus, that controls virtually all other glands in the body through the release of hormones.

Plasma: the fluid part of the blood, after removal of red and white cells; plasma devoid of clotting factors is known as serum.

Plasticity: the ability of neurons or groups of neurons to acquire new functions.

Platelets: cell fragments in the blood that play an essential role in blood clotting and wound repair.

Poliomyelitis: a viral disease that attacks motor neurons, often resulting in paralysis and muscular atrophy.

Process: an axon or a dendrite extending from the cell body of a neuron.

Protein: a molecule consisting of possibly thousands of amino acids linked together and folded to form a distinct shape that determines the protein's function. Proteins are the fundamental components of the body and play an essential role in all biological processes.

Receptor: a protein molecule on the surface of a cell to which complementary molecules, such as neurotransmitters and growth factors, can bind.

Schwann cells: cells that envelop and produce the myelin sheath around nerve fibers of the peripheral nervous system.

Spleen: a lymphoid organ in the abdomen that serves as a filter for blood, a production site for antibodies, and the major site for dismantling worn red blood cells.

Stem cell: a regenerating cell that produces daughter cells that may differentiate into specific types of cells.

Synapse: a narrow gap, less than a thousandth of a millimeter across, between the axon terminal of the presynaptic, or sending, neuron and a dendrite or the cell body of the postsynaptic, or receiving, neuron.

Telomeres: DNA segments at the ends of chromosome chains that carry no vital information and are thought to play a role in monitoring the number of times a cell may divide.

Thyroid gland: a gland in the neck that secretes hormones involved in the regulation of metabolic rate.

T lymphocyte: also called a T cell, one of several types of lymphocytes that are key players in the immune response.

Tumor: tissue growing abnormally. Tumors are either benign—growing locally—or malignant—that is, cancerous, invading surrounding tissue and sometimes spreading to distant tissue.

Vein: a blood vessel that conveys blood toward the heart.

White blood cell: any of a group of nearly colorless immune cells, including lymphocytes and phagocytes, that fight infection and digest cell debris. White blood cells migrate into tissues in order to perform their functions.

BIBLIOGRAPHY

BOOKS

Alberts, Bruce, et al. *Molecular Biology of the Cell* (2d ed.). New York: Garland, 1989.

Björklund, Anders. "Brain Implants." In *The Science of Mind*, by Kenneth A. Klivington. Cambridge, Mass.: MIT Press, 1989.

Bloom, Floyd E., and Arlyne Lazerson. *Brain, Mind, and Behavior* (2d ed.). New York: W. H. Freeman, 1988.

Buckman, Robert, and Karl Sabbagh. *Magic or Medicine: An Investigation of Healing and Healers*. Toronto: Key Porter Books, 1993.

Burgess, Jeremy, Michael Marten, and Rosemary Taylor. *Under the Microscope: A Hidden World Revealed*. Cambridge, England: Cambridge University Press, 1987.

Chopra, Deepak. *Quantum Healing: Exploring the Frontiers of Mind/Body Medicine*. New York: Bantam, 1989.

Cohen, I. Kelman, Robert F. Diegelmann, and William J. Lindblad (eds.). *Wound Healing: Biochemical and Clinical Aspects*. Philadelphia: W. B. Saunders, 1992.

Cohn, Victor. *Sister Kenny: The Woman Who Challenged the Doctors*. Minneapolis: University of Minnesota Press, 1975.

Columbia University College of Physicians and Surgeons Complete Home Medical Guide. New York: Crown, 1985.

Cotran, Ramzi S., Vinay Kumar, and Stanley L. Robbins. *Robbins Pathologic Basis of Disease* (4th ed.). Philadelphia: W. B. Saunders, 1989.

Cranton, Elmer M., and Arline Brecher. *Bypassing Bypass*. New York: Stein and Day, 1984.

Davis, Goode P., Jr., and Edwards Park. *The Heart: The Living Pump*. Washington, D.C.: U.S. News Books, 1981.

DeFelipe, Javier, and Edward G. Jones. *Cajal's Degeneration and Regeneration of the Nervous System*. Translated by Raoul M. May. New York: Oxford University Press, 1991.

Dinsmore, Charles E. (ed.). *A History of Regeneration Research: Milestones in the Evolution of a Science*. New York: Cambridge University Press, 1991.

Fewkes, Jessica L., Mack L. Cheney, and Sheldon V. Pollack. *Illustrated Atlas of Cutaneous Surgery*. Philadelphia: J. B. Lippincott, 1992.

Fisher, Arthur. *The Healthy Heart* (Library of Health series). Alexandria, Va.: Time-Life Books, 1981.

Gillispie, Charles Coulston (ed.). *Dictionary of Scientific Biography* (Vol. 11). New York: Charles Scribner's Sons, 1970.

Goleman, Daniel, and Joel Gurin (eds.). *Mind/Body Medicine: How to Use Your Mind* for Better Health. Yonkers, N.Y.: Consumer Reports Books, 1993.

Gordon, James S., Dennis T. Jaffe, and David E. Bresler (eds.). Mind, Body, and Health. New York: Human Sciences Press, 1984.

Goss, Richard J.:
The Physiology of Growth. New York: Academic Press, 1978.
Principles of Regeneration. New York: Academic Press, 1969.

Gotto, Antonio M., Jr., et al. Atherosclerosis. Kalamazoo, Mich.: Upjohn, 1977.

Grundy, Scott M. Cholesterol and Atherosclerosis: Diagnosis and Treatment. New York: Gower Medical Publishing, 1990.

Guinness, Alma E. (ed.). ABC's of the Human Body. Pleasantville, N.Y.: The Reader's Digest Association, 1987.

Ham, Arthur W. Histology (6th ed.). Philadelphia: J. B. Lippincott, 1969.

Heppenstall, R. Bruce (ed.). Fracture Treatment and Healing. Philadelphia: W. B. Saunders, 1980.

Hogan, Michael John, Jorge A. Alvarado, and Joan Esperson Weddell. Histology of the Human Eye: An Atlas and Textbook. Philadelphia: W. B. Saunders, 1971.

The Incredible Machine. Washington, D.C.: The National Geographic Society, 1986.

Johnson, Kurt E. Histology and Cell Biology (2d ed.). Malvern, Pa.: Harwal, 1991.

Junqueira, L. Carlos, José Carneiro, Robert O. Kelley. Basic Histology (7th ed.). Norwalk, Conn.: Appleton and Lange, 1992.

Lentz, Thomas L. Cell Fine Structure. Philadelphia: W. B. Saunders, 1971.

Levi-Montalcini, Rita. In Praise of Imperfection. Translated by Luigi Attardi. New York: Basic Books, 1988.

McGoon, Michael D. Mayo Clinic Heart Book: The Ultimate Guide to Heart Health. New York: William Morrow, 1993.

McGraw-Hill Encyclopedia of Science and Technology (Vol. 14, 7th ed.). New York: McGraw-Hill, 1992.

Marieb, Elaine N. Essentials of Human Anatomy and Physiology (4th ed.). Redwood City, Calif.: Benjamin/Cummings, 1994.

Mind and Brain (Journey Through the Mind and Body series). Alexandria, Va.: Time-Life Books, 1993.

Moschella, Samuel L., and Harry J. Hurley. Dermatology (3d ed.). Philadelphia: W. B. Saunders, 1992.

Moyers, Bill. Healing and the Mind. New York: Doubleday, 1993.

Page, Jake. Blood: The River of Life. Washington, D.C.: U.S. News Books, 1981.

Price, Sylvia Anderson, and Lorraine McCarty Wilson. Pathophysiology: Clinical Concepts of Disease Processes. New York: McGraw-Hill, 1978.

Purves, Dale, and Jeff W. Lichtman. Principles of Neural Development. Sunderland, Mass.: Sinauer Associates, 1985.

Ramón y Cajal, Santiago. Histologie du Système Nerveux. Madrid: Instituto Ramón y Cajal, 1955.

Richards, R. N., and G. E. Meharg. Cosmetic and Medical Electrolysis and Temporary Hair Removal. Toronto: Medric, 1991.

Rockwood, Charles A., David P. Green, and Robert W. Bucholz (eds.). Rockwood and Green's Fractures in Adults (3d ed.). Philadelphia: J. B. Lippincott, 1991.

Ross, John, Jr., and Robert A. O'Rourke. Understanding the Heart and Its Diseases. New York: McGraw-Hill, 1976.

Ross, Michael H., Edward J. Reith, and Lynn J. Romrell. Histology: A Text and Atlas (2d ed.). Baltimore: Williams and Wilkins, 1989.

Ruoslahti, Erkki. "Integrins as Receptors for Extracellular Matrix." In Cell Biology of Extracellular Matrix, edited by Elizabeth D.

Hay. New York: Plenum Press, 1991.

St. Aubyn, Lorna (ed.). Healing. London: Heinemann, 1983.

Schaefer, Ernst J. High-Density Lipoproteins and Coronary Heart Disease. New York: Gower Medical Publishing, 1990.

Sinclair, David. Human Growth after Birth. New York: Oxford University Press, 1985.

Smith, Chris A., and Edward J. Wood. Cell Biology. New York: Chapman and Hall, 1992.

Thoenen, Hans, et al. "Nerve Growth Factor." In Growth Factors in Biology and Medicine, Ciba Foundation Symposium 116. New York: John Wiley and Sons, 1985.

Thomas, Lewis. The Lives of a Cell: Notes of a Biology Watcher. New York: Bantam Books, 1974.

Tomei, L. David, and Frederick O. Cope (eds.). Apoptosis: The Molecular Basis of Cell Death. Cold Spring Harbor, N.Y.: Cold Spring Harbor Laboratory Press, 1991.

Tortora, Gerard J., and Sandra Reynolds Grabowski. Principles of Anatomy and Physiology (7th ed.). New York: HarperCollins College Publishers, 1993.

Vander, Arthur J., James H. Sherman, and Dorothy S. Luciano. Human Physiology (5th ed.). New York: McGraw-Hill, 1990.

Weiss, Leon (ed.). Histology: Cell and Tissue Biology (5th ed.). New York: Elsevier Biomedical, 1983.

PERIODICALS

Allman, William F. "Detecting a Brain Killer." U.S. News and World Report, Sept. 13, 1993.

Alper, Joseph. "Boning Up: Newly Isolated Proteins Heal Bad Breaks." Science, Jan. 21, 1994.

Altman, Lawrence K. "New Recommendations on Clot-Busting Drugs for Heart Victims." New York Times, Feb. 8, 1994.

Angier, Natalie. "Biologists Decipher Body's Signals for Repairing Wounds." *New York Times*, Nov. 9, 1993.

Araton, Harvey. "Varying Perceptions of Byrd's Recovery." *New York Times*, Aug. 8, 1993.

"Atherosclerosis: Getting Clear." *Harvard Health Letter*, Jan. 1994.

Baker, Sherry. "Internal Medicine." *Omni*, Jan. 1991.

Barinaga, Marcia:
"The Brain Remaps Its Own Contours." *Science*, Oct. 9, 1992.
"Cell Suicide: By ICE, Not Fire." *Science*, Feb. 11, 1994.
"Neuroscientists Track Nerve Development." *Science*, Nov. 10, 1989.

Barnes, Deborah E. "Damage-Limitation Exercises." *Nature*, Sept. 3, 1992.

Björklund, Anders. "A Question of Making It Work." *Nature*, Jan. 13, 1994.

Blakeslee, Sandra. "Missing Limbs, Still Atingle, Are Clues to Changes in the Brain." *New York Times*, Nov. 10, 1992.

Bower, Bruce. "Stressed-Out Platelets Secrete Hazards." *Science News*, Dec. 18/25, 1993.

Brown, Michael S., and Joseph L. Goldstein:
"How LDL Receptors Influence Cholesterol and Atherosclerosis." *Scientific American*, Nov. 1984.
"Receiving Windows for the Cell." *Science Year*, 1980.

Brownlee, Shannon:
"The Cellular Battlefield." *U.S. News and World Report*, Mar. 28, 1994.
"The Secret Dialogue." *U.S. News and World Report*, Sept. 9, 1991.
"Untangling the Skein of Dementia." *U.S. News and World Report*, Nov. 22, 1993.

Bruno, Richard L. "Post-Polio Sequelae: Research and Treatment in the Second Decade." *Orthopedics*, Nov. 1991.

Bruno, Richard L., et al. "The Pathophysiology of Post-Polio Fatigue." *Annals of the New York Academy of Sciences*, May 1994.

Burgess, Wilson H., and Thomas Maciag. "The Heparin-Binding (Fibroblast) Growth Factor Family of Proteins." *Annual Review of Biochemistry*, 1989, Vol. 58, pp. 575-606.

Byrd, Dennis. "Walking on Air." *People*, Sept. 13, 1993.

Clark, Matt. "Heart Attacks." *Newsweek*, Feb. 8, 1988.

Clarkson, Thomas B., et al. "Remodeling of Coronary Arteries in Human and Non-human Primates." *Journal of the American Medical Association*, Jan. 26, 1994.

Cotton, Paul. "Eventual Central Nervous System Regeneration?" *Journal of the American Medical Association*, Oct. 23/30, 1991.

Dautry-Varsat, Alice, and Harvey F. Lodish. "How Receptors Bring Proteins and Particles into Cells." *Scientific American*, May 1984.

"Deathless Tissues." *New York Times*, July 3, 1914.

Deuel, Thomas F. "Polypeptide Growth Factors: Roles in Normal and Abnormal Cell Growth." *Annual Review in Cell Biology*, 1987, Vol. 3, pp. 443-492.

Dexter, T. Michael, and Harry White. "Growth without Inflation." *Nature*, Mar. 29, 1990.

"Dr. Carrel's Miracles in Surgery Win Nobel Prize." *New York Times*, Oct. 13, 1912.

Drexler, Madeline. "Healing the Spinal Cord." *Boston Globe*, Mar. 27, 1994.

Elliott, Laura. "Mending a Heart." *Washingtonian*, Dec. 1993.

Eskenazi, Gerald. "Byrd Gets Movement in His Legs." *New York Times*, Dec. 6, 1992.

Ewin, Dabney M.:
"Emergency Room Hypnosis for the Burned Patient." *American Journal of Clinical Hypnosis*, July 1986.
"Hypnotherapy for Warts (Verruca Vulgaris): 41 Consecutive Cases with 33 Cures." *American Journal of Clinical Hypnosis*, July 1992.

Ezzell, Carol:
"Adult Neurons: Not Too Old to Divide." *Science News*, Apr. 4, 1992.
"Fetal Tissue Grafts Reverse Parkinson's." *Science News*, Aug. 29, 1992.
"Paving the Way for Spinal Cord Repair." *Science News*, Apr. 25, 1992.
"Skin Cells Bridge Injured Spinal Cords." *Science News*, Nov. 7, 1992.

Fackelmann, Kathy A.:
"Blood Substances Linked to Heart Disease." *Science News*, Nov. 20, 1993.
"Mutant Gene Offers Cholesterol Resistance." *Science News*, Nov. 20, 1993.

Folkman, Judah, and Michael Klagsbrun. "Angiogenic Factors." *Science*, Jan. 23, 1987.

"The Fountain of Youth." *New York Times*, Sept. 5, 1913.

Friend, Tim. " 'Fusion Proteins' May Be Medical Savior as Clot-Busters." *USA Today*, Nov. 16, 1993.

Goss, Richard J.:
"Prospects for Regeneration in Man." *Clinical Orthopaedics and Related Research*, Sept. 1980.
"Why Mammals Don't Regenerate—Or Do They?" *News in Physiological Sciences*, June 1987.

Hamilton, David P. "Severed Spines Healed in Rats, Researchers Say." *Wall Street Journal*, Jan. 13, 1994.

Hayflick, Leonard. "The Cell Biology of Human Aging." *Scientific American*, Jan. 1980.

"Heart Valves: They Have to Work." *Heartbeat*, Winter 1992.

Henig, Robin Marantz. "For Many Young

Blacks, Pediatric Neurosurgeon Is a Folk Hero." *New York Times*, June 8, 1993.

Hilts, Philip J. "Cells May Bear Mark of Each Cancer Agent." *New York Times*, Jan. 18, 1994.

Hopkins, James M., and Richard P. Bunge. "Regeneration of Axons from Adult Human Retina *in Vitro*." *Experimental Neurology*, 1991, Vol. 112, pp. 243-251.

Hynes, Richard O. "Fibronectins." *Scientific American*, June 1986.

Jackson, Anthony, et al. "Heat Shock Induces the Release of Fibroblast Growth Factor 1 from NIH 3T3 Cells." *Proceedings of the National Academy of Sciences*, Nov. 1992.

Kolata, Gina:
"Scientists Decipher Mysterious Process of Signaling in Cells." *New York Times*, June 22, 1993.
"Success Reported Using Fetal Tissue to Repair a Brain." *New York Times*, Nov. 24, 1992.

Kotulak, Ronald. "Casting New Light on the Brain." *Washington Post*, Aug. 31, 1993.

Krarup, Christian, Joseph Upton, and Mark A. Creager. "Nerve Regeneration and Reinnervation after Limb Amputation and Replantation: Clinical and Psychological Findings." *Muscle and Nerve*, Apr. 1990.

Lavker, Robert M., et al.:
"Hair Follicle Stem Cells: Their Location, Role in Hair Cycle, and Involvement in Skin Tumor Formation." *Journal of Investigative Dermatology*, July 1993.
"Stem Cells of Pelage, Vibrissae, and Eyelash Follicles: The Hair Cycle and Tumor Formation." *Annals of the New York Academy of Sciences*, Dec. 26, 1991.

Levi-Montalcini, Rita, and Pietro Calissano. "The Nerve Growth Factor." *Scientific American*, June 1979.

Levine, Joe. "Lives of Spirit and Dedication." *Time*, Oct. 27, 1986.

McGill, Henry C., Jr. "Arteries Too Good to Kill." *Journal of the American Medical Association*, Jan. 26, 1994.

McLean, John W., et al. "cDNA Sequence of Human Apolipoprotein(a) Is Homologous to Plasminogen." *Nature*, Nov. 12, 1987.

Maier, Jeanette A. M., et al. "Extension of the Life-Span of Human Endothelial Cells by an Interleukin-1α Antisense Oligomer." *Science*, Sept. 28, 1990.

Marx, Jean:
"Holding the Line against Heart Disease." *Research News*, June 22, 1990.
"NGF and Alzheimer's: Hopes and Fears." *Science*, Jan. 26, 1990.

Melzack, Ronald. "Phantom Limbs." *Scientific American*, April 1992.

Miller, Julie Ann. "Grow, Nerves, Grow." *Science News*, Mar. 29, 1986.

Monastersky, Richard. "Extending Cell Life Yields Clues to Growth." *Science News*, Sept. 29, 1990.

Monmaney, Terence. "The Cholesterol Connection." *Newsweek*, Feb. 8, 1988.

Morrow, J., and Rick Wolff. "Wired for a Miracle." *Health*, May 1991.

Moyzis, Robert K. "The Human Telomere." *Scientific American*, Aug. 1991.

Nabel, Elizabeth G., et al. "Recombinant Fibroblast Growth Factor-1 Promotes Intimal Hyperplasia and Angiogenesis in Arteries *in Vivo*." *Nature*, Apr. 29, 1993.

Napier, Kristine. "Understanding Cholesterol Once and for All." *American Health*, Nov. 1993.

Null, Gary. "Chelation Therapy: One of Medicine's Best-Kept Secrets?" *Omni*, Nov. 1993.

Oliwenstein, Lori. "Striking a Nerve." *Discover*, Dec. 1991.

Onifer, Stephen M., Scott R. Whittemore, and Vicky R. Holets. "Variable Morphological Differentiation of a Raphé-Derived Neuronal Cell Line Following Transplantation into the Adult Rat CNS." *Experimental Neurology*, 1993, Vol. 122, pp. 130-142.

Palca, Joseph. "Fetal Tissue Transplants Remain Off Limits." *Science*, Nov. 10, 1989.

Pendick, Daniel. "Gene Finding Gives Clues to DNA Repair." *Science News*, May 15, 1993.

Pennisi, Elizabeth. "Monitoring the Movements of Nerves." *Science News*, July 31, 1993.

Pons, Tim P., et al. "Massive Cortical Reorganization after Sensory Deafferentation in Adult Macaques." *Science*, June 28, 1991.

Pons, Tim P., Preston E. Garraghty, and Mortimer Mishkin. "Plasticity in Non-primary Somatosensory Cortex of Adult Monkeys." In *Post-Legion Neural Plasticity*, edited by H. Flohr. Berlin: Springer-Verlag, 1988.

Potera, Carol. "Limbering Up the Arteries." *American Health*, Jan./Feb. 1994.

Raff, Martin C. "Social Controls on Cell Survival and Cell Death." *Nature*, Apr. 2, 1992.

Raff, Martin C., et al. "Programmed Cell Death and the Control of Cell Survival: Lessons from the Nervous System." *Science*, Oct. 29, 1993.

Rensberger, Boyce. "Cancer's 'Immortality' May Depend on Enzyme." *Washington Post*, Apr. 12, 1994.

Reynolds, Brent A., and Samuel Weiss. "Generation of Neurons and Astrocytes from Isolated Cells of the Adult Mammalian Central Nervous System." *Science*, Mar. 27, 1992.

Rogers, Malcolm, and Peter Reich. "Psychological Intervention with Surgical Patients: Evaluation Outcome." *Advances* in *Psychosomatic Medicine*, 1986, Vol. 15, pp. 23-50.

Rosen, Ora M. "After Insulin Binds." *Science*, Sept. 18, 1987.

Ross, Russell, Elaine W. Raines, and Daniel F. Bowen-Pope. "The Biology of Platelet-Derived Growth Factor." *Cell*, July 18, 1986.

Rusting, Ricki L. "Why Do We Age?" *Scientific American*, Dec. 1992.

Scherer, Ron. "Peelable Wool Not Shear Fantasy." *Christian Science Monitor*, Apr. 17, 1991.

Skerrett, P. J. " 'Matrix Algebra' Heals Life's Wounds." *Science*, May 24, 1991.

Smith, Timothy W.:
"Byrd's Landscape Is Faith and Fortitude." *New York Times*, Mar. 12, 1993.
"Byrd's Spine Is Stabilized in 7 Hours of Surgery." *New York Times*, Dec. 3, 1992.

Sporn, Michael B., and Anita B. Roberts. "Transforming Growth Factor-β." *Journal of the American Medical Association*, Aug. 18, 1989.

Steinberg, Daniel. "Antioxidants and Atherosclerosis." *Circulation*, Sept. 1991.

Swaab, D. F. "Brain Aging and Alzheimer's Disease, 'Wear and Tear' versus 'Use It or Lose It.' " *Neurobiology of Aging*, 1991, Vol. 12, pp. 317-324.

Thomas, Kenneth A., and Guillermo Gimenez-Gallego. "Fibroblast Growth Factors: Broad Spectrum Mitogens with Potent Angiogenic Activity." *Trends in Biochemical Science*, Feb. 1986.

Thompson, John A., et al. "Heparin-Binding Growth Factor I Induces the Formation of Organoid Neovascular Structures *in Vivo*." *Proceedings of the National Academy of Sciences*, Oct. 1989.

Travis, John:
"Army Targets a Potential Vaccine against Cholesterol." *Science*, Dec. 24, 1993.
"New Optimism Blooms for Developing Treatments." *Science*, Oct. 9, 1992.

Ubell, Earl. "When Is Heart Surgery Really Called For?" *Parade*, Mar. 13, 1994.

Vidal-Sanz, Manuel, et al. "Axonal Regeneration and Synapse Formation in the Superior Colliculus by Retinal Ganglion Cells in the Adult Rat." *Journal of Neuroscience*, Sept. 1987.

Wallis, Claudia. "Filtering Out Killer Cholesterol." *Time*, Feb. 10, 1986.

Wang, John L., and Yen-Ming Hsu. "Negative Regulators of Cell Growth." *Trends in Biochemical Science*, Jan. 1986.

Weiss, Rick:
"Antibodies Enhance Spinal Nerve Regrowth." *Science News*, Jan. 20, 1990.
"New Alzheimer's Theory Advances." *Washington Post*, Nov. 8, 1993.

Welch, William J. "How Cells Respond to Stress." *Scientific American*, May 1993.

"What Lies under the Skin Predicts Cancer Risk." *Johns Hopkins Magazine*, Apr. 1993.

Williams, Gwyn T., et al. "Haemopoietic Colony Stimulating Factors Promote Cell Survival by Suppressing Apoptosis." *Nature*, Jan. 4, 1990.

Winter, Ruth. "A Dose of Nature." *Health*, July/Aug. 1990.

Young, Richard W. "Visual Cells." *Scientific American*, Oct. 1970.

Zhan, Xi, et al. "Long Term Growth Factor Exposure and Differential Tyrosine Phosphorylation Are Required for DNA Synthesis in BALB/c 3T3 Cells." *Journal of Biological Chemistry*, May 5, 1993.

Zucker, Marjorie B. "The Functioning of Blood Platelets." *Scientific American*, June 1980.

OTHER SOURCES

"Atherosclerosis Revealed." Slide-lecture program. New York: Pfizer Labs, 1991.

"Blood: Bearer of Life and Death." Report.

Chevy Chase, Md.: Howard Hughes Medical Institute, 1993.

Cohen, Stanley. "Epidermal Growth Factor." Nobel lecture. Stockholm, Sweden: Dec. 8, 1986.

"Heart and Stroke Facts: 1994 Statistical Supplement." Dallas: American Heart Association, 1993.

"The Heart of Healing, Program 1: What You Believe." TBS television production. New York: Turner Home Entertainment, Sept. 1993.

"The Heart of Healing, Program 2: How You Change." TBS television production. New York: Turner Home Entertainment, Sept. 1993.

"The Human Heart: A Living Pump." Bethesda, Md.: National Institutes of Health, 1978.

"In Search of the Secrets of Aging." NIH Publication No. 93-2756. Bethesda, Md.: National Institutes of Health, May 1993.

"Nutritional Aspects of Ambulatory Practice." Hoffman-LaRoche advertisement in *Journal of the American Medical Association*, Jan. 26, 1994.

"Report of the Expert Panel on Blood Cholesterol Levels in Children and Adolescents." NIH Publication No. 91-2732. Bethesda, Md.: National Institutes of Health, Sept. 1991.

Schindler, Lydia Woods. "The Immune System—How It Works." NIH Publication No. 92-3229. Bethesda, Md.: National Institutes of Health, June 1992.

"Society for Neuroscience Conference." Notes from press conferences. Washington, D.C.: Society for Neuroscience, Nov. 7-12, 1993.

"Triglyceride, High Density Lipoprotein, and Coronary Heart Disease." NIH Consensus Development Conference, Bethesda, Md.: Feb. 26-28, 1992.

INDEX

ACKNOWLEDGMENTS

The editors of *Repair and Renewal* would like to thank these individuals for their valuable contributions:

Albert J. Aguayo, Montreal General Hospital, Quebec, Canada; J. José Bonner, Indiana University, Bloomington; Garth Bray, Montreal General Hospital, Quebec, Canada; Bernard S. Brucker, University of Miami School of Medicine; Richard L. Bruno, Kessler Institute for Rehabilitation, Inc., Saddle Brook, N.J.; Dabney Ewin, Tulane University, New Orleans; Nancy M. Frick, Harvest Center, Hackensack, N.J.; James Gordon, The Center for Mind-Body Medicine, Washington, D.C.; Richard J. Goss, Brown University, Providence, R.I.; Christian Haudenschild, American Red Cross, Rockville, Md.; Gunilla Hedesund, Bonnierförlagen, Stockholm; R. Bruce Heppenstall, University of Pennsylvania School of Medicine, Philadelphia; Bob Jacobs, Colorado College, Colorado Springs; Julie Meyne, Los Alamos National Laboratory, Los Alamos, N.Mex.; Stanley Miller, The Johns Hopkins Medical Institutions, Baltimore; Pietro Motta, Università La Sapienza, Rome; Charles Rader, Gillette Research Institute, Gaithersburg, Md.; Douglas Rosing, Bethesda, Md.; Douglas Shander, Gillette Research Institute, Gaithersburg, Md.; Allen L. Van Beek, Centennial Lakes Medical Center, Edina, Minn.; Peter van Mier, Washington University School of Medicine, St. Louis, Mo.; Steven Vazquez, The Health Institute of North Texas, Hurst; Samuel Weiss, University of Calgary, Alberta, Canada; Louise Williams, National Heart, Lung and Blood Institute, Bethesda, Md.

PICTURE CREDITS

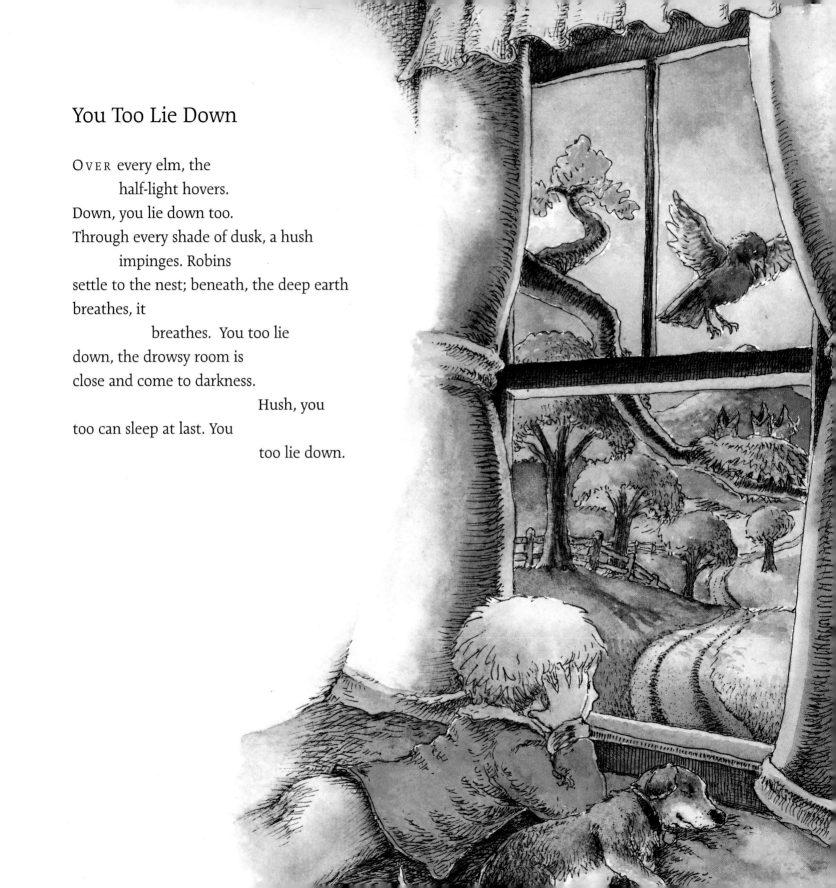

You Too Lie Down

OVER every elm, the
        half-light hovers.
Down, you lie down too.
Through every shade of dusk, a hush
        impinges. Robins
settle to the nest; beneath, the deep earth
breathes, it
            breathes. You too lie
down, the drowsy room is
close and come to darkness.
                Hush, you
too can sleep at last. You
                too lie down.

Blue Balloon

N OBODY noticed,
    And nobody knew,
How lonely my heart
    In its little house grew,

When my friend went away,
    Yes, my friend went away—
My very best friend
    Went away to stay.

    With a hullabaloo in a blue balloon:
    Sing hey for my very best friend.

Now no one has noticed,
    And nobody knows,
How giddy my heart
    In its little house grows,

For it happened today,
    Yes, it happened today—
My very best friend
    Came home to stay!

    With a hullabaloo in a blue balloon:
    Sing hey for my very best friend!

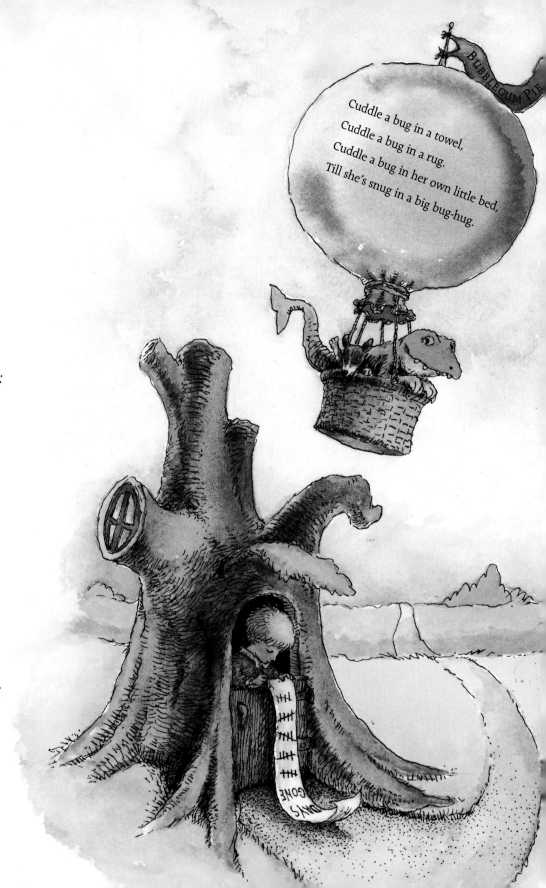

Cuddle a bug in a towel,
Cuddle a bug in a rug.
Cuddle a bug in her own little bed,
Till she's snug in a big bug-hug.

Lavender and Bergamot

SWEET perfume in my garden grows:
Lavender and bergamot, jasmine, rose,

Sandalwood and juniper, ylang-ylang—
Balm for the bee, and the heart's deep pang.

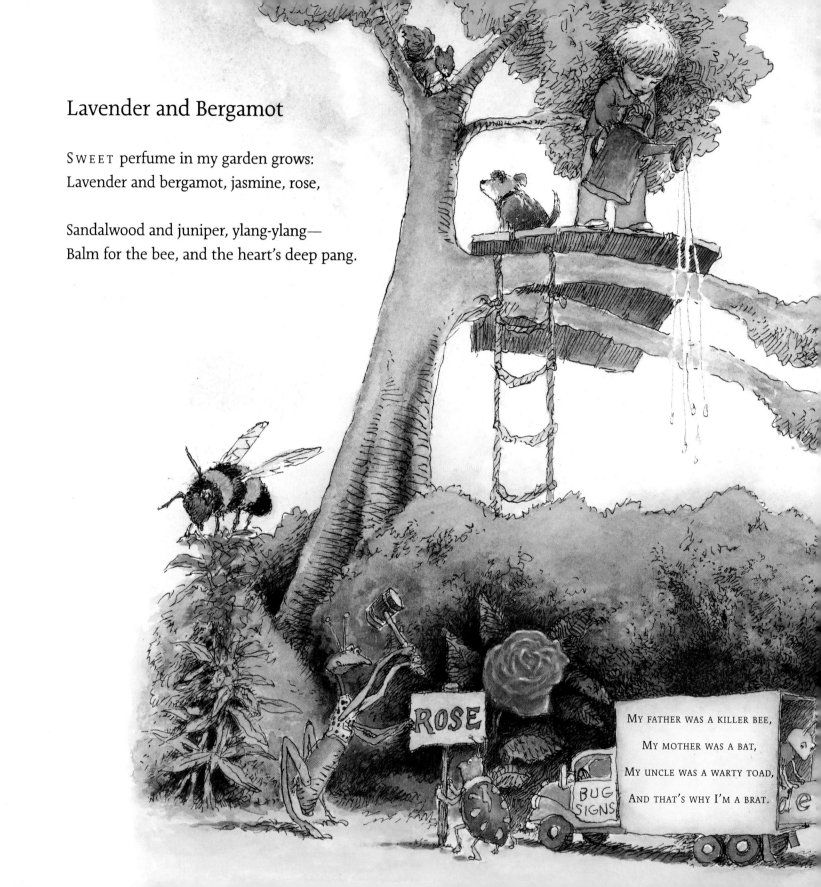

ROSE

MY FATHER WAS A KILLER BEE,
MY MOTHER WAS A BAT,
MY UNCLE WAS A WARTY TOAD,
AND THAT'S WHY I'M A BRAT.

BUG SIGNS

If Lonesome Was a Pot of Gold

IF LONESOME was a pot of gold,
    I'd be a millionaire.
If missing you was party time,
    I wouldn't have a care.

And if a flock of memories
    Could make a person sing,
I'd be an all-night radio
    And play like anything.

(It's not as though I dream about
    The things we used to do;
It's only morning, noon, and night
    I sit and think of you.)

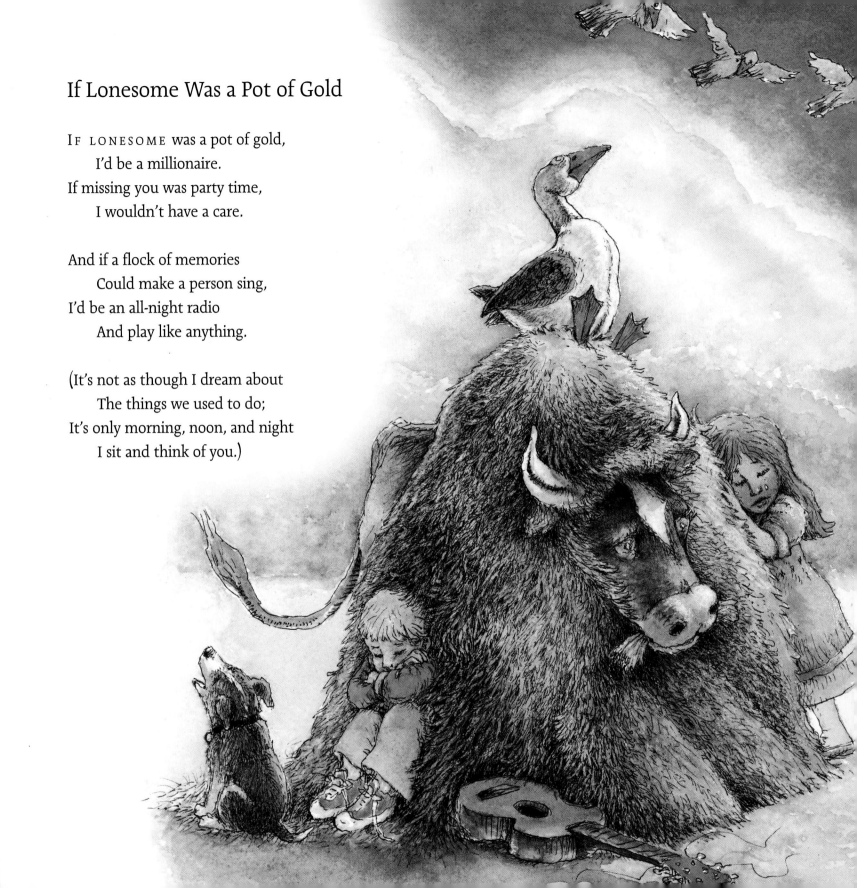

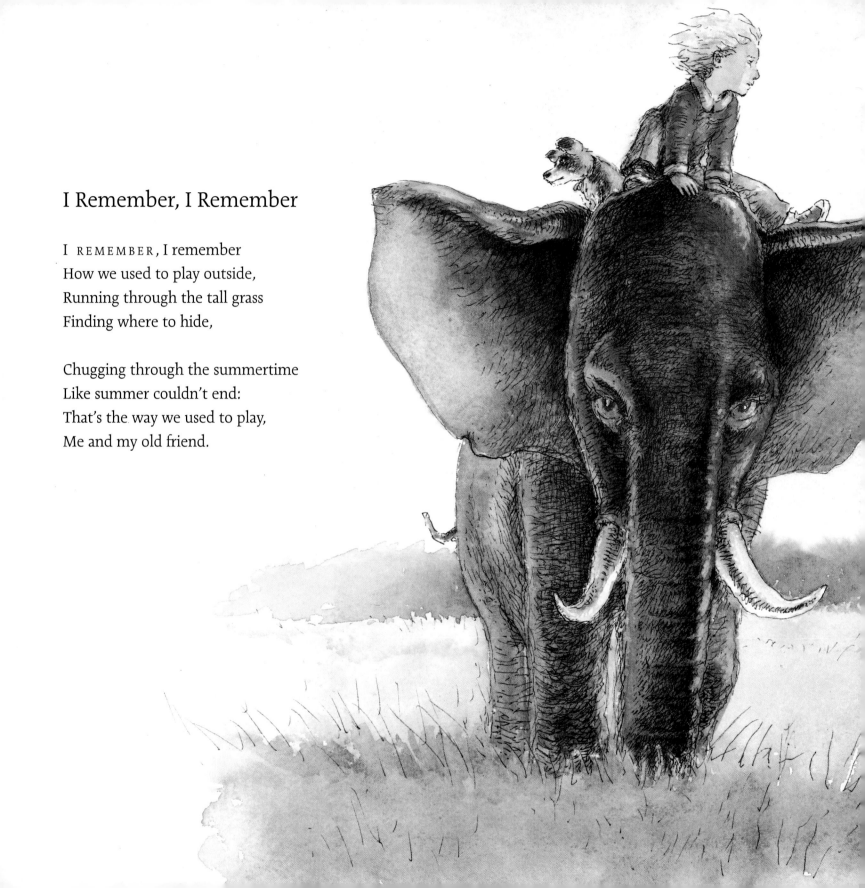

I Remember, I Remember

I REMEMBER, I remember
How we used to play outside,
Running through the tall grass
Finding where to hide,

Chugging through the summertime
Like summer couldn't end:
That's the way we used to play,
Me and my old friend.

My friend said, "It's too late-late-late,
Till morning you must wait-wait-wait."
So then we fell asleep-sleep-sleep
And lay in slumber deep-deep-deep.

But in the night a thief-thief-thief
To my dismay and grief-grief-grief
Made off with that TV-vee-vee,
So I never got to see-see-see . . .

Well, now I sit alone-lone-lone
Inside my little home-home-home,
And in the evening glow-glow-glow
I watch the radio-o-o.

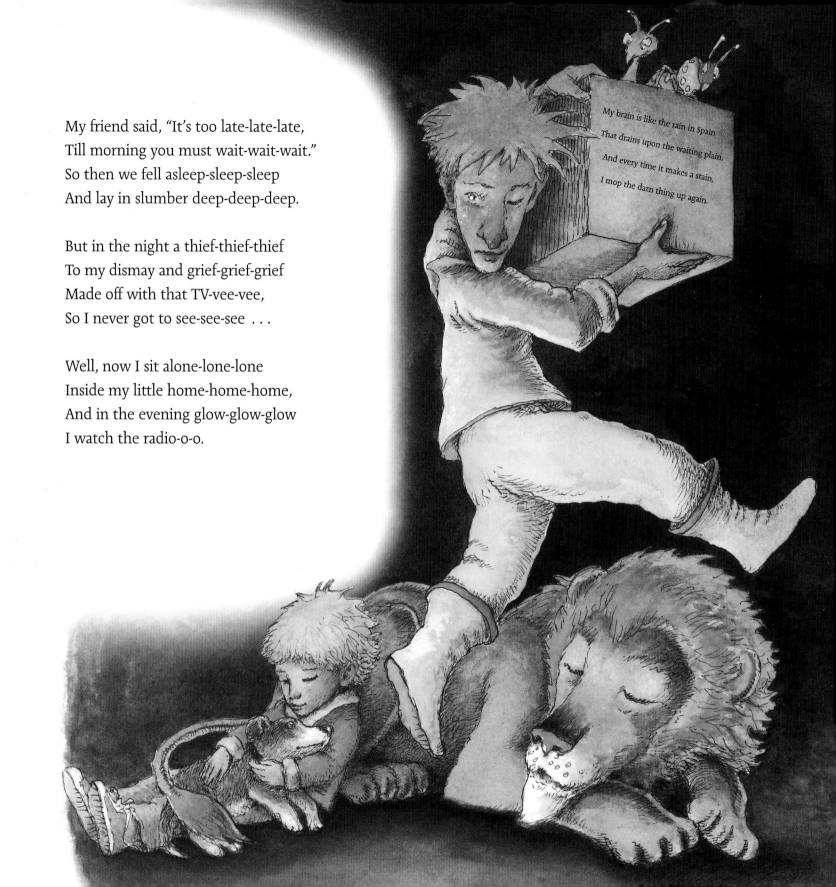

My brain is like the rain in Spain
That drains upon the waiting plain.
And every time it makes a stain,
I mop the darn thing up again.

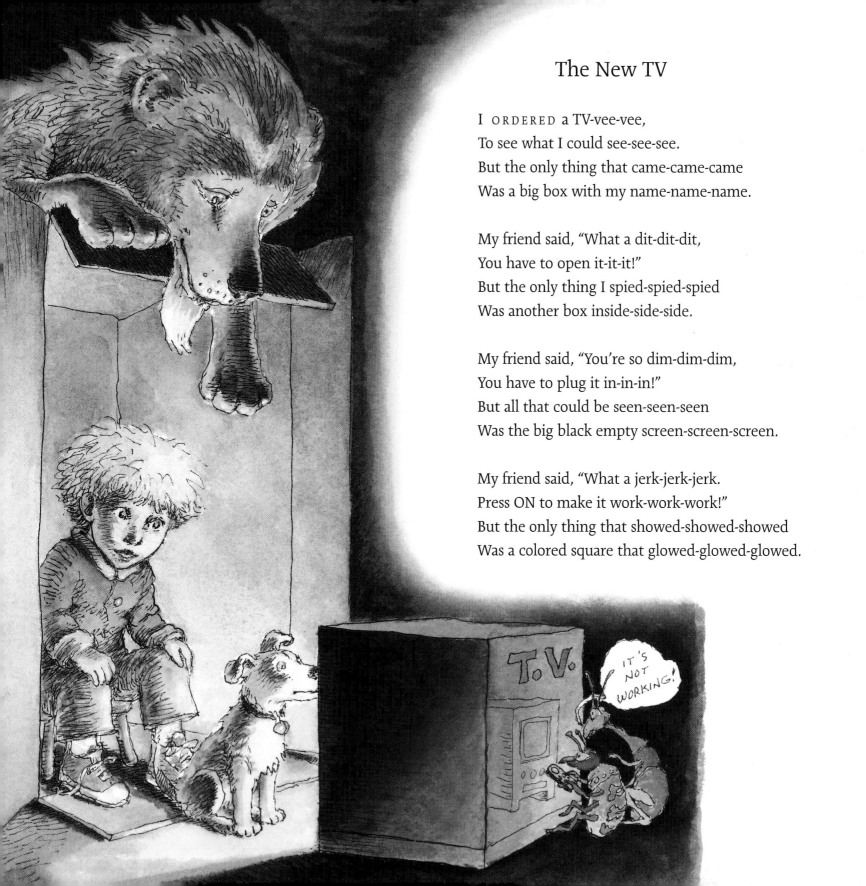

The New TV

I ORDERED a TV-vee-vee,
To see what I could see-see-see.
But the only thing that came-came-came
Was a big box with my name-name-name.

My friend said, "What a dit-dit-dit,
You have to open it-it-it!"
But the only thing I spied-spied-spied
Was another box inside-side-side.

My friend said, "You're so dim-dim-dim,
You have to plug it in-in-in!"
But all that could be seen-seen-seen
Was the big black empty screen-screen-screen.

My friend said, "What a jerk-jerk-jerk.
Press ON to make it work-work-work!"
But the only thing that showed-showed-showed
Was a colored square that glowed-glowed-glowed.

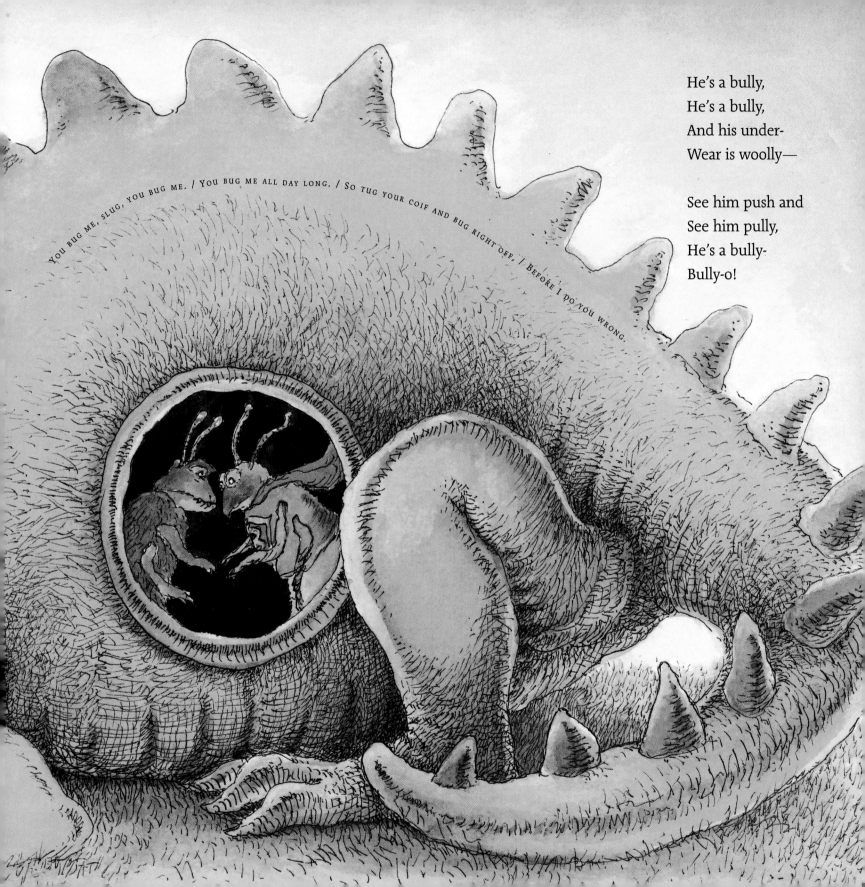

He's a bully,
He's a bully,
And his under-
Wear is woolly—

See him push and
See him pully,
He's a bully-
Bully-o!

YOU BUG ME, SLUG, YOU BUG ME. / YOU BUG ME ALL DAY LONG. / SO TUG YOUR COIF AND BUG RIGHT OFF, / BEFORE I DO YOU WRONG.

The Bully

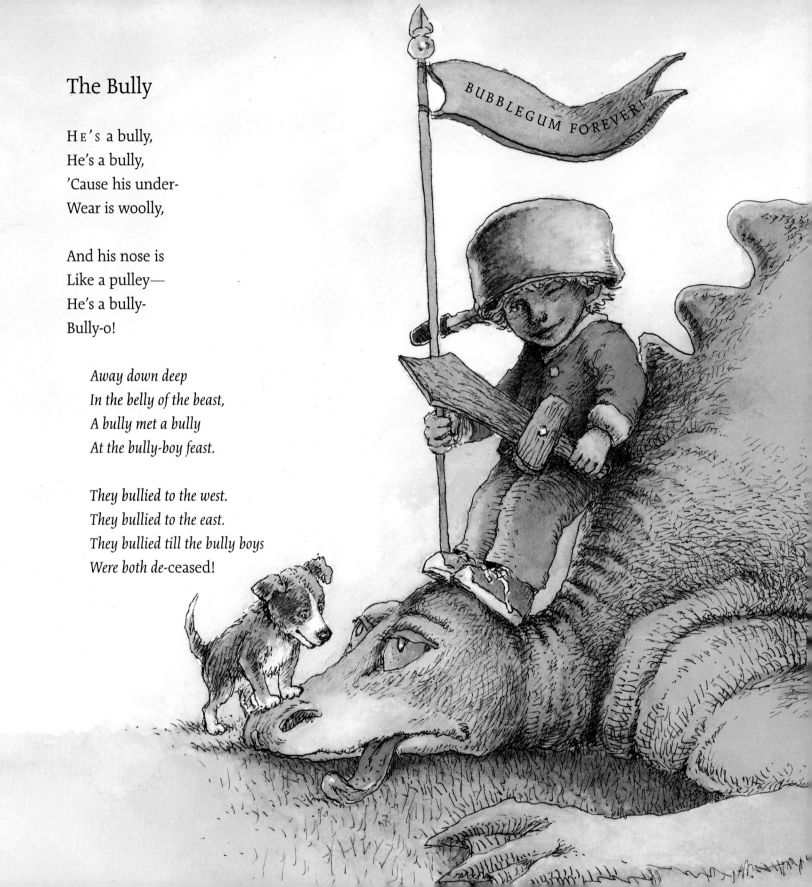

HE'S a bully,
He's a bully,
'Cause his under-
Wear is woolly,

And his nose is
Like a pulley—
He's a bully-
Bully-o!

Away down deep
In the belly of the beast,
A bully met a bully
At the bully-boy feast.

They bullied to the west.
They bullied to the east.
They bullied till the bully boys
Were both de-ceased!

BUBBLEGUM FOREVER!

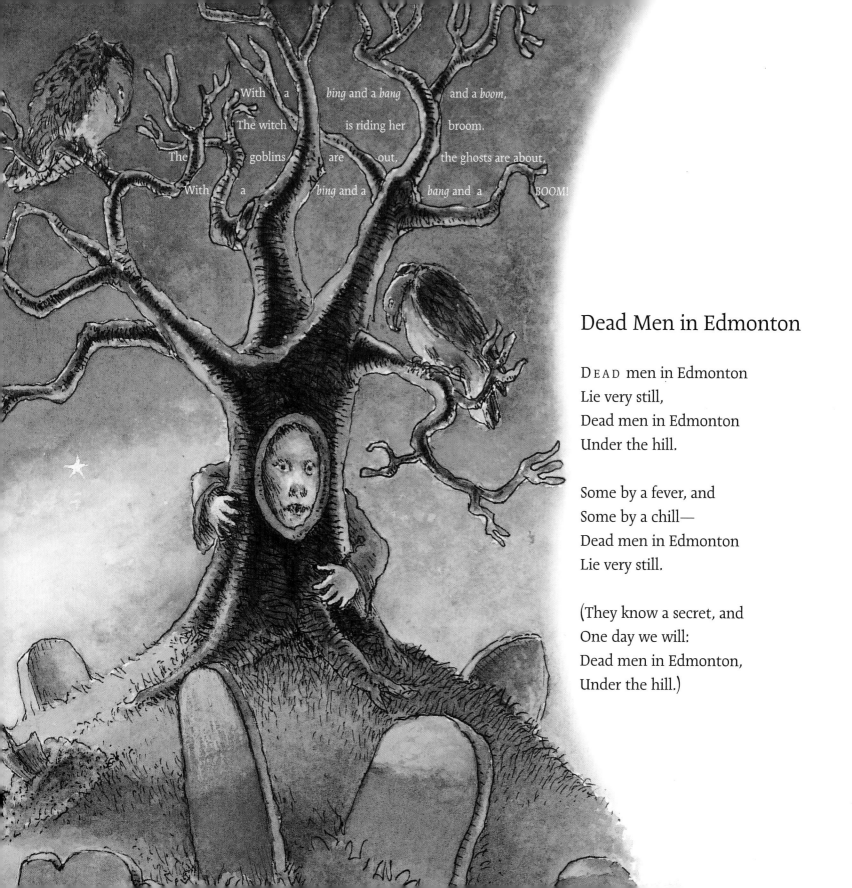

With a *bing* and a *bang* and a *boom*,
The witch is riding her broom.
The goblins are out, the ghosts are about,
With a *bing* and a *bang* and a BOOM!

Dead Men in Edmonton

DEAD men in Edmonton
Lie very still,
Dead men in Edmonton
Under the hill.

Some by a fever, and
Some by a chill—
Dead men in Edmonton
Lie very still.

(They know a secret, and
One day we will:
Dead men in Edmonton,
Under the hill.)

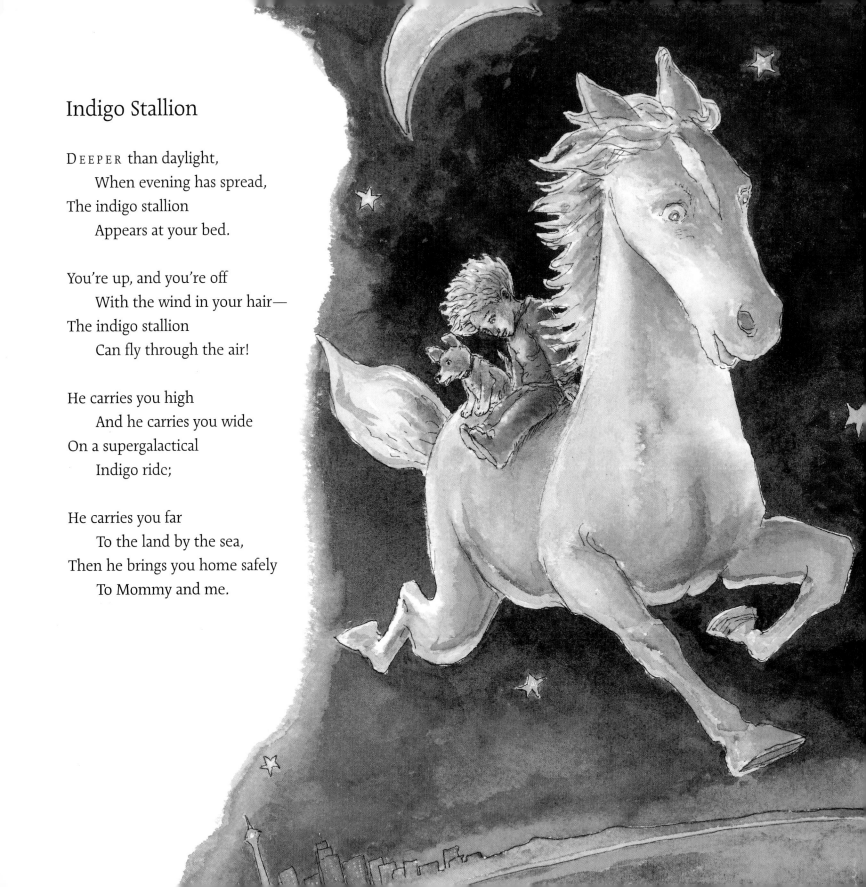

Indigo Stallion

DEEPER than daylight,
  When evening has spread,
The indigo stallion
  Appears at your bed.

You're up, and you're off
  With the wind in your hair—
The indigo stallion
  Can fly through the air!

He carries you high
  And he carries you wide
On a supergalactical
  Indigo ride;

He carries you far
  To the land by the sea,
Then he brings you home safely
  To Mommy and me.

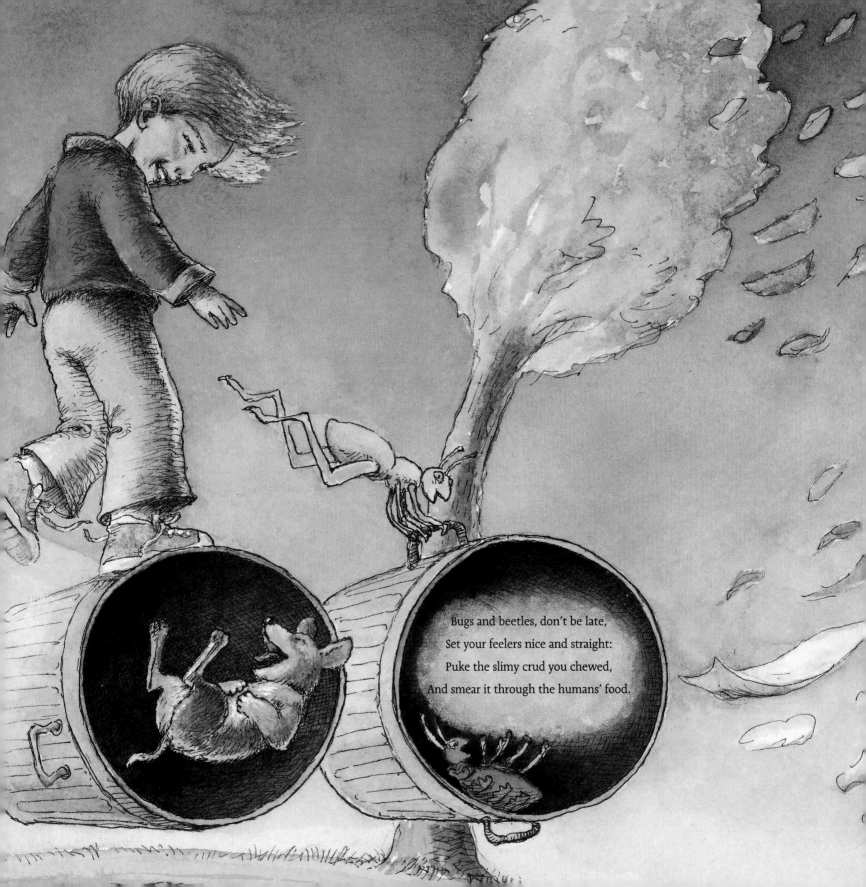

Bugs and beetles, don't be late,
Set your feelers nice and straight:
Puke the slimy crud you chewed,
And smear it through the humans' food.

The Tantrum

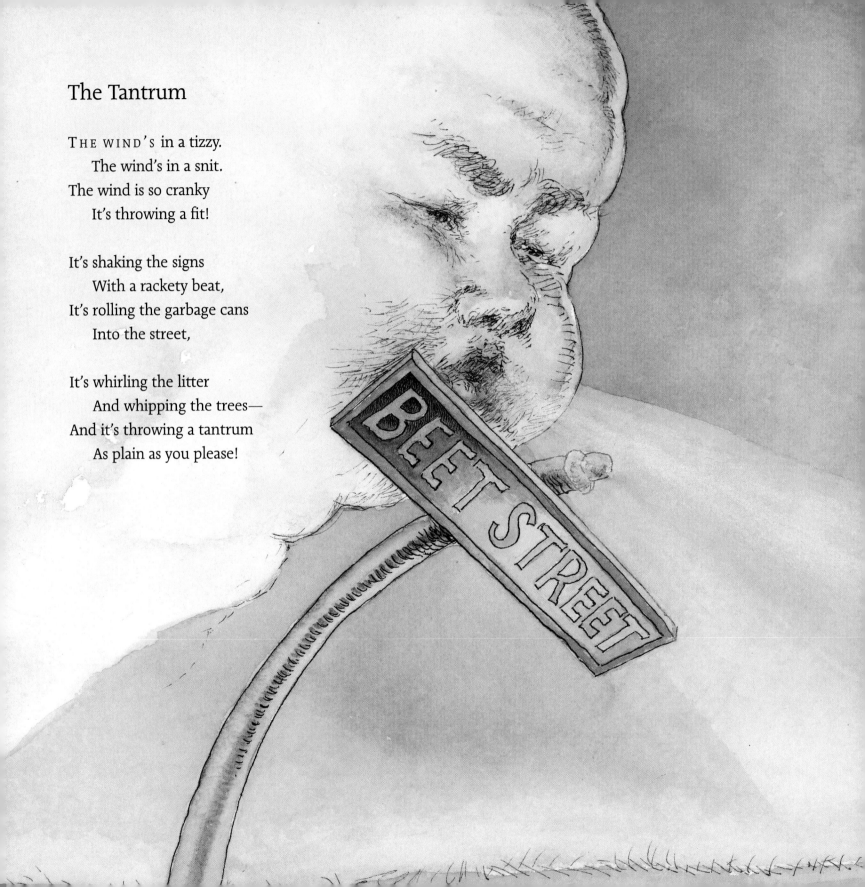

The wind's in a tizzy.
　　The wind's in a snit.
The wind is so cranky
　　It's throwing a fit!

It's shaking the signs
　　With a rackety beat,
It's rolling the garbage cans
　　Into the street,

It's whirling the litter
　　And whipping the trees—
And it's throwing a tantrum
　　As plain as you please!

The Faithful Donut

(*Slowly, with feeding*)

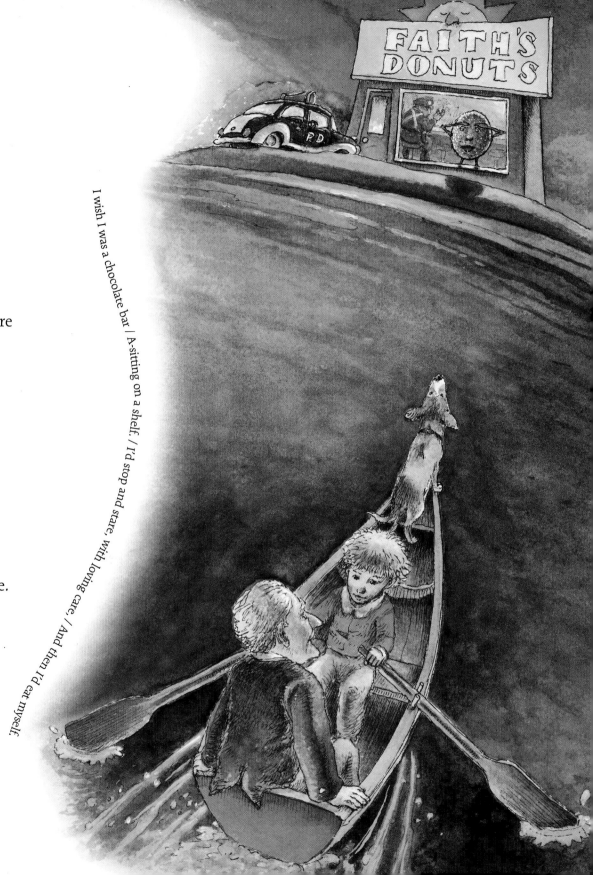

FAR across the ocean,
    Far across the sea,
A faithful jelly donut
    Is waiting just for me.

Its sugar shines with longing,
    Its jelly glows with tears;
My donut has been waiting there
    For twenty-seven years.

O faithful jelly donut,
    I beg you don't despair!
My teeth are in Toronto, but
    My heart is with you there.

And I will cross the ocean,
    And I will cross the sea,
And I will crush you to my lips.
    And make you one with me.

I wish I was a chocolate bar / A-sitting on a shelf. / I'd stop and stare, with loving care, / And then I'd eat myself.

Doctor Bop

THE BAND was playing dixie
The band was playing swing
But Doctor Bop was rocking
With a boogie-woogie thing.

They told him play some dixie
They told him play some swing
But Doctor Bop just wouldn't stop
That boogie-woogie thing—

'Cause he had hot stuff, cool stuff
Good old break-the-rules stuff
Stuff with jelly, stuff with jam
Boogie-woogie stuff with a sis-boom-bam!

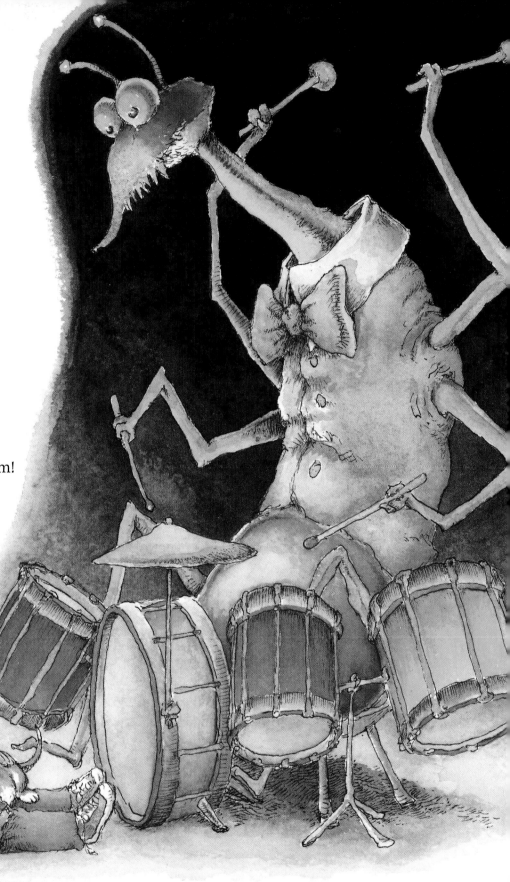

The Waves

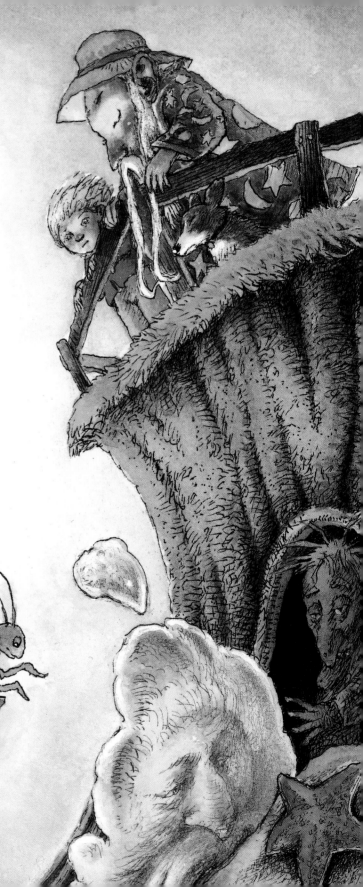

THEY'RE old, they're old, they're very old,
　　As old as ever more,
The long blue slap and the sucking waves
　　That pound against the shore.

And starfish and anemones
　　Go trundling to and fro,
Like starfish and anemones
　　A million years ago.

And the waves roll in, and the tides roll in,
　　And the sea rolls in each day.
And people for a thousand years
　　Have heard the ocean say,

We're old, we're old, we're very old,
　　As old as ever more,
The long blue slap and the sucking waves
　　That pound against the shore.

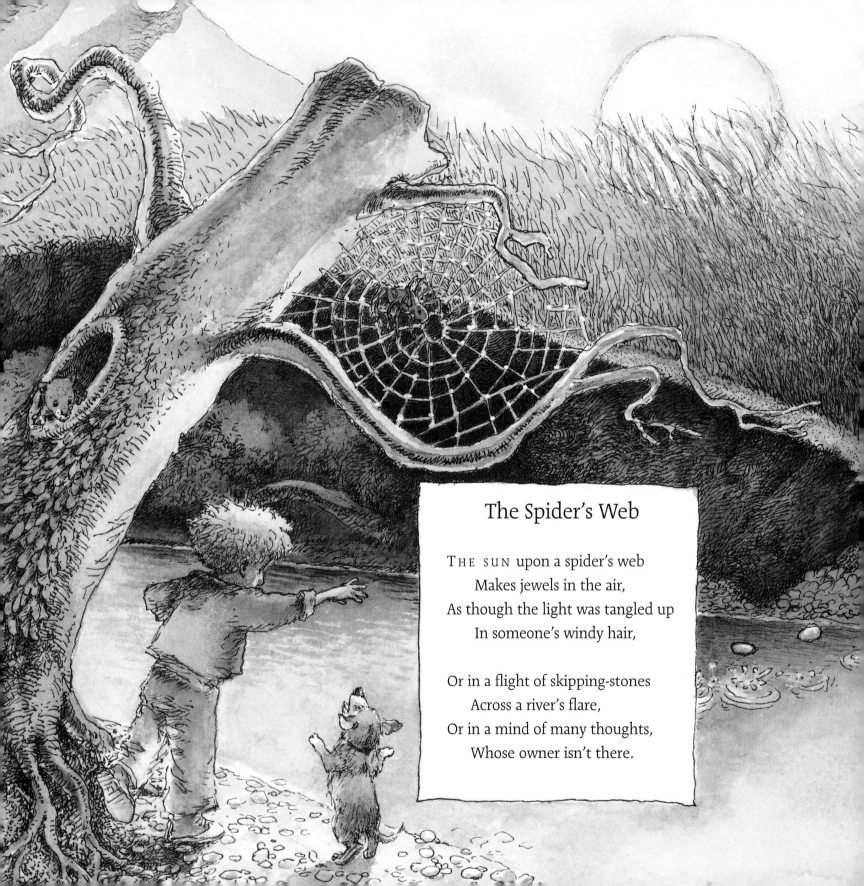

The Spider's Web

THE SUN upon a spider's web
Makes jewels in the air,
As though the light was tangled up
In someone's windy hair,

Or in a flight of skipping-stones
Across a river's flare,
Or in a mind of many thoughts,
Whose owner isn't there.

The King of Calabogie

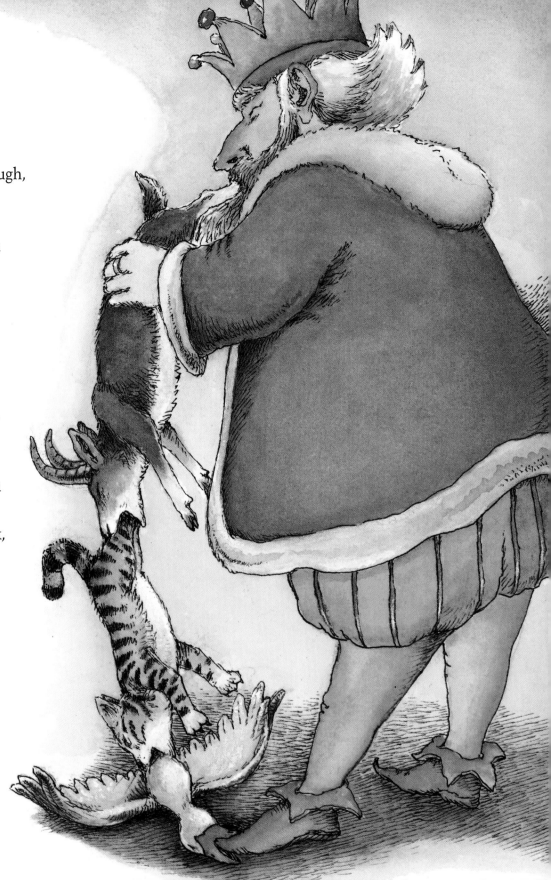

THE KING of Calabogie
Had a tickle in his throat.
He coughed a long and mighty cough,
And up came—a goat!

The goat the king provoked began
To butt His Highness flat.
It horked a long and mighty hork,
And up came—a cat!

The cat the goat begat began
To guzzle apple juice.
It burped a long and mighty burp,
And up came—a goose!

The goose the cat produced began
To flap like anything.
It honked a long and mighty honk,
And up came—a king!

Pollywog Dreams

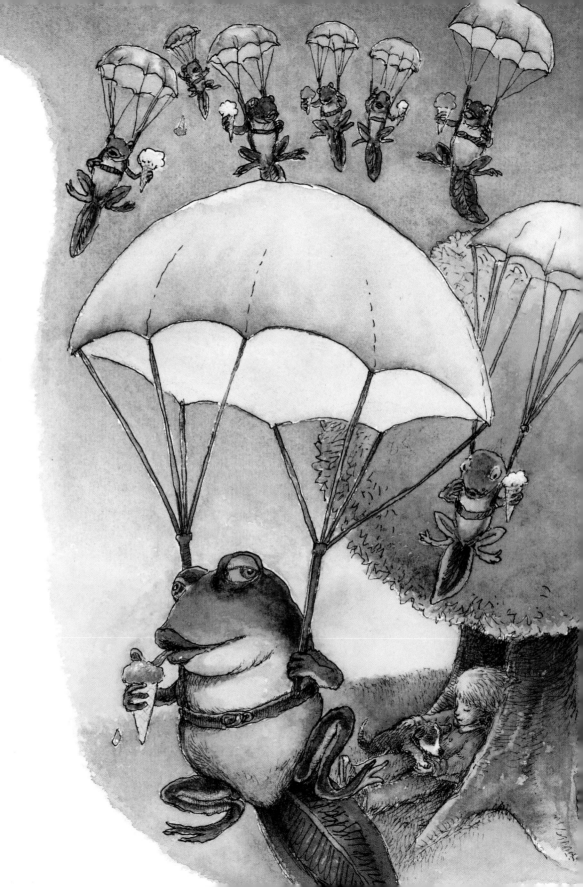

POLLYWOGS
    In parachutes
Are drifting through
    My dream—
Pollywogs
    In parachutes,
With pink and white
    Ice cream.

They move in cloud
    Formation
As they curtsey
    One, two, three—
Pollywogs
    In parachutes,
Above the maple
    Tree.

They never guess
    I'm dreaming them,
But in my dream
    I see
That pollywogs
    In parachutes
Are also dreaming
    Me.

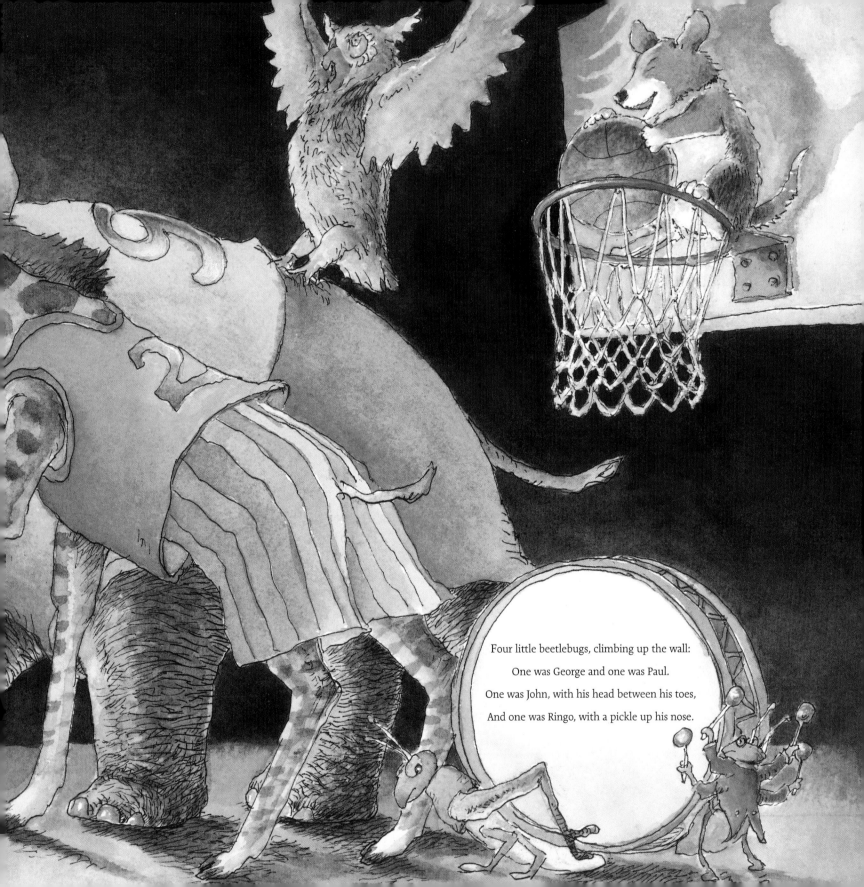

Four little beetlebugs, climbing up the wall:
One was George and one was Paul.
One was John, with his head between his toes,
And one was Ringo, with a pickle up his nose.

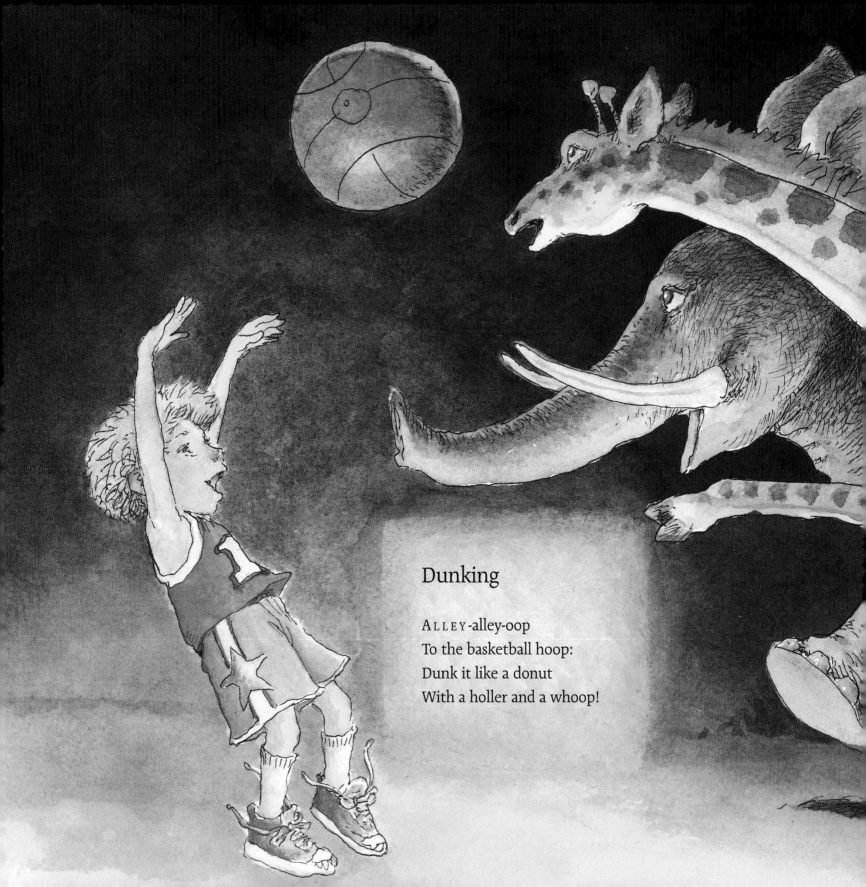

Dunking

ALLEY-alley-oop
To the basketball hoop:
Dunk it like a donut
With a holler and a whoop!

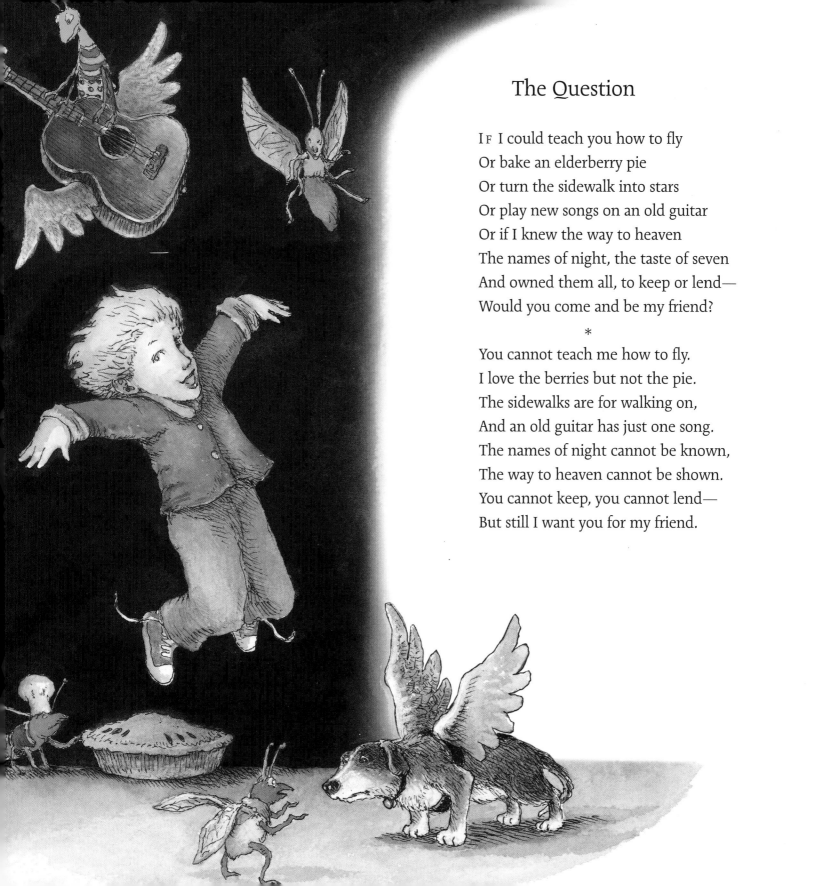

The Question

IF I could teach you how to fly
Or bake an elderberry pie
Or turn the sidewalk into stars
Or play new songs on an old guitar
Or if I knew the way to heaven
The names of night, the taste of seven
And owned them all, to keep or lend—
Would you come and be my friend?

*

You cannot teach me how to fly.
I love the berries but not the pie.
The sidewalks are for walking on,
And an old guitar has just one song.
The names of night cannot be known,
The way to heaven cannot be shown.
You cannot keep, you cannot lend—
But still I want you for my friend.

Goober and Guck

GOOBER and guck,
Goober and guck,
We're making a sandwich
Of goober and guck.

It won't make you healthy
Or bring you good luck,
But gobble it down and
You'll quack like a duck;

You'll quack like a duck and
You'll smell like a truck—
So eat your nice sandwich
Of goober and guck!

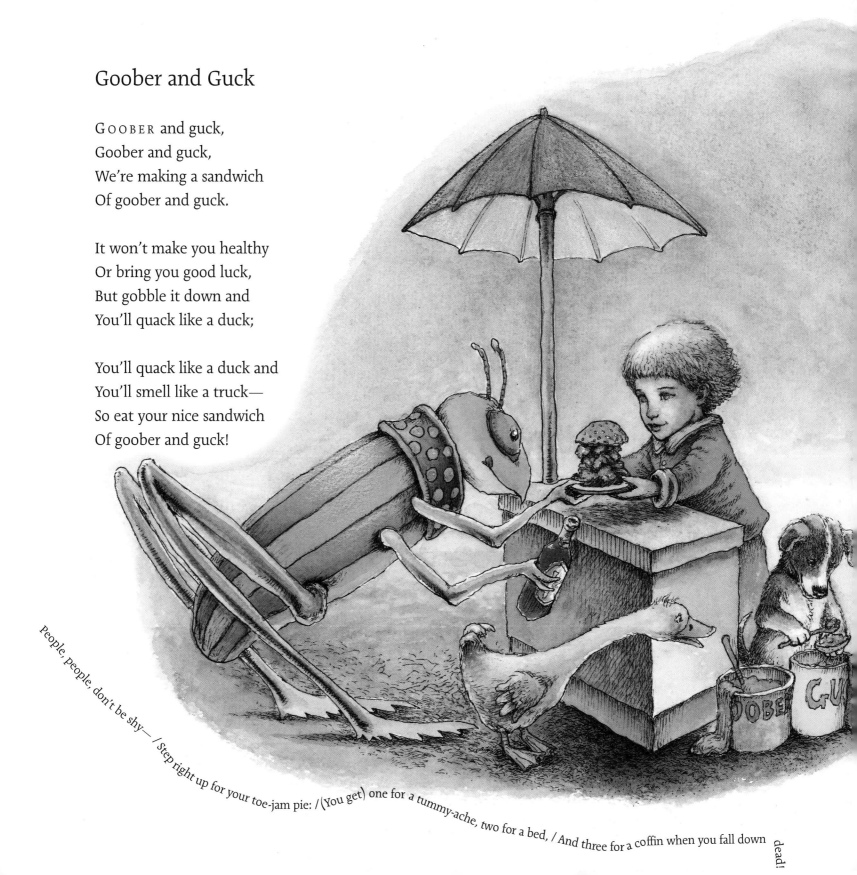

People, people, don't be shy— / Step right up for your toe-jam pie: / (You get) one for a tummy-ache, two for a bed, / And three for a coffin when you fall down dead!

Dipsy-doodle through the lane,
Turn around and *Charge!* again,

Till the bad guys in dismay
Spread their wings and fly away . . .

Through the city, block on block,
A pair of mighty hunters stalk.

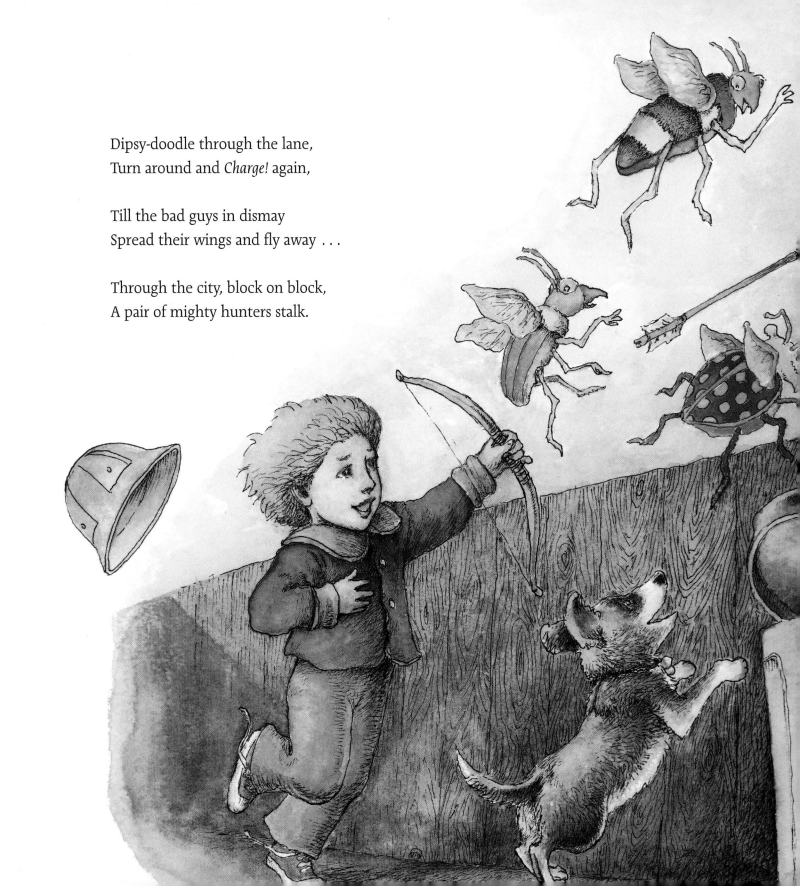

Mighty Hunters

THROUGH the city, block on block,
A pair of mighty hunters stalk.

Down the alley—hush! beware!
Tracking bad guys to their lair.

Past the hideout—not a peep!
Where the bad guys strut and creep.

Now it's time for an attack:
Holler *Charge!* and drive them back.

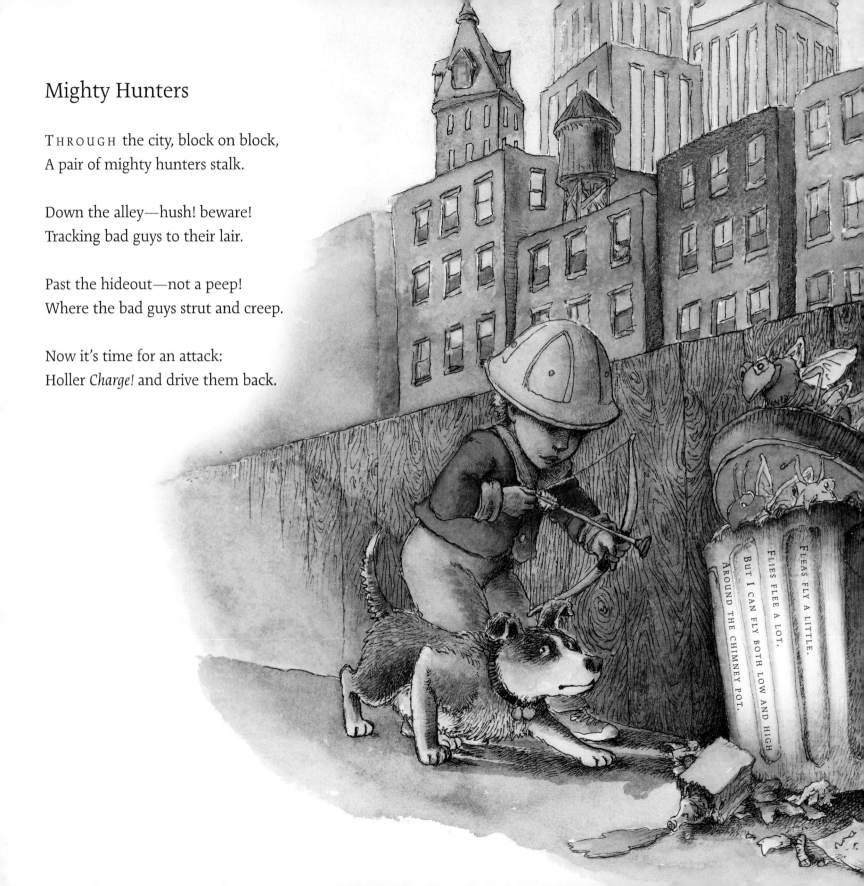

FLEAS FLY A LITTLE.
FLIES FLEE A LOT.
BUT I CAN FLY BOTH LOW AND HIGH
AROUND THE CHIMNEY POT.

The Movies

TAKE me to the movies,
Take me to the show,
Take me to the pictures
Where the big kids go.

I think we're gonna laugh,
I think we're gonna cry,
I think we're gonna love it
When the time flies by.

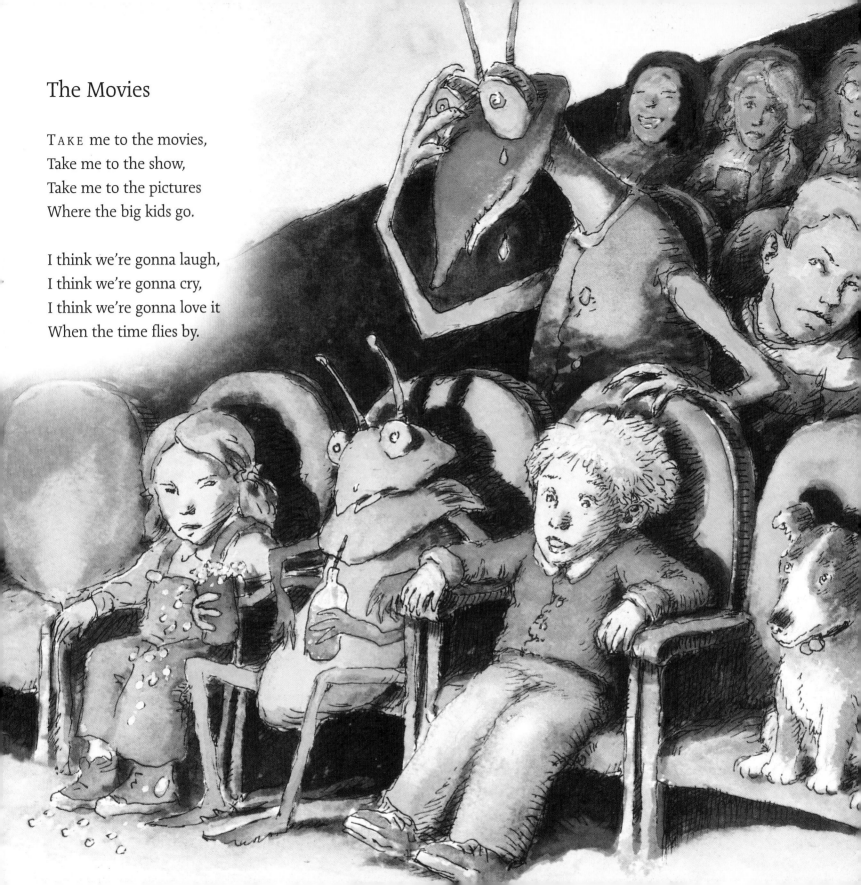

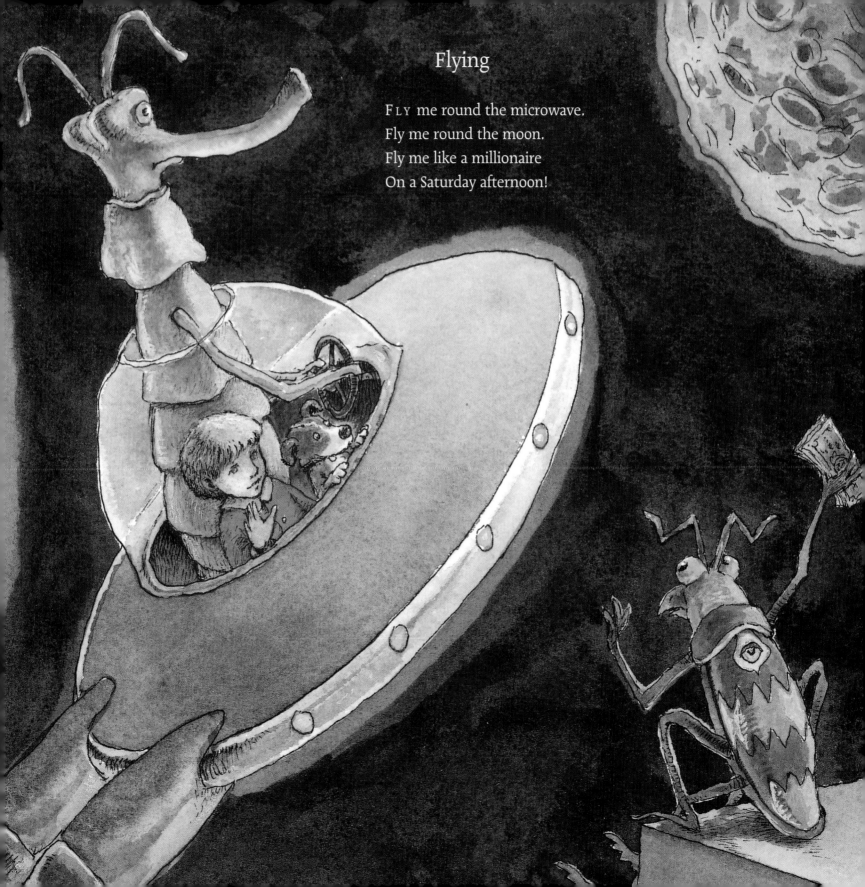

Flying

FLY me round the microwave.
Fly me round the moon.
Fly me like a millionaire
On a Saturday afternoon!

The Rocking Chair

I LOVE to rock
  In the rocking chair.
I rock rock rock
  And I just don't care.

I rock around the block
  In my underwear;
Then I rock back home
  In the rocking chair.

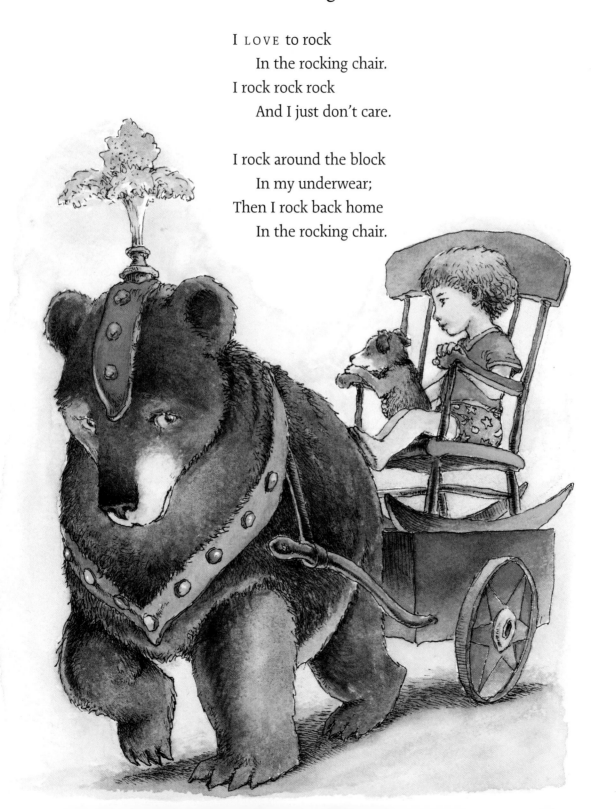

Good Morning

W H E N I woke up, my heart was high.
The sun was hot in the bright blue sky.
The bees were buzzing, and I knew why—
'Cause I had a friend to play with!

Well it's one-ery, two-ery, hickory, dock:
Dogs can dance and bugs can talk.
There's tons of secrets around the block—
And I have a friend to play with!

Round and around in the neighborhood,
The day goes by like a daytime should.
So tickle my tummy and I'll be good—
'Cause I've got a friend to play with!

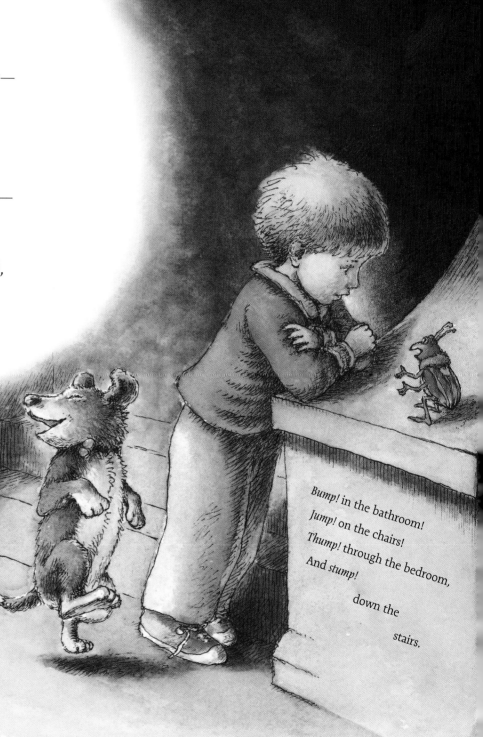

Bump! in the bathroom!
Jump! on the chairs!
Thump! through the bedroom,
And stump!

down the

stairs.

Bubblegum Delicious

poems by Dennis Lee

pictures by David McPhail

HarperCollins*Publishers*

Library of Congress Cataloging-in-Publication Data

Lee , Dennis.

Bubblegum delicious / by Dennis Lee ; pictures by David McPhail

p.   cm.

ISBN 0-06-029773-5 — ISBN 0-06-623709-2 (lib. bdg.)

1. Children's poetry, Canadian.   [1. Canadian Poetry]   I. McPhail, David M., ill.   II. Title.

PR9199.3.L387 B8 2001   00-047266

811'.54—dc21   CIP

                                                                                        AC

1 2 3 4 5 6 7 8 9 10

❖

First HarperCollins Edition, 2001

Originally published by Key Porter Books, Canada

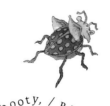

Bless my booty, / Bless my soul— / Here comes bratty / Bug patrol!

Bubblegum Delicious

Wrap you up in bubble wrap,
Wrap you up in gum,
Wrap you up in wonderful
Cause you're the special one!

BUBBLEGUM delicious,
Bubblegum delight,
Bubblegum de-lovely in the
Middle of the night.

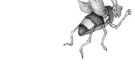

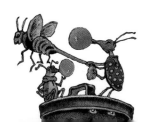

Contents

The Recipe Booklet that accompanies this volume has been designed for use in the kitchen. It contains all of the 49 recipes printed here plus 54 more. It also has a wipe-clean cover and a spiral binding so that it can either stand up or lie flat when open.

One Book for a Multitude of Delightful Cuisines

In Georgia, the nation where I was born (it is now a republic of the Soviet Union), men learn to cook and to cook well. Some foods, like our *mtswadi* or grilled meats, were—and for that matter still are—cooked *only* by men. It is the men who prepare the food for the big parties given when a whole village celebrates a holiday. In my own village, my father and two of his friends had the special duty and pleasure of preparing wedding feasts and they taught me to cook our traditional Georgian dishes as soon as I could handle a knife.

Later in my youth I went to Russia as an apprentice—actually, a boy-of-all-work—to a professional swordmaker, and since he was a man who liked to eat and to have his friends around him at his table, I learned rather more about cooking than I really wanted to know at the time. But it turned out to be just as well that I did, for eating has been in style longer than swords.

As a grown man in the Czar's army during World War I, I came to know and love the food of the various parts of the Russian Empire in which I was stationed. And remembering a Georgian proverb, "Cooks never die of starvation," I learned to prepare as many of these dishes as I could. When I arrived in the United States without money or any command of the language, I found work in a restaurant; what had begun as a hobby became my business.

In the course of time I married an American girl, and my Georgian-American friends warned me that I must forget my "old country dishes." "No more *borshch*, no *shashlyk*, no *bliny*," they said. "Now you will eat baked beans, barbecued spare ribs and apple pie for the rest of your life."

As it turned out, I did not get those good American dishes often enough. My wife preferred the "old country dishes," and set about learning how to cook them. Over the years our friends here—many of them immigrants from Russia, the Ukraine, the Baltic and the Caucasus—and the friends we made on visits to the Soviet Union generously shared their treasured recipes with her, and spent many patient hours demonstrating the preparation of their regional dishes.

When we came to plan the contents of this volume, the extraordinary range of these regional dishes presented a problem. I was reminded of the old saying "Two Russians—three points of view," except in our case it was "One Russian cookbook—a multitude of cuisines." Russia, or more correctly the Soviet Union or the U.S.S.R., is not only an immense country but a diverse one. Within its borders live people of some 110 different nationalities, each with a distinct language and apparently a distinct cuisine (if you have your own word for soup, it seems to me, you will probably have your own way of making it).

How to choose from such a bountiful array of fine food? We solved the problem by selecting the gastronomic regions we like best: Great Russia; the Baltic Republics of Estonia, Latvia, and Lithuania; the Ukraine; Armenia and Georgia in the Caucasus; and the four states of Central Asia together with neighboring Kazakhstan. From the best and most characteristic dishes of each region, we selected the foods that we most like to cook, to eat and to serve our friends.

If I am asked—and I will be—why we did not mention, say, *omul* fish from Lake Baikal, or *borshch* from some crossroads village in Siberia, or asparagus au gratin exactly as prepared by the Grand Duke Sergei's chef in 1903, I will answer with another Russian proverb: "In matters of taste one has neither brother nor friend."

A second question is more complex and will be more difficult to answer. Will the many cuisines of the Soviet Union survive, or must they—along with the cultures that sustain them—succumb to Russianization? No cuisine is constant. Countries borrow and lend dishes; wars, invasions and political alliances influence any cuisine. Yet I believe that the regions that preserved their culinary independence when they were parts of Russia's empire will continue to do so as republics of the Soviet federation. Modern education and mass communications tend to lessen regional differences—but they also give people a new awareness of the distinctive form and meaning of their culture and a determination to preserve its best features.

This has happened, I believe, in Georgia, to take the case I know best. Great changes have taken place there in the last 50 years, but my native country has not been Russianized. Our traditional customs, our ways of eating and drinking still prevail and the table remains the symbol of the home. And I can report that the determination to cherish and preserve a national style in literature and art, in fashion and food, was manifest in every republic we visited in behalf of this volume.

Paradoxically, the part of the Soviet Union that has suffered most influence and change in its eating habits is the very Republic, called Russia, from which the country gets its familiar name. The days when *borshch*, *kasha*, cabbage and beets formed the basic diet of Russia are gone. The most popular restaurants in Moscow, Leningrad and other large cities now specialize in the cuisine of some non-Russian republic—Armenia, Georgia, Uzbekistan or the Ukraine. Indeed, I noted "minority" dishes on almost every restaurant menu, and certain Georgian dishes, such as chicken *tabaka*, green beans with nuts, and spitted lamb, have become standard Russian fare. In their markets Russians are eagerly buying foods most of them scarcely knew by name a generation ago—pomegranates, figs, citrus fruits and melons from the Caucasus and Central Asia; cheese, fish, chocolates and cakes from the Baltic Republics; fresh and preserved vegetables from the Ukraine; and canned game from Siberia.

To the foregoing reflections I must add a final note. In the pages that follow, I wrote the section on Georgia and Armenia; the rest of the text was written by my wife. But it was together that we visited the places we describe, and we again thank all those who welcomed us to their homes and hospitable tables. We hope we shall sit together with them all again and drink a toast for peace in the world.   —*George Papashvily*

I

The Bygone Days of the Czars

The first thing a traveler to the Soviet Union must learn is how to answer questions—from friends, from acquaintances, and even from complete strangers—questions that express not casual curiosity but true concern. In Anglo-Saxon countries reserve may be a form of courtesy; in Russia it verges on rudeness. Share a table in a restaurant, a bench in the park, a seat on a plane, and the inevitable question follows, a conversation develops, then an audience gathers and the conversation expands into a conference.

We arrived in Leningrad late one morning, and as soon as I unpacked I went at once to the "buffet," the small refreshment room located on every floor (or every second or third floor) in most Russian hotels. It was a cozy place with just enough room for a tiny kitchen, a glass display case, a counter, and four or five tables. There, I knew, we could drink an early tea or a late coffee, eat a thick piece of rosy ham or a wedge of cheese with a good bread at any hour of the day and most of the night. We could also order, if such was our pleasure, a more substantial meal—hearty *borshch*, beef Stroganov, *kasha*—sent up from the hotel kitchen below. Wine, extra glasses, and a plate of appetizers would be at hand in case unexpected guests knocked at our door, and gift boxes of chocolates if we went visiting.

The buffet also acts as a central clearing house for news. Is the new ballerina as good as her notices? Who received the basket of yellow roses carried through the hall this morning and why? Are the Laplanders in the lobby an official delegation, a party of tourists, or a basketball team? The patrons of the buffet know the answers.

I had heard disquieting reports that new hotels in the Soviet Union had

A gold and silver samovar *(opposite)*, made in 1866 for Czarevich (Crown Prince) Alexander, later Czar Alexander III, is a symbolic relic of Imperial Russia. The two interlocked "A's" beneath the imperial crown on the samovar are the initials of the Czarevich's given name, Alexander Alexandrovich. The silver tea-glass holder was designed and made during the same decade, in the then-popular bound-raffia motif.

8

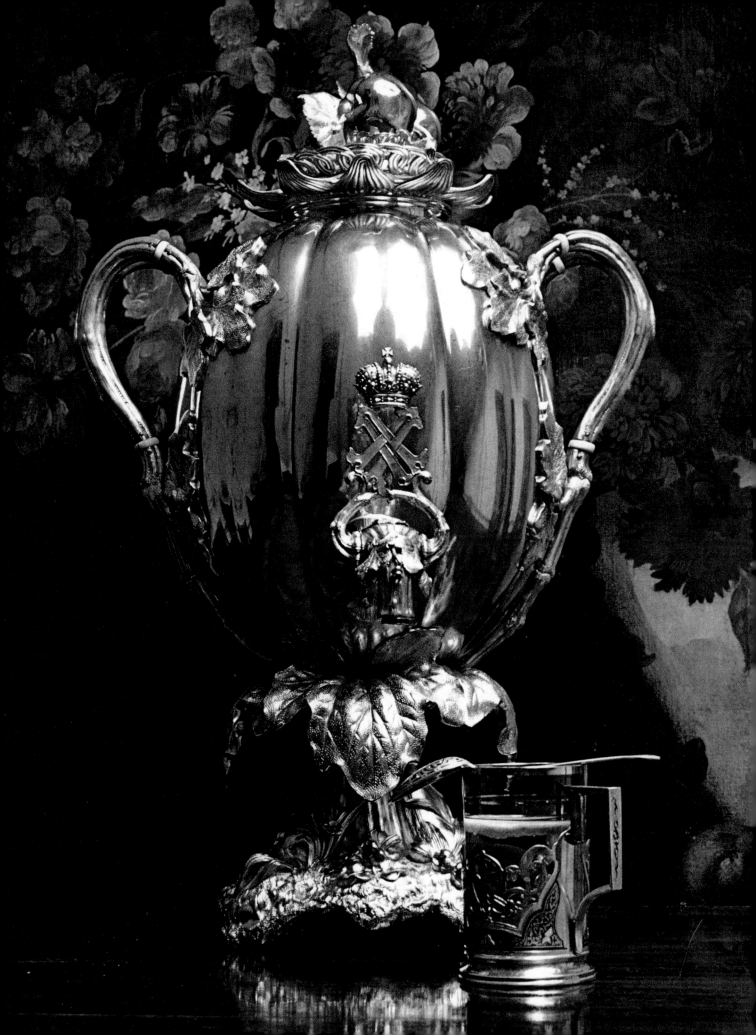

begun to provide room service, and the reports proved true—but happily, the buffet at our hotel survived unchanged. The rosy-cheeked woman behind the counter still wore a filigreed plastic diadem on her curls; the samovar hissed, the tea glasses glittered, the napkins folded into cones stood at starched attention. All the tables were full, but an extra chair was found and a place made for me between a young girl and an elderly woman, tall, erect, handsomely dressed in a well-cut black suit.

The hostess set down my tea, with two ice-blue sugar cubes in the saucer.

"You are a tourist?" It was a statement rather than a question.

"Yes."

"From the U.S.A.?"

"Yes."

"It must be a wonderful place."

The rise and fall of the Soviet political barometer never seems to affect the interest in all things American. Now came the questions.

"Do you sometimes see Indians?"

"What is considered Mr. Louis Armstrong's best album?"

"Do apples grow in the United States?"

I gave the usual answers.

"Excuse me, but why do you speak Russian with a Georgian accent?"

"I suppose it is because I learned Russian from my husband, and he is a Georgian."

"A Georgian!"

We explored the details of my husband's parentage, his early life, his emigration to the United States, our meeting, our marriage, our family.

"And is he here, too?"

"Yes, but just now he is visiting the museum. He is a sculptor."

A hum of approbation greeted this announcement. In the Soviet Union artists are accorded the honors once bestowed upon grand dukes.

"And your profession?"

"A writer."

"Of what nature are your works?"

I gave a short backlist of titles.

"And now you are writing . . .?"

"A book on food and cooking—on Russian cooking."

A moment of silence followed while my audience considered this.

"But I think," said the buffet hostess, "most people here already know how to cook."

"Oh, I am sure they do, but, you see, the book I am writing is not for Russians. It is initially for Americans."

"For Americans! So *they* will know how *we* cook!" Smiles and nods of mutual esteem were exchanged between tables. Immediately from every side I was told where I would find the very best food.

"Right here in Leningrad you must try our partridge with sour cream, and *rassolnik* soup with pickled cucumbers, and chicken and *sudak* fish baked in a crust so flaky that . . ."

"Moscow!" said a man across the table. "You must go to Moscow for cabbage soup, and sturgeon in aspic with horseradish, and *kotlety pozharskie* and . . ."

"And what about chicken Kiev?" asked the young girl on my right. "One touch with your fork and a fountain of golden butter spurts out. I'm *from* Kiev, and I know."

A man at the corner table passed a folded paper across to me. "In Odessa try this restaurant. It is very small, and if too many people discover it, it will be overcrowded, but the cooks there make a mushroom appetizer with cream and just a touch of black pepper. I had three portions last time I was there." He blew a kiss in what I took to be the general direction of Odessa.

I was also entreated to go to Tallinn ("smoked lamb, ivory apples, cold raspberry soup"); to Riga *("minoga* fish with mustard and vinegar, and don't forget the liqueur made of cream"); to Vilnius ("crayfish, and the grilled sausage with the sharp sauce, and the porcupine cake with almond quills").

A man stepped into the buffet and asked for mineral water. Before the bottle was uncapped he was made aware of the problem and gave his opinion.

"Samarkand! Red poppies, turquoise domes—and everywhere, everywhere the fragrance of orchards in bloom and sticks of lamb broiling on grills in the streets. You will never forget it." He smiled blissfully at the memory.

"Isn't Samarkand rather far?" I asked.

Several voices assured me it was very near Georgia ("green beans with pounded nuts, fried cheese, corn bread") where I was going anyway. Other adjacent localities seemed to include Alma Ata ("be sure to try the steamed meat dumplings they call *manty*"); Erevan ("rose-petal jelly, trout fresh from Lake Sevan") and Batum ("sturgeon with a sauce of pomegranates").

"I think you will find," the girl from Kiev told me, "that we Russians know how to eat well."

"But we know how to go hungry, too." The woman sitting next to me, who turned out to be a doctor completing 40 years of service, spoke quietly. "I was here in Leningrad through all the 900 days of the siege. We shall never forget when a piece of bread this size"—with her finger she drew an exact four-inch square on the tablecloth—"meant the difference between life and death."

The man from Odessa nodded. "Then and many, many times before."

"My grandfather was a baker all his life," said the man across the table, "and he never went to school. I once read him a passage from a book that said at the Battle of Such and Such, General So and So made history. 'Fool's words,' my grandfather said. He picked up a loaf hot from his oven. 'Bread, or the lack of it—*that* is what makes history.' An intelligent man, my grandfather, and an artist at *pirozhki*."

The man from Odessa motioned to the buffet hostess. "Be so kind as to serve us all champagne. I think we should have a toast."

"And to go with it, please," said the baker's grandson, "just a few slices of tongue and a bit of that smoked sturgeon and some caviar. Talking about food is hungry work."

When the glasses were filled and the plates distributed, the man from Odessa rose. "When you write this book, please tell Americans for me"—he looked around the room—"for all of us, that we hope they enjoy our table, and say, too, that we wish them *'Na zdorovie!'* " (To your health!)

The Russians do know how to eat. And they also know how to go hungry. Both facts stem from the realities of geography and history. Seen from the air the Soviet Union looks exactly as the schoolbooks promised. It *is* flat, *is* immense, a limitless plain of forest and field only slightly mountain-

Continued on page 14

11

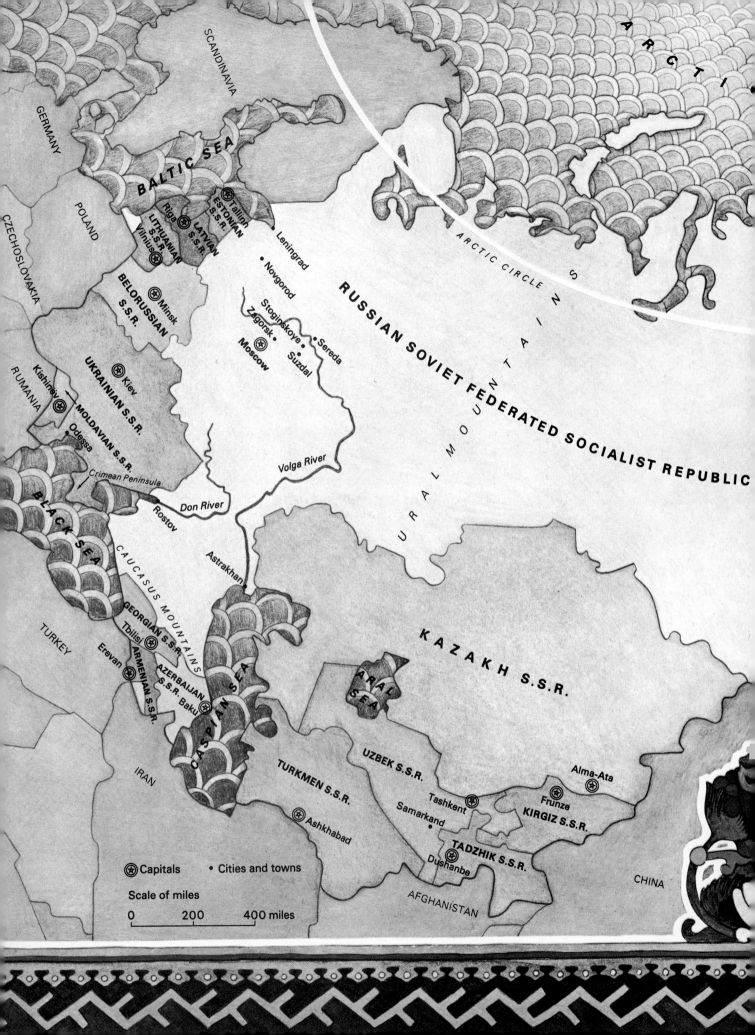

SCANDINAVIA

ARCTI

ARCTIC CIRCLE

GERMANY

BALTIC SEA

RUSSIAN SOVIET FEDERATED SOCIALIST REPUBLIC

POLAND

Tallinn
ESTONIAN
S.S.R.
Riga
LATVIAN
S.S.R.
LITHUANIAN
S.S.R.
Vilnius

CZECHOSLOVAKIA

BELORUSSIAN
S.S.R.
Minsk

Leningrad

Novgorod

Stoginskoye
Zagorsk
Sereda
Moscow
Suzdal

UKRAINIAN S.S.R.
Kiev

RUMANIA

Kishinev
MOLDAVIAN S.S.R.
Odessa

Crimean Peninsula

BLACK SEA

Rostov

Don River

Volga River

Astrakhan

URAL MOUNTAINS

CAUCASUS MOUNTAINS

KAZAKH S.S.R.

TURKEY

GEORGIAN S.S.R.
Tbilisi
Erevan
ARMENIAN S.S.R.
AZERBAIJAN
S.S.R. Baku

CASPIAN SEA

IRAN

ARAL
SEA

TURKMEN S.S.R.

UZBEK S.S.R.

Alma-Ata

Tashkent
Frunze
Samarkand
KIRGIZ S.S.R.

Ashkhabad

TADZHIK S.S.R.
Dushanbe

AFGHANISTAN

CHINA

⊛ Capitals   • Cities and towns

Scale of miles

0   200   400 miles

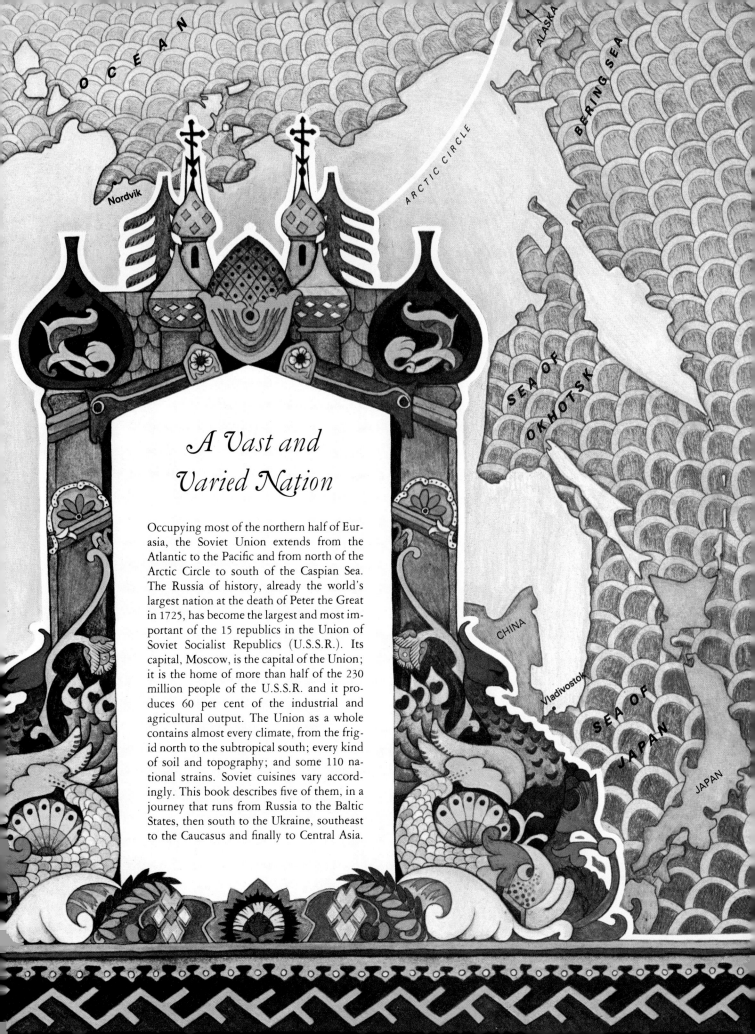

A Vast and Varied Nation

Occupying most of the northern half of Eurasia, the Soviet Union extends from the Atlantic to the Pacific and from north of the Arctic Circle to south of the Caspian Sea. The Russia of history, already the world's largest nation at the death of Peter the Great in 1725, has become the largest and most important of the 15 republics in the Union of Soviet Socialist Republics (U.S.S.R.). Its capital, Moscow, is the capital of the Union; it is the home of more than half of the 230 million people of the U.S.S.R. and it produces 60 per cent of the industrial and agricultural output. The Union as a whole contains almost every climate, from the frigid north to the subtropical south; every kind of soil and topography; and some 110 national strains. Soviet cuisines vary accordingly. This book describes five of them, in a journey that runs from Russia to the Baltic States, then south to the Ukraine, southeast to the Caucasus and finally to Central Asia.

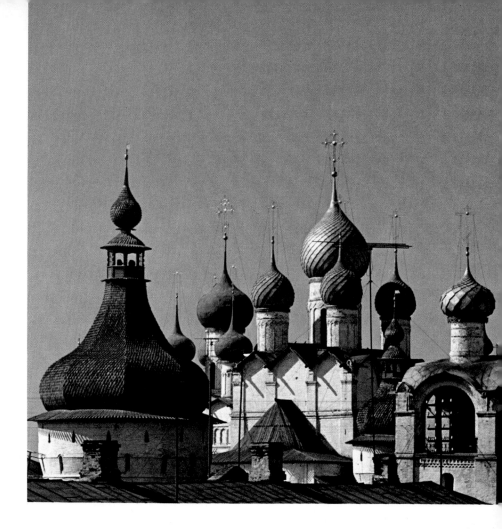

The onion domes of Byzantine-inspired structures, surmounted by ornamented Russian Orthodox crosses, soar above Rostov's 17th Century Kremlin, or citadel. In earlier times this complex of buildings, which also contains government offices and a palace, was frequently visited by Russia's czars; today its endless galleries and passageways, restored to their former glory by the Soviet state, are a major attraction for tourists from all over the world.

wrinkled, that stretches beyond horizons, beyond time, beyond belief. The scale and span of the country constantly surprise the visitor, even when he remembers that this largest of all nations covers one sixth of the inhabited globe, has more than 8.5 million square miles and spreads over two continents. From the town of Nordvik, the most northerly in the world, to Ashkabad near the southern border is 3,000 miles; when the sun sets in Liepaya on the Baltic a new day has dawned in eastern Siberia.

This immensity encompasses a wide range of climates and highly diverse terrains, not all of them benign. More than three fourths of the Soviet Union lies north of the fiftieth parallel (roughly the latitude of the United States-Canadian border), and since few warm ocean currents temper the cold and no east-west mountain chains break the arctic winds, winters in much of the nation are long and bitter. As in Alaska, small fruits, melons and vegetables can be raised during the brief, bright summer, but in this submarginal land where crop yields are generally small and undependable, famines have been all too frequent.

Happily the semiarable and nonarable regions—the tundra in the north, the burning rocks and sands of Central Asia and Kazakhstan, the Pripet marshes—are balanced by others like the fertile black-earth steppes of the Ukraine, and the lush pastures of the Baltic Republics. In the subtropical zone of Transcaucasia, glossy tea bushes and golden citrus fruits flourish. The Soviet forest belt contains more than a quarter of all the trees on earth, and game—woodcock, grouse, hare, elk, deer and bear—abounds.

14

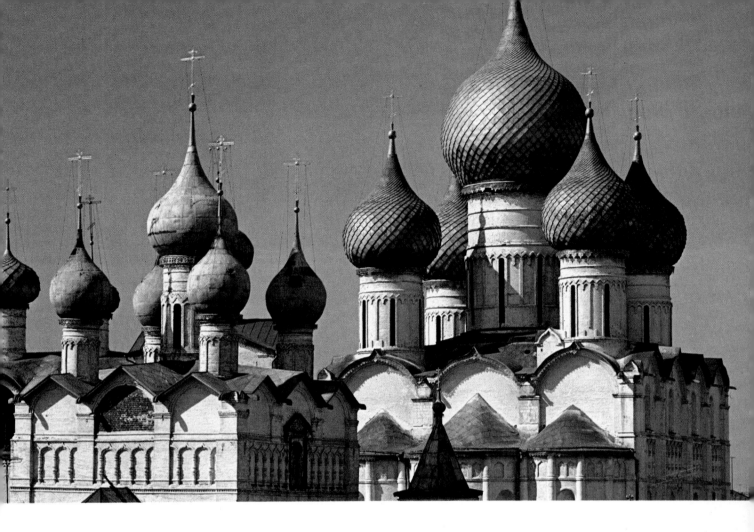

The Soviet Union is rich in water as well, with shores on 12 seas, a quarter of a million lakes including the world's largest (the Caspian) and deepest (Lake Baikal), and an unsurpassed network of rivers totaling two million miles. From these waters come more than a hundred different edible fish, including sturgeon, pike, carp, bream, trout, *sudak* and salmon.

Sharing this bounty are some 230 million people of many and varied nationalities—Latvians, Lithuanians and Estonians along the Baltic; Armenians, Georgians and Azerbaijanians in the Caucasus; Uzbeks, Turkomens, Kazakhs, Kirghiz and Tadzhiks of Central Asia; Slavs of the Ukraine, central Russia and Byelorussia—each with a language, a culture, a tradition and a cuisine distinctly its own. Since more than half the people are Slavs, Slavic cookery predominates. Rich, robust and plenteous, it is designed to nourish the spirit as well as the flesh. The heaped dish, the crowded table, the pressing hospitality that strangers have sometimes taken as a sign of ostentation—or worse, mere voracity—is actually an assertion of life, an answer to the ancient specter of hunger forever lurking outside the door.

For Slavs food has always been a symbol. Their pagan ancestors worshipped the sun, and honored their god at the spring solstice by cooking and eating his image—a thin, round golden batter cake fried in golden butter. The same meltingly delicious *bliny* are still served today.

These early Slavs had a few domestic animals and raised some grains, but they were probably not overly fastidious. They ate where and how they could, supplementing their own efforts with nature's gifts—the game, hon-

15

ey, nuts, and mushrooms of their great forests, and fish taken from the uncounted rivers. Often, undoubtedly, they went hungry.

Early chronicles offer little more of gastronomic interest, but at a few points the darkness lifts a bit. Russia's first ruler was a Viking named Rurik, a half-legendary figure who came with a band of Norsemen from Scandinavia in 862 A.D. to rule the city-state of Novgorod. According to tradition, he introduced Slavs to the cookery of his homeland—rich cream sauces and the "queen cake," a meringue-covered confection of apples and cherries baked between two layers of sweet pastry.

One of Rurik's successors, Vladimir, changed his country's food habits more significantly when he became a communicant of the Greek Orthodox Church in 988. Along with the Orthodox creed, there came to Russia an elaborate church calendar of fast days and feasts, marked respectively by new meatless dishes and formalized revelry. (The chronicles say that Vladimir really preferred Islam until he discovered that alcohol was forbidden to the Faithful. "The joy of Russia is drinking," he said. "She cannot do without it.")

Subsequent invasions by Mongols influenced every aspect of Russian life, including food habits. The barbarians pillaged and destroyed, but they also showed the Slavs how to broil meat, to make yoghurt, *kumys* (a mildly alcoholic drink) and curd cheese from soured or fermented milks; and, most important of all, to preserve cabbage in salt brine, producing sauerkraut, which became a basic Russian food. The Mongols, too, taught Russians the pleasure of tea, and gave them the samovar to bubble on through the centuries.

The invaders were finally driven out in the 16th Century, during the reign of Ivan the Terrible. Ivan is remembered primarily for his violence and cruelty, but he was also a man of refined tastes who enjoyed celebrations and ceremony, music and chess, rich raiment and fine food, and who tried to turn his nobles from their coarse and barbarous ways. On one occasion he invited 300 guests to a dinner served in separate courses. First came five game dishes—roast peacock in full plumage, spiced swan, cranes seasoned with ginger, guinea fowl with cinnamon, and creamed ducks. Three bouillons and three thick soups followed. The main course was a whole calf, a whole sheep, several quarters of beef, and the loins of a bear and a reindeer. For dessert a huge pudding molded in the shape of Ivan's palace, the Kremlin, was borne in by lackeys clad in white satin liveries edged with sable.

Unimpressed by this glimpse of gentility, most of Ivan's nobles kept to

A succession of lusty, strong-willed monarchs ruled Russia from the Ninth Century onward. Rurik, a Viking invader, was the half-legendary founder of the first Russian dynasty. His most notable successors in both historical and culinary importance were Ivan IV (the Terrible), Peter I (the Great) and Catherine II (the Great), each of whom reigned at a time that marked a turning point in the development of Russian culture and cuisine.

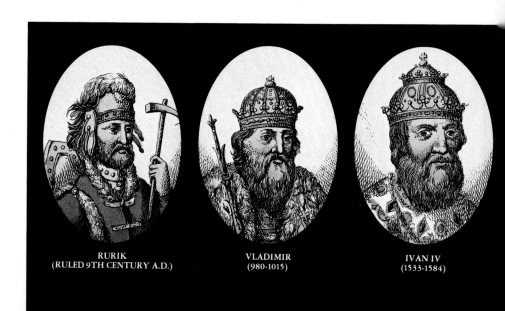

RURIK
(RULED 9TH CENTURY A.D.)

VLADIMIR
(980-1015)

IVAN IV
(1533-1584)

their old ways. They sometimes had an entire meal set out at once—boned geese, roasted hazel hens, a whole carp, gallons of *ukha* (a fish soup), pounds of caviar, fried spine of sturgeon, cakes, fruits and preserves. While their food was served in jewel-studded vessels of gold or silver, such incidentals as forks, knives and napkins were not provided for the guests (though each diner was welcome to his part of the tablecloth as an all-purpose serviette). A plate, if it appeared at all, might be shared by two or three diners. Guests dipped into bowls with their hands, gnawed on joints, let bones drop to the floor, dripped streams of sauce and grease onto their rich robes, spooned soup from a common pot, licked their fingers, belched, spit, and drank wine, mead and spirits until they collapsed in a drunken stupor.

Only men attended such festivities. Upper-class women spent their lives in the *terem,* a separate, secluded section of the house. A husband might command his wife to appear briefly as an honored guest at dinner, but usually she saw no one outside her immediate family. She wore an elaborate coif and a veil that covered much of her face, she used fantastic cosmetics (painting the teeth black was popular), grew fat, and seldom left home except to attend church in a closed carriage or litter.

Such was Russian society until the close of the 17th Century, when Peter the Great came to the throne, determined to modernize his country and his subjects. The new Czar was a strange and complex man, coarse, violent and often sadistic, but intelligent, curious and always willing to try something new. In France he sampled the soldiers' soup, and a smacking mouthful was all he needed to pronounce it excellent. He noted the recipe and hired a French cook to come to Russia. In Holland he liked Dutch cheese and bread so much that he learned how to make them himself, and he adopted the Dutch custom of serving fruit preserves with meat.

In Russia Peter built a new capital, St. Petersburg (now Leningrad), on the marshy islands at the mouth of the Neva River, and made it as beautiful as any city in Europe. He ordered noble families to move there from Moscow and then, in one royal ukase after another, imposed the refinements of Western society on his unwilling subjects. Under the threat of heavy taxes, men were ordered to cut their beards and long hair. Women were ordered to adopt new coiffures and discard the face veil. The *terem* was abolished. In the future husbands *and* wives would appear together, both in modern dress (and the ladies' gowns were to be daringly *décolleté),* at *assemblées* in the pal-

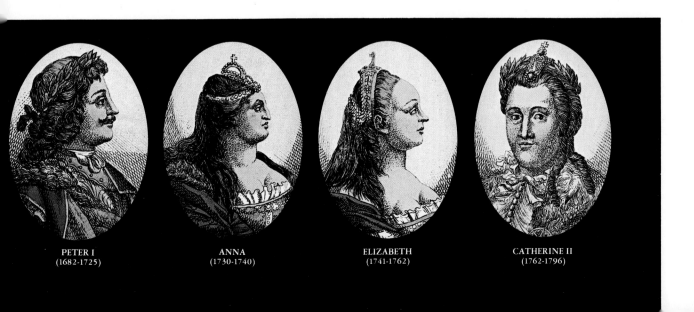

PETER I
(1682-1725)

ANNA
(1730-1740)

ELIZABETH
(1741-1762)

CATHERINE II
(1762-1796)

ace. "An *assemblée*," the ukase explained, "is a French term which cannot be expressed by any single Russian word. It implies a number of persons who have gathered together . . . to pass the time agreeably."

When the guests gathered, they stood in petrified silence while refreshments were served. In a frenzy of hospitality, the Czar rushed from room to room pressing tea, cake and chocolates upon the ladies, vodka and beer upon the men. After these treats the entire company was taught to dance.

The *assemblées* were only the beginning. Members of the court were ordered to give and attend dinners and balls; learn foreign languages; buy silks, brocades and porcelains; refurnish their palaces and celebrate weddings, holidays and similar occasions in a manner worthy of their position, their nation and their enlightened monarch. Timorously they obeyed, and found it was not so difficult to grow accustomed to luxurious living.

In 1730, five years after Peter's death, his niece Anna ascended the throne. She had lived most of her life in the Baltic provinces, subsisting on a pittance, and was so stingy that, according to one of the Baltic barons, "she has been known to count the apples on a tree for fear that her gardeners would cheat her." (He added: "I wish that barbaric Russia joy of her.") Once she was Empress, her balls and banquets became the talk of Europe.

For a "country picnic" for 300, Anna had a pavilion of green silk supported by pillars of real flowers set up in the imperial garden. In winter she had the dining room of her palace lined with orange trees in fragrant bloom, and delicacies of every kind were spread before her guests.

In 1740, during the 10th year of her reign, Anna collapsed at the table during one of her great dinners and died soon afterward, to be succeeded by her cousin Elizabeth, a gay and frivolous woman even more fond of food and drink. Elizabeth conferred upon her chef the military rank and salary of brigadier—and often infuriated him by demanding such "common" dishes as fish pie, pickled pork, and nettle soup. When she received a present, she liked it to be edible. Her favorites at court (gossip ran their number into the hundreds), expressed their eternal devotion in Périgord and Versailles pâtés, truffles, sweetmeats, exotic fruits and rare wines.

By the late 18th Century, during the reign of Catherine the Great, the pleasures of the table preoccupied the nobility. Catherine, who came to the throne in 1762, was German by birth and a hard-working, abstemious woman. But the fact that she had bread and coffee for breakfast and meat and soup for dinner (she considered supper unnecessary) did not influence her court to follow her example. The Youssoupoff family, who were richer than the ruling Romanovs (or so the Empress claimed), had so many formal dining rooms that they could use a different one every night of the week, and enough gold and silver plates to serve a thousand guests. One Youssoupoff prince ordered part of the Sèvres factory, workmen included, imported from France and set it up on one of his estates. Other families garbed their armies of lackeys in a different livery for each course at dinner—cream satin and silver for the fish, crimson velvet with gold facings for the meat.

Fortunes were spent on a single dinner—fresh oysters at a rouble apiece for a thousand guests (at the time, a good craftsman was lucky to earn 30 roubles in a year;) Astrakhan melons carried 1,000 miles by carriage; dwarf cherry trees, hung with ripe fruit, in golden pots for a midwinter table decoration.

Continued on page 24

Opulent Art for the Nobility's Tables

Over the centuries, members of the Russian nobility stocked their palaces with masterpieces of applied art in the form of priceless tableware. Silversmiths and enamelers, summoned from every part of Europe, created jewellike utensils, plates and vessels in traditional Russian shapes and with traditional Russian motifs. This gilded silver and enamel dish, for example, with its raised medallion bearing the double monogram of Czar Alexander III and his Czarina, is derived from the Russian "bread and salt" dishes offered to guests as symbols of hospitality. Drinking vessels also reflect old Russian themes; the birdlike shape of the ceremonial *kovsh (lower left, overleaf)* dates from prehistoric times.

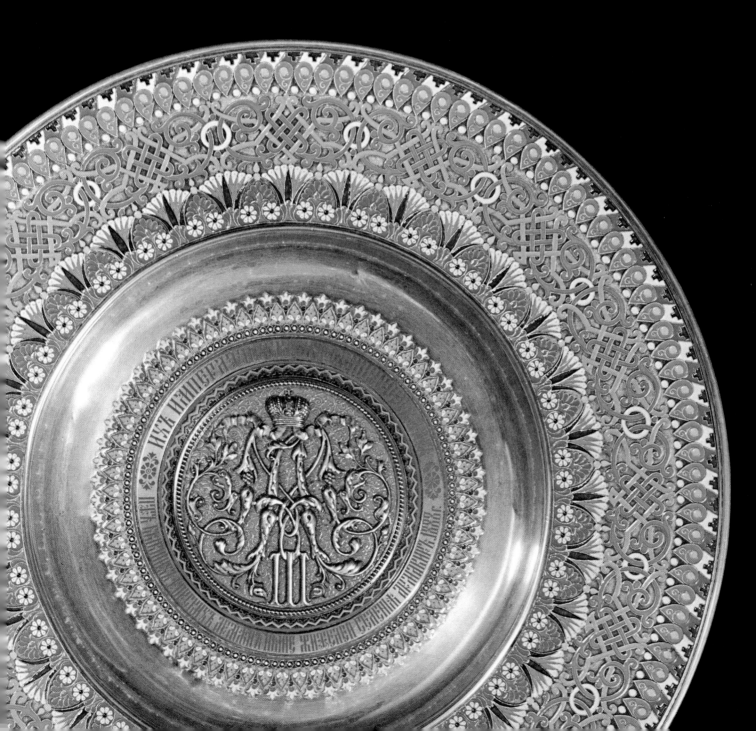

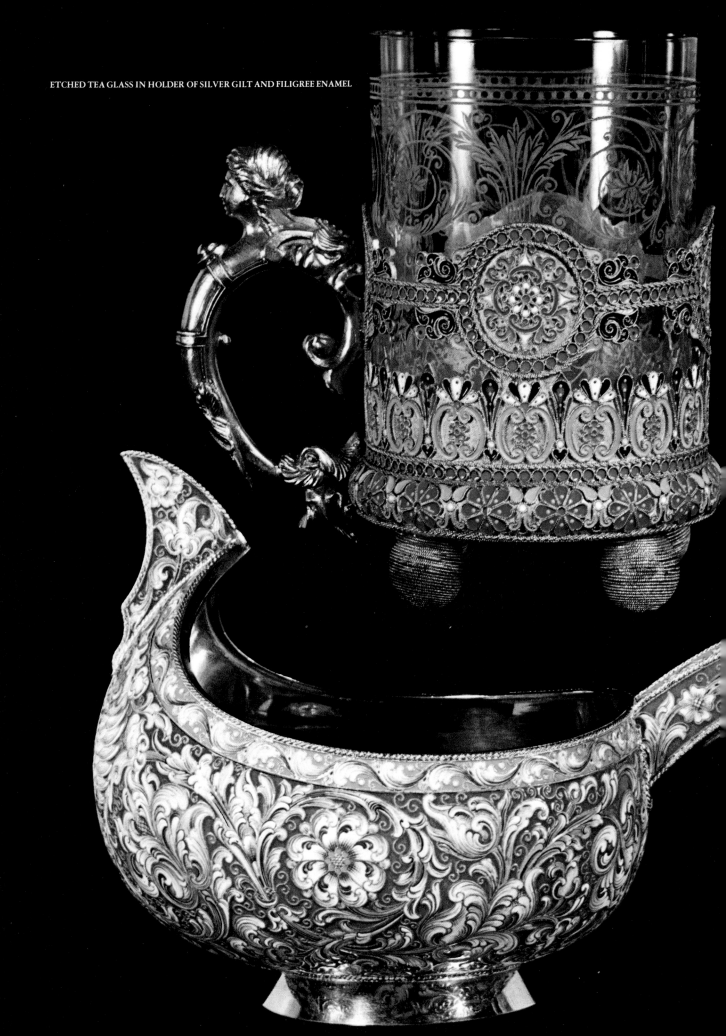

ETCHED TEA GLASS IN HOLDER OF SILVER GILT AND FILIGREE ENAMEL

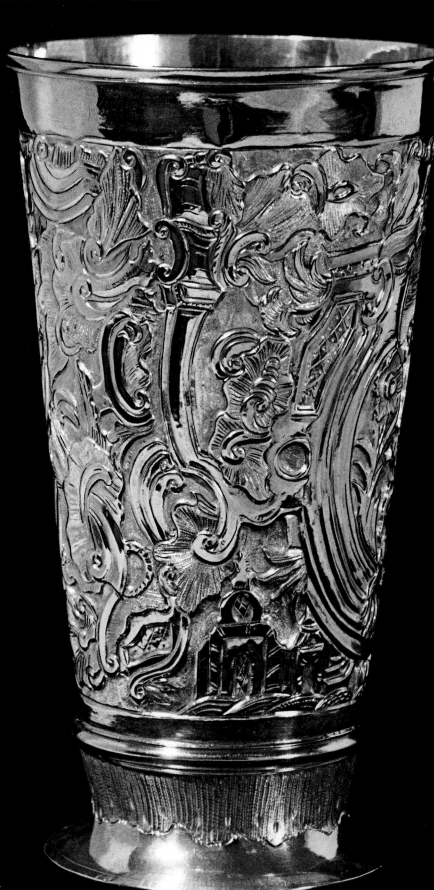

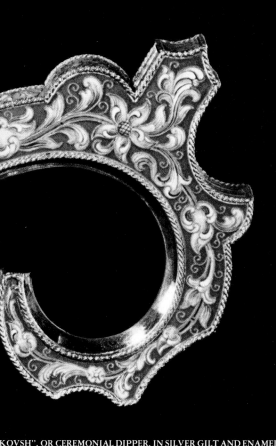

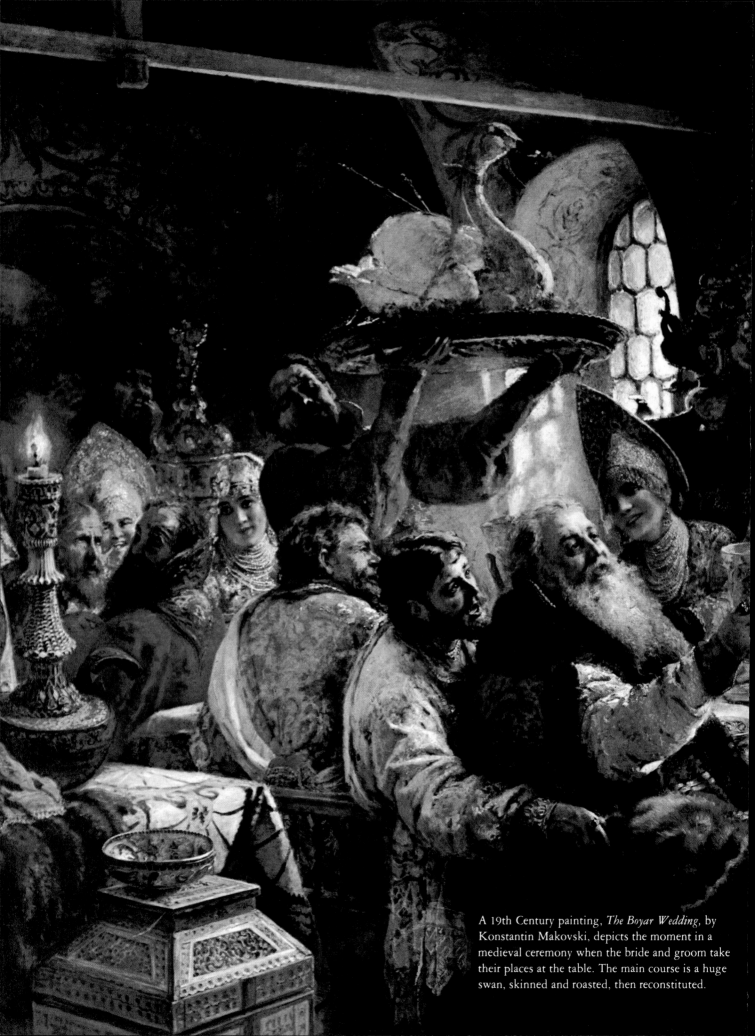

A 19th Century painting, *The Boyar Wedding*, by Konstantin Makovski, depicts the moment in a medieval ceremony when the bride and groom take their places at the table. The main course is a huge swan, skinned and roasted, then reconstituted.

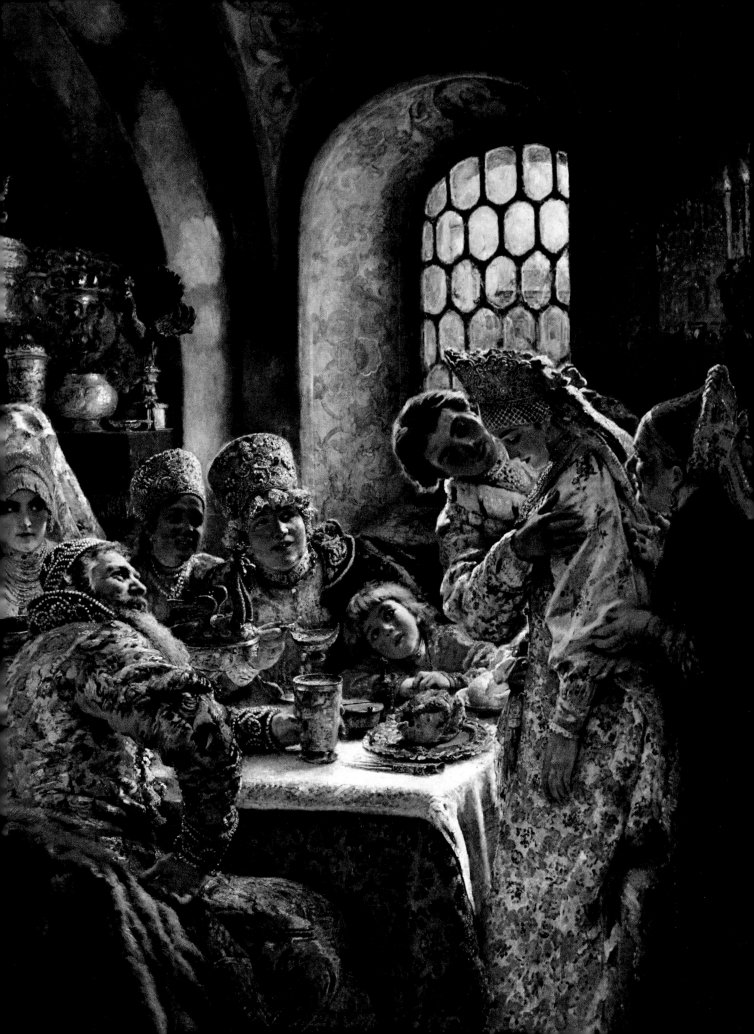

Every distinguished household had a French or Swiss chef, who was well paid and well treated lest he be enticed to another kitchen. One famous gourmet planned to assure himself of an uninterrupted lifetime of *grande cuisine* by sending one of his serfs to Paris to be professionally trained. The serf learned his trade—and some new ideas from the French Revolution, then in progress. He wrote back to his master, "I shall stay in France and you, sir, may make your own sauces or go without."

From the early 19th Century upper-class society, particularly in St. Petersburg, affected foreign manners and clothes, spoke French almost exclusively (and Russian, if at all, with an artificial accent), hired German tutors, Parisian governesses and English nurses, and sent the family laundry to Western Europe to be laundered. But this all-pervasive snobbery changed the basic cuisine very little. Russian foodstuffs, climate and customs did not adapt to continental standards. Chefs came and went, a few new dishes were introduced, a few old ones improved, but generally the traditional table seemed to suit Russians best. By the middle of the century that table and the foods that appeared upon it were stabilized in what is often considered the finest cuisine in Russian history. From that time until the outbreak of World War I, Russians of nobility and wealth passed their day in an elaborate ritual of four distinct meals, coming to a climax in a feast of small dishes—the famous *zakuska* —and a splendid dinner. Let us follow such a day from meal to meal.

The day began with tea, a strong essence made in a china pot and diluted in the cup to the desired strength with briskly boiling water from the samovar, an ornate brass urn heated by a charcoal fire in a vertical tube at the center. Milk was sometimes added, and a bit of sugar broken from the loaf with a small silver pincer. Women drank their tea from a cup, men from a glass set in an engraved or filigreed metal holder with a handle. With the tea went sweet buns, plain rolls, or bread with butter and perhaps a slice of cheese.

Around noon a simple lunch was prepared, usually fish or meat and a vegetable with, perhaps, a plain pudding for dessert. Often only the women and children of the family appeared at the table. The men were lunching at some male stronghold—at the club, at the officers' mess, or at a restaurant. In Moscow, the restaurant might be Testov's, for oblong pies stuffed with gelatinous sturgeon spine, eggs and mushrooms; or the Slaviansky Bazaar, for clear, rich, deep orange sterlet soup; or the Moscovi Traktir, for *kotlety pozharskie* of minced chicken.

Dinner, the main meal of the day, could be eaten at any time from late afternoon to mid-evening. It began with *zakuska*, an array of "small bites" accompanied by vodka, set out in advance on a table in the hall, the parlor or an alcove in the reception room. In some households particularly in Moscow which was considered more "Russian" than St. Petersburg, the *zakuska* table was a permanent fixture, constantly replenished, always available.

Because *zakuska* is so typically Russian an institution, it is worth special attention. The custom probably originated in country houses on vast estates, to which guests came over long distances on bad roads, often in sub-zero weather. People might arrive at any hour, frequently unexpected, usually hungry. *Zakuska* offered a practical way to give them sustenance and keep them in good spirits until dinner could be prepared.

As time passed, the *zakuska* grew increasingly lavish, with more and

In the heyday of imperial power and wealth even a summer residence like this royal house at Pavlovsk, near St. Petersburg, was stocked with priceless tableware. The china service shown in small part on a table in the throne room consisted of 4,000 pieces, all designed and manufactured at the Czar's own factory in the early 19th Century. The equally elaborate crystal service was imported from England.

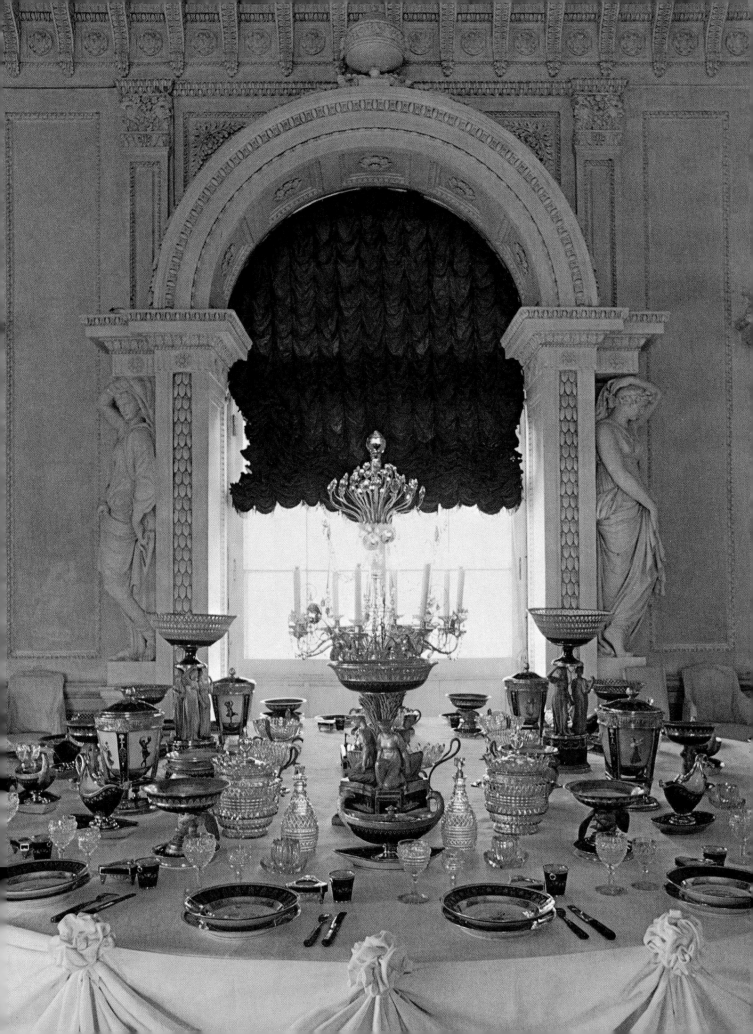

varied dishes. It became commonplace for visitors from abroad to mistake it for the full dinner and partake so heartily they could not eat the meal that followed. By the last decades of the 19th Century the composition and content of the *zakuska* table had evolved from a culinary exercise into an esoteric art form that embraced the techniques of mosaic, collage, sculpture, easel painting and taxidermy. Each dish was lavishly decorated—a wreath of turnip rosebuds for the pâté, carrot daisies blooming in the aspic, sweet-butter lilies for the bread, a silver chain of onion rings encircling a herring, scallions transmuted into white peacocks spreading green fantails.

An overall plan combining both functional and aesthetic principles was worked out for the table, which was usually oval and placed so that guests might circle it comfortably while sampling the scores of dishes. Some foods, such as the fish, cheeses and meats, were more or less grouped together; others, such as pickles and breads, were set at several convenient points. To keep within this framework and yet achieve a balance of taste, texture and color—so that the dark smoked eel was close to the pink salmon, the hard, thin sausage beside a creamy ivory cheese, a bowl of crisp green pickles near the golden sprats—called for a discerning eye and a skilled hand.

The most important item on the table was caviar, offered in a variety and an amount that indicated both the host's solvency and the guests' consequence. (One noble family had a cut-glass barrel that held 20 kilograms —about 45 pounds—and was refilled daily.) It was served from a crystal dish with a silver spoon, since base metals impaired the flavor.

In earlier times the roes of many kinds of fish—shad, mullet, whiting, codfish, catfish—had been considered delicacies. By the 19th Century, however, fashions in food had changed and the most popular were the roe of four species of sturgeon, called caviar from the Turkish word for roe, *khavyah.*

From the Volga sterlet came the rarest of all caviars—a golden roe that was traditionally reserved for the imperial table. Of the three other sturgeons from which roe is taken, the *Beluga,* largest in size, produces the largest eggs, which may vary after processing from almost black to grey, touched by a pearly lustre. *Sevruga* and *Osetrova* sturgeon, smaller both in body and in the size of their eggs, sometimes yield a darker roe. While the large grey Beluga egg was (and is) generally considered the choicest caviar available, the quality of caviar depends not only on the variety of sturgeon, but also on the individual fish—its age, genetic composition, food supply, environment—and on the treatment of the roe.

For the finest caviar, the roe is sieved by hand to remove membranes and is lightly salted (the Russian word for the best grade, *malossol,* means just that —lightly salted). Less choice roes are more heavily salted and pressed into bricks called *Pausnaia.* Freezing permanently destroys the cellular composition of the roe used in producing caviar, and at temperatures above 45° caviar soon spoils. Today, caviar is generally pasteurized and vacuum-packed in glass and tin, but in earlier times its transportation to Moscow and St. Petersburg required containers that had to be carefully warmed in winter and iced in summer.

Black caviar was usually served on small pieces of white bread, often toasted very dry in a low oven. Red "caviar"—actually the roe of salmon—was a little hearty for a formal *zakuska,* but spread generously on a large slice of buttered pumpernickel and sprinkled with minced scallion tops and finely chopped egg yolks it made a fine between-meal snack.

No *zakuska* table was complete without salted, young, fat, first-run herring. It might be served in a mustard sauce or in sour cream, or the whole fish might be scored diagonally, dressed with oil and vinegar, and served with the head and tail left on. The choice of other fish was almost limitless—eel, smoked or jellied; sprats in oil; tiny silver pilchards, painstakingly boned; anchovies pounded with sweet butter to a paste; sardines; sweet river crayfish and sturgeon and salmon, served either in thin slices of smoked fillet or as the whole fish in an amber aspic clarified with caviar.

From caviar and fish, the *zakuska* sampler could move on to meat and vegetables. *Pashtet*, a kind of pâté, might be based upon chicken, calf liver, boned pheasant, or hare. The meat was simmered with wine, herbs and vegetables until tender, then sieved, seasoned, baked in or out of a crust, mellowed a day or two, and served cold. There was usually game on the table, such as grouse or partridge in aspic; other meats might include smoked tongue, ham, sausages of wild fowl or liver, a quivering mold of *kholodets* (diced pork, in a natural jelly) and on special occasions a whole suckling pig, roasted and boned. Nearby stood a pot of mustard and a bowl of freshly grated horseradish, both so potent that one taste would make a guest weep, smack the crown of his head in agonized appreciation, and taste again.

Vegetables were often converted into "caviars." One such favorite was eggplant baked in the skin, then mashed with finely chopped onions, seasoned with oil and lemon juice and fresh coriander. Another was prepared from crushed dried mushrooms soaked in wine, simmered in sweet butter with onions, parsley, and a hint of garlic. And adding color and piquancy were pickles, dilled cucumbers, green tomatoes, pearl onions, whole pickled mushrooms, tart plums, melon rind and crisp white apples.

In the early years of the 20th Century, it became fashionable in some circles to have a substantial *zakuska*, attend the theater, and then eat a late supper. At that time, hot dishes were added to the *zakuska* table: *bitki*, which are tiny highly seasoned meatballs; veal kidneys in Madeira; chicken livers in sour cream; small Vienna sausages in pungent tomato sauce; and *forshmak*, a dish in which herring, boiled potatoes, onions and apples are baked together in sour cream and become, through some gastronomic alchemy, deliciously compatible.

Crowning the table was a selection from some 15 or 20 kinds of vodka, both crystal clear and jewel-toned. Clear vodka, always served in the original bottle, was well chilled, then poured into a small glass that held less than a half ounce. Properly, it was never sipped, but taken in one quick swallow, followed by a bite of caviar or *pashtet*, then another glass of vodka, a taste of herring, and vodka again in a kind of point-counterpoint rhythm. The best clear vodka, called Krasnaia Golovka or "red cap," was also the base for many flavored vodkas prepared at home and served from decanters. One of the simplest and best, *zubrovka*, was made by steeping two or three stalks of buffalo grass in a bottle of vodka, and had the color of new hay and the taste of a June morning. Other favorites were *rubinovaia*, brilliant orange and slightly astringent from berries of the mountain ash; litmus vodka, colored mauve and flavored with the faint earthiness of truffles by the litmus li-

Overleaf: A *zakuska* table features a platter of sturgeon in aspic, in the foreground, flanked by pots of red and black caviar. Three more cold appetizers dominate the center of the table—a chicken-based *salat Olivier*, a *pashtet* (pâté) of liver and a plate of pickled herring—and the silver casserole of kidneys in Madeira sauce provides a hot dish. Ranged around these major dishes are a variety of appetite-teasers: three kinds of bread, a bowl of fruit, pickles and pickled mushrooms, and a full assortment of vodkas.

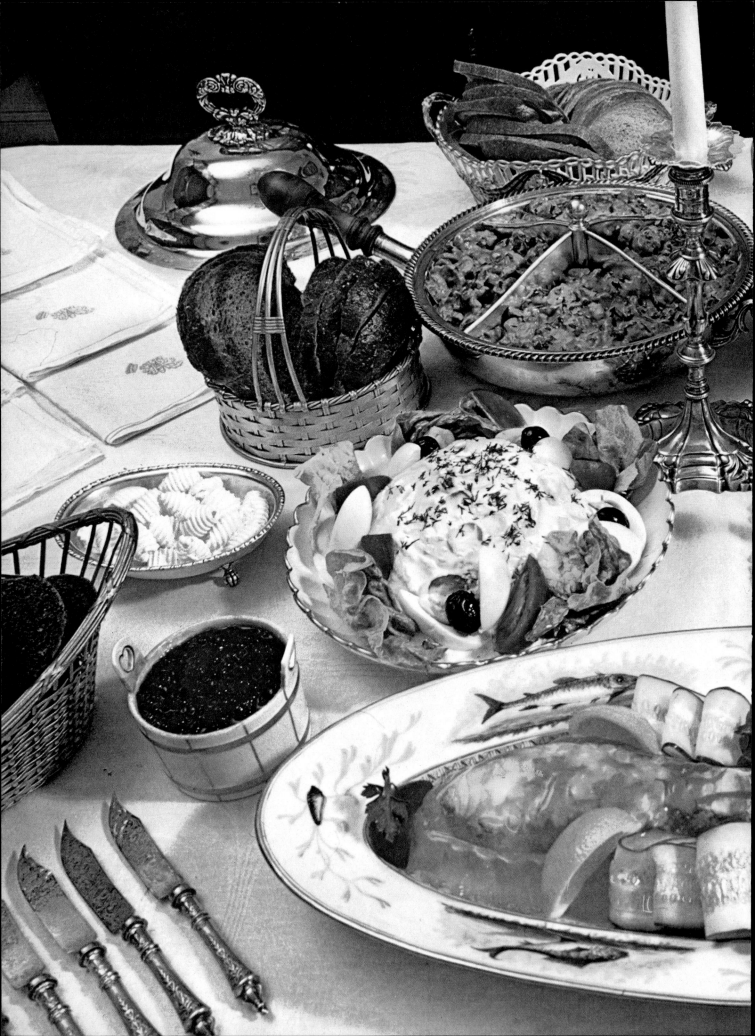

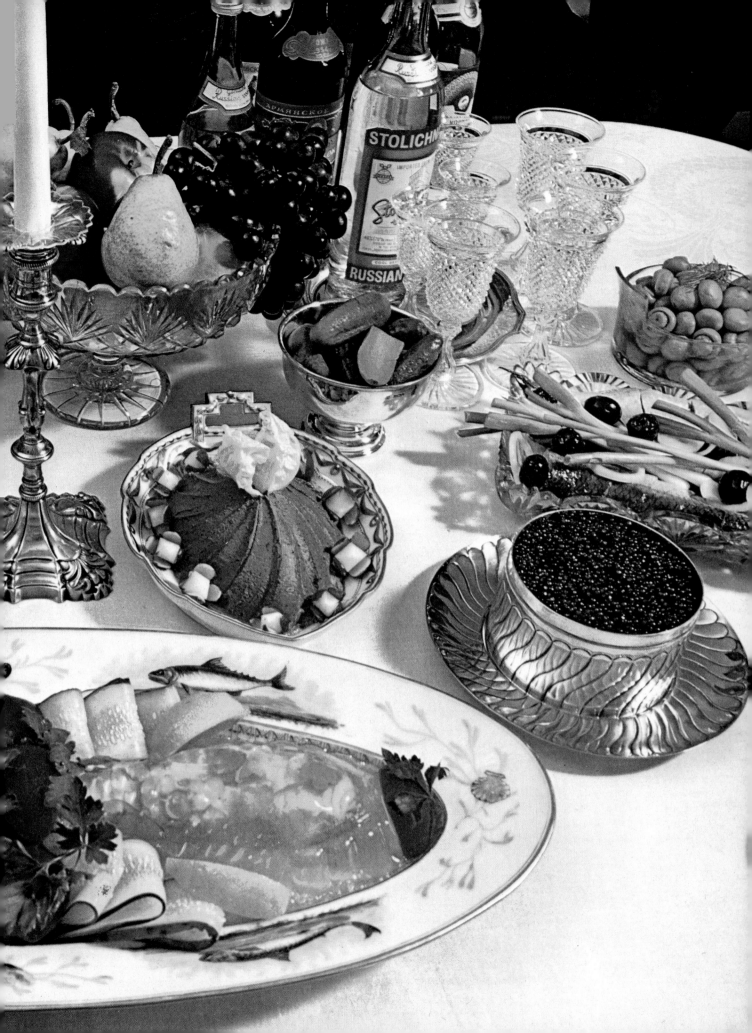

chen; lemon vodka, which got its flavor and color from a long curl of peel pared off a single fruit; *smarodinovka*, ruby hued, with a lightly bitter aftertaste from an infusion of black currant leaves or shoots; and *pertsovka*, fortified with black pepper. Women usually took sherry rather than vodka. Men who ate and drank a great deal often finished their *zakuska* with a glass of English ale, which was thought to restore appetite and sobriety.

After an hour or so around the *zakuska* table, guests were summoned to the flower-banked dining room and took their places around an enormous, elaborately decorated table. It was customary to have a centerpiece of fruits arranged in epergnes, flanked by cake stands, candelabra, sculptured figures and ornamented salt dishes, all in gold and silver.

Dinner began with soup. Usually three were offered, one cold, such as *botvinia* (sorrel with salmon or sturgeon), or *okroshka* (cucumbers, game and herbs in *kvas* and cream); the other two hot, perhaps *Bagration* (cream of veal poured over spinach or asparagus tips), the fish soup called *ukha*, red bouillon with quenelles, or chicken consommé with tiny dumplings. A guest normally chose only one, occasionally a second. Cream soups were served with croutons; other soups with *pirozhki*, small finger-length pasties, or with *pychki*, fritters so light and dry that one could be picked up without soiling a white kid glove. *Pirozhki* and *pychki* both had fillings appropriate to the soup they accompanied—minced fish, meat, mushrooms, hard-boiled eggs, or cheese.

The order in which the other dishes followed varied considerably. There was customarily a fish course, possibly sturgeon cooked in a rich creamy tomato sauce, crayfish soufflé, or pike stuffed with rice and gelatinous sturgeon spine. The game, depending on the season, might be hazel hen, partridge slightly resinous from a diet of juniper berries, or pheasant. Roasts were often served in pairs, and might include saddle of wild goat, white veal from Archangel, or Astrakhan mutton, all accompanied by pickled or salted fruits. The vegetables—succulent all-white asparagus three inches thick, tiny peas, cucumbers braised in dill butter, or leeks in parsley sauce—were served as a separate course.

Elaborate desserts ended the dinner. There might be a frozen cream flavored with whortleberries, strawberries or raspberries; an apple charlotte of tart apples and black bread crumbs *(Recipe Index);* a *gurev kasha*, caramel glazed farina pudding, studded with candied fruits and nuts *(Recipe Index);* or a *charlottka*, created by that towering figure of *la grande cuisine*, the Frenchman Antonin Carême, who served as chef to Czar Alexander I, the only true gourmet the Romanovs ever produced.

In some houses sherry, Madeira, and port were offered after the soup, white wines with fish, red wines with meat, and Málaga, Muscat and Tokay with dessert. Often, however, champagne (particularly Abrau-Durso champagne from the Caucasus, the favorite wine of the last Czar, Nicholas II) was served with every course.

Two or three hours after dinner was disposed of, the fourth and final meal was taken—*vecherny tchai*, or evening tea. Cold cuts, cheeses, sweet cordials, small cakes and candied fruits were brought into the drawing room, and the crowded day of formidable upper-class eating ended as it began with boiling hot tea from the samovar.

Two luscious desserts exemplify a classic ingenuity in elaborating originally simple dishes. The cream-filled charlotte russe in the foreground, bordered by ladyfingers and served with a raspberry sauce, is a refinement of the more modest apple charlotte in the background, in which fresh applesauce is surrounded by strips of crisp bread and served with an apricot sauce. Recipes for both the desserts and the fruit sauces are given on the following pages.

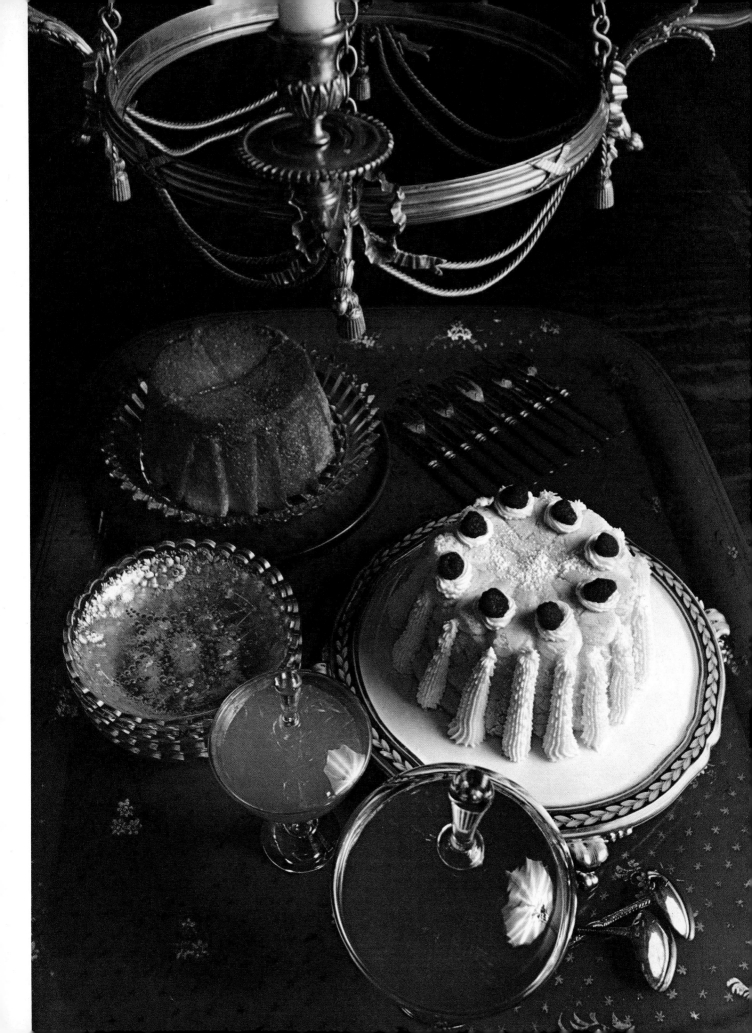

To serve 8

1 tablespoon unsalted butter, softened

½ pound plus 3 tablespoons unsalted butter, clarified *(see tabaka, page 171)*

16 slices (½ inch thick) homemade-style white bread, trimmed of all crusts

5 pounds tart red apples, peeled, cored and thinly sliced (5 quarts)

1 cup sugar

⅓ cup water

1 teaspoon cinnamon

APRICOT SAUCE

1½ cups apricot preserves (12 ounces)

2 tablespoons cold water

¼ cup applejack or Calvados

Babka Yablochnaya
APPLE CHARLOTTE WITH APRICOT SAUCE

With a pastry brush, lightly coat the bottom and sides of a 1½-quart, 3- to 3½-inch-deep charlotte or other straight-sided mold with the tablespoon of softened butter.

Pour all but 3 tablespoons of the clarified butter into a large bowl. With a sharp knife, cut 3 slices of the bread into 6 triangles by slicing them in half diagonally. Cut another 7 slices of the bread in half. One at a time, briefly dip the bread triangles into the bowl of clarified butter and lay them side by side in the bottom of the mold. With a small, sharp knife, trim the triangles so that their points meet in the middle and no spaces show between the slices. Now dip the bread halves in the butter and stand them upright around the sides of the mold, overlapping them slightly. The bread will rise slightly above the top of the mold.

Cut another 3 slices of the bread into 1-inch squares. Heat the 3 reserved tablespoons of clarified butter in a heavy 10- to 12-inch skillet set over high heat and drop in the bread squares. Turning them about constantly with a wooden spoon, cook the squares for 2 to 3 minutes, until they are lightly and evenly colored on all sides. Remove the browned bread squares from the pan with a slotted spoon and set aside.

In a 4-quart casserole combine the apples, sugar and water. Bring to a boil over high heat, then cover tightly, reduce the heat to low, and simmer 30 minutes, or until the apples are tender and show no resistance when pierced with the tip of a sharp knife. Uncover and cook over high heat, stirring frequently, for about 15 minutes, or until most of the liquid has evaporated and the apples become a thick, coarse purée. Stir in the cinnamon and refrigerate the purée until well chilled.

When ready to assemble and bake the dessert, stir the browned bread squares into the thick apple purée and pour the mixture into the prepared mold. Do not be concerned if the filling rises above the rim of the mold; the apple purée will subside as it bakes.

Preheat the oven to 375°. Cut 2 of the remaining slices of bread in half, dip them in the butter and place them on top of the filling. Cut the remaining slice into narrow strips, dip them into the butter and arrange them around the top to cover the exposed areas.

Bake in the center of the oven for 1 hour, or until the bread is golden brown. Cool for 30 minutes at room temperature, then invert a flat serving platter on top and, grasping the plate and mold firmly together, turn them over. Let the mold rest in this fashion for another 30 minutes before gently lifting it off the cake.

APRICOT SAUCE: With the back of a large spoon rub the apricot preserves through a fine sieve set over a 1-quart saucepan. Add the water and cook over moderate heat for about 10 minutes, stirring constantly until the sauce is thick enough to run sluggishly off a spoon when it is lifted from the pan. Off the heat stir in the applejack or Calvados.

Either pour the sauce over the top and sides of the unmolded apple charlotte, or serve it separately in a bowl.

Charlottka

CHARLOTTE RUSSE: LADYFINGERS MOLD WITH CREAM FILLING

Trim 12 of the ladyfinger halves, tapering them slightly at one end. Arrange these halves, side by side, curved sides down, on the bottom of a 1-quart charlotte mold with the tapered ends meeting in the center. Stand the remaining ladyfingers, curved side out, side by side around the inside of the mold; if possible, avoid leaving any open spaces between them.

Beat the egg yolks briefly in a mixing bowl with a whisk or an electric or rotary mixer. Still beating, gradually add the sugar, and continue to beat until the mixture is thick and pale yellow and runs sluggishly off the beater when lifted from the bowl. In a small saucepan, warm the milk and vanilla bean over moderate heat until bubbles appear around the edges of the pan. Remove the bean and slowly pour the hot milk into the eggs, beating constantly. Cook over low heat, stirring constantly, until the mixture thickens into a custard heavy enough to coat a spoon. Do not let it boil or it will curdle.

Off the heat, stir in the softened gelatin. When it has completely dissolved, strain the custard through a fine sieve set over a large bowl. With a whisk or rotary or electric beater, whip together the sour cream and heavy cream until the mixture forms stiff peaks on the beater when it is lifted out of the bowl. Fill half a large pot with ice cubes and cover them with 2 inches of water, set the bowl of custard into the pot and stir the custard with a metal spoon for at least 5 minutes, or until it is quite cold and just beginning to thicken to a syrupy consistency. With a rubber spatula, gently fold the whipped cream into the custard. (If by some mischance the cream-and-custard mixture is lumpy, beat it with a whisk until smooth.) Pour the mixture into the prepared mold, smooth the top with a spatula, cover with plastic wrap and refrigerate for 4 or 5 hours.

RASPBERRY PURÉE: Rub the raspberries with the back of a large spoon through a fine sieve set over a mixing bowl. Stir in the sugar and kirsch, cover tightly with plastic wrap, and refrigerate until ready to serve.

To unmold the charlotte russe, invert a flat serving plate on top of the mold and, grasping the plate and mold firmly together, turn them over. Gently remove the mold and serve the dessert with a bowl of the raspberry purée.

To serve 6

12 to 16 ladyfingers, split in half
  lengthwise
4 large egg yolks
½ cup sugar
1 cup milk
A 2-inch piece of vanilla bean
2 level teaspoons unflavored gelatin,
  softened in ¼ cup cold water
½ cup chilled sour cream
½ cup chilled heavy cream

RASPBERRY PURÉE
2 ten-ounce packages frozen
  raspberries, defrosted and
  thoroughly drained
2 tablespoons superfine sugar
1 tablespoon kirsch or any other
  type of cherry-flavored brandy.

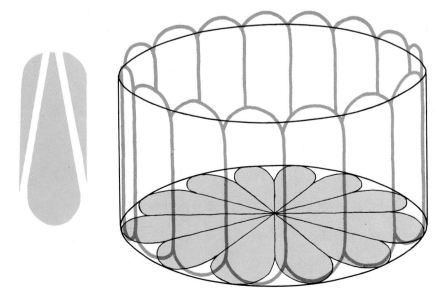

To line a straight-sided mold for *charlottka* (charlotte russe, *recipe above),* trim 12 ladyfingers, tapering them at one end as shown at far left so that the pointed tips will meet in the middle when the ladyfingers are arranged on the bottom of the mold. Stand the remaining ladyfingers side by side around the inside of the mold, overlapping slightly to avoid leaving open spaces between them.

To serve 6 to 8

FISH STOCK AND FISH

6 cups cold water

4 pounds fish trimmings: spines, heads and tails from any white-fleshed fish

2 medium carrots, scraped

4 sprigs parsley

2 stalks celery with leaves, coarsely chopped

¼ cup white wine vinegar

1 bay leaf

8 whole cloves

1 tablespoon salt

4 fresh sturgeon or halibut steaks, cut 1 inch thick and weighing about 8 ounces each

ASPIC

2 packages unflavored gelatin

½ cup water

4 egg whites

To serve 6 to 8

1 cup red wine vinegar

2 whole cloves

½ cup cold water

5 whole black peppercorns

½ bay leaf

2 teaspoons salt

2 cloves garlic, peeled and crushed with the flat of a knife or cleaver

1 pound small, fresh white mushrooms

1 tablespoon vegetable oil

Osetrina Zalivnaya
FISH IN ASPIC

In a 2- to 3-quart enameled or stainless-steel casserole, combine 6 cups of cold water with the fish trimmings, carrots, parsley, celery, vinegar, bay leaf, cloves and salt. Bring to a boil over high heat, then reduce the heat to low and partially cover the pot. Simmer the stock undisturbed for 1 hour.

Remove the carrots with a slotted spoon and set them aside. Strain the stock through a fine sieve set over a 3- to 4-quart enameled or stainless-steel casserole, pressing down on the vegetables and trimmings with the back of a large spoon to extract all their juices before discarding them. Bring the stock to a boil over high heat and add the fish steaks. Cover the pot, reduce the heat to low, and simmer gently for 8 minutes, or until the fish is firm to the touch. Do not overcook. With a slotted spoon, transfer the fish to a platter and cut each steak in half.

There should be 4 cups of stock in the pot. If there is less, add cold water; if more, boil rapidly uncovered until it has reduced to 4 cups.

ASPIC: Pour the gelatin into the cold water and let it soften for 5 minutes. Meanwhile, beat the egg whites to a froth. Bring the stock to a boil over high heat and stir in the softened gelatin and egg whites. Stirring constantly with a whisk, boil until the aspic begins to froth and rise. When it almost threatens to overflow the pan remove it from the heat and let it rest for 5 minutes. Then pour the entire contents of the pan into a cheesecloth-lined sieve set over a deep bowl. Let the aspic drain through slowly without disturbing it at all. Discard the contents of the sieve and taste the aspic for seasoning. It should be quite definite in flavor and will doubtless need more salt.

Cut the carrots into ¼-inch slices and arrange them in concentric circles in the bottom of a 2-quart charlotte or a similar mold about 3 inches deep. A teaspoon at a time, sprinkle the carrots evenly with the aspic and continue adding the aspic by the teaspoon until the carrots are half submerged, but not floating in the liquid. Place the mold in the refrigerator without dislodging the design and chill for at least 1 hour, or until the aspic is firm. By this time, the remaining aspic should be cool. Arrange half of the fish in a single layer on the aspic in the mold and pour in just enough aspic to submerge them. Refrigerate for at least 1 hour, or until the aspic is firm, then arrange the remaining fish on top and cover with the remaining aspic. Refrigerate for 2 hours, or until firm.

To unmold the aspic, run a sharp knife around the sides of the dish and dip the bottom in hot water for a few seconds. Place a flat, shallow platter upside down over the dish and, grasping both firmly together, invert the two. Rap the platter on a table and the aspic should slide out easily. Serve as a first course or a light luncheon dish, or as part of a *zakuska* table.

Marinovannye Griby
PICKLED MUSHROOMS

In a 1½- to 2-quart enameled or stainless-steel saucepan, combine the red wine vinegar, whole cloves, water, peppercorns, bay leaf, salt and crushed garlic. Bring to a boil over high heat, drop in the mushrooms, and reduce the heat to low. Simmer uncovered, for 10 minutes, stirring the mushrooms occasionally, then cool to room temperature.

Remove the garlic from the marinade and pour the entire contents of the pan into a 1-quart jar. Slowly pour the vegetable oil on top, secure the top with plastic wrap, and cover the jar tightly. Marinate the mushrooms in the refrigerator for at least one week.

Serve the pickled mushrooms as part of a *zakuska* table, or as a piquant accompaniment to meat or fish.

Pashtet
LIVER PÂTÉ

In a heavy 10- to 12-inch skillet, heat the oil over high heat until a light haze forms above it. Drop in the calf or beef liver and, stirring constantly, fry until the pieces are golden brown. With a rubber spatula scrape the liver into a mixing bowl.

Melt the 2 tablespoons of butter in the same skillet and add the carrot and onions. Cook uncovered over moderate heat, stirring occasionally, until the vegetables are soft but not brown, then add them to the liver in the bowl. Stir in the chopped parsley and put the entire mixture through the finest blade of a meat grinder.

With a large spoon, beat in the salt, pepper and nutmeg, then beat in the 8 tablespoons of butter, 1 tablespoon at a time. Purée the mixture through the finest blade of a food mill and taste for seasoning. Spoon the pâté into a 1- to 1½-quart mold, smooth the top and cover with plastic wrap. Refrigerate for at least 8 hours, or until firm.

Serve the pâté directly from the mold or, if you prefer, unmold the pâté in the following fashion: Run a knife around the edge of the mold and invert a flat plate on top. Grasp the plate and mold firmly together and turn them over. The pâté should slide out easily. Surround the pâté with the hard-cooked egg halves and serve as a first course, in an open sandwich, or on the *zakuska* table.

To serve 6 to 8

¼ cup vegetable oil
1 pound calf's or baby beef liver, carefully trimmed and cut into ½-inch dice
2 tablespoons unsalted butter
1 carrot, scraped and coarsely chopped
1 cup coarsely chopped onions
1 tablespoon finely chopped parsley
1½ teaspoons salt
⅛ teaspoon finely ground black pepper
⅛ teaspoon ground nutmeg
8 tablespoons unsalted butter, softened (¼-pound stick)
4 hard-cooked eggs, peeled and halved

Pochki v Madere
KIDNEYS IN MADEIRA SAUCE

Cut the kidneys crosswise into ½-inch-thick slices. Dip the slices in flour one at a time and shake them vigorously to rid them of any excess flour. Melt the butter in a 10- to 12-inch enameled or stainless-steel skillet over high heat. When the butter begins to brown, drop in the kidneys, and stirring them frequently, cook 2 or 3 minutes on each side, or until they are lightly browned.

With a slotted spoon or tongs, transfer the kidneys to a heated plate and pour the Madeira into the pan. Raise the heat to high and boil briskly, meanwhile scraping in any brown particles clinging to the bottom of the pan. Continue to boil briskly, uncovered, until the wine has cooked down to about ½ cup. Reduce the heat to low and, with a whisk, beat in the sour cream, a tablespoon at a time. Return the kidneys to the pan, stir to coat them thoroughly with the sauce, and simmer another minute or so to heat them through. Sprinkle with salt and pepper, taste for seasoning, and serve at once, as a first course or on a *zakuska* table.

To serve 4

4 veal kidneys, trimmed of their knobs of fat
¼ cup all-purpose flour
4 tablespoons butter
1 cup Madeira wine
6 tablespoons sour cream
2 teaspoons salt
¼ teaspoon freshly ground black pepper

Bef Stroganov

SAUTÉED BEEF WITH MUSHROOMS AND ONIONS IN SOUR-CREAM SAUCE

Created in the late 19th Century for a Russian count, "bef Stroganov" has become one of the world's famous dishes. The recipe that follows is the classic Russian version. The numerous European and American variations called beef Stroganov do not in any sense reproduce the dish as it was originally made.

To serve 4 to 6

1 tablespoon powdered mustard
1 tablespoon sugar
2 teaspoons salt
4 to 5 tablespoons vegetable oil
4 cups thinly sliced onions separated
    into rings
1 pound fresh mushrooms, thinly
    sliced lengthwise
2 pounds fillet of beef, trimmed of
    all fat
1 teaspoon freshly ground black
    pepper
1 pint sour cream

In a small bowl combine the mustard, 1½ teaspoons of the sugar, a pinch of the salt and enough hot water (perhaps a tablespoon) to form a thick paste. Let the mustard rest at room temperature for about 15 minutes.

Heat 2 tablespoons of the oil in a heavy 10- to 12-inch skillet over high heat until a light haze forms above it. Drop in the onions and mushrooms, cover the pan, and reduce the heat to low. Stirring from time to time, simmer 20 to 30 minutes, or until the vegetables are soft. Drain them in a sieve, discard the liquid and return the mixture to the skillet.

With a large, sharp knife cut the fillet across the grain into ¼-inch-wide rounds. Lay each round on a board and slice it with the grain into ¼-inch-wide strips. Heat 2 tablespoons of oil in another heavy 10- to 12-inch skillet over high heat until very hot but not smoking. Drop in half the meat and, tossing the strips constantly with a large spoon, fry for 2 minutes or so until the meat is lightly browned. With a slotted spoon transfer the meat to the vegetables in the other skillet and fry the remaining meat similarly, adding additional oil if necessary. When all the meat has been combined with the vegetables, stir in the remaining salt, pepper and the mustard paste. Stir in the sour cream, a tablespoon at a time, then add the remaining ½ teaspoon of sugar and reduce the heat to low. Cover the pan and simmer 2 or 3 minutes, or until the sauce is heated through. Taste for seasoning.

To serve *bef Stroganov*, transfer the contents of the pan to a heated serving platter and, if you like, scatter straw potatoes *(Recipe Index)* over the top.

Salat Olivier

TART CHICKEN SALAD WITH SOUR-CREAM DRESSING

To serve 6

2 whole chicken breasts, about ¾
    pound each
1 large onion, peeled and quartered
2 teaspoons salt
½ cup coarsely chopped, drained,
    sour dill pickles
4 boiled new potatoes, cooled,
    peeled, and thinly sliced
3 hard-cooked eggs, peeled and
    thinly sliced
⅛ teaspoon white pepper
¾ cup mayonnaise, freshly made or
    a good unsweetened commercial
    variety
¾ cup sour cream
2 tablespoons capers, drained,
    washed, and patted dry with paper
    towels
1 tablespoon finely cut fresh dill
    leaves
6 green olives
1 medium tomato, peeled *(see borshch
    ukraïnsky, page 141)* and cut
    lengthwise into eighths
1 small head Boston lettuce, the
    leaves separated, washed and dried
    with paper towels

In a heavy 2- to 3-quart pot, combine the chicken, onion and 1 teaspoon of the salt. Cover with about 1½ quarts of cold water and bring to a boil uncovered over high heat, skimming off the fat and scum as it rises to the surface. Partially cover the pan, reduce the heat to low, and simmer about 10 minutes, or until the chicken is tender. Remove the chicken from the pot and with a small, sharp knife, remove and discard the skin and cut the meat away from the bones. Cut the chicken meat into strips about ½ inch wide and combine them in a large mixing bowl with the pickles, potatoes and eggs. Sprinkle with the remaining teaspoon of salt and ⅛ teaspoon of white pepper. In a small bowl, beat together the mayonnaise and sour cream, and stir half of it into the salad. Taste for seasoning.

To serve *salat Olivier* in the traditional Russian manner, shape the salad into a pyramid in the middle of a serving platter. Mask with the remaining sour-cream-and-mayonnaise dressing and sprinkle it with capers and dill. Decorate with olives, tomatoes and lettuce leaves.

Bef Stroganov, created by a French chef, is a blend of favorite Russian foods—fine beef, plump mushrooms, yellow onions—served in a spicy sour-cream sauce and customarily strewn with crisp straw potatoes.

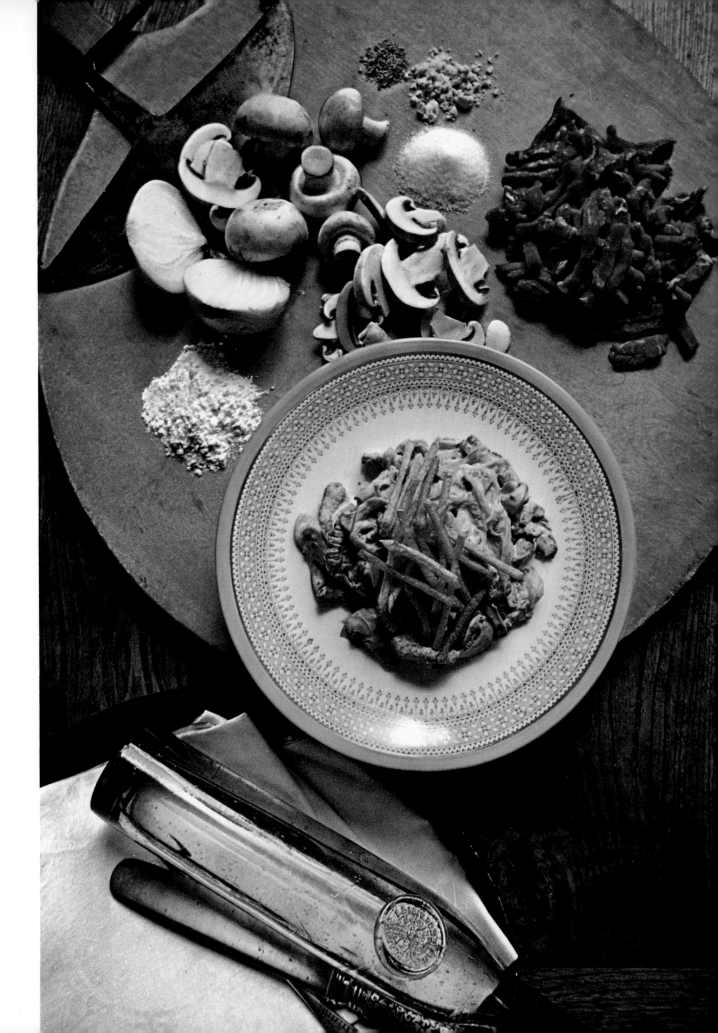

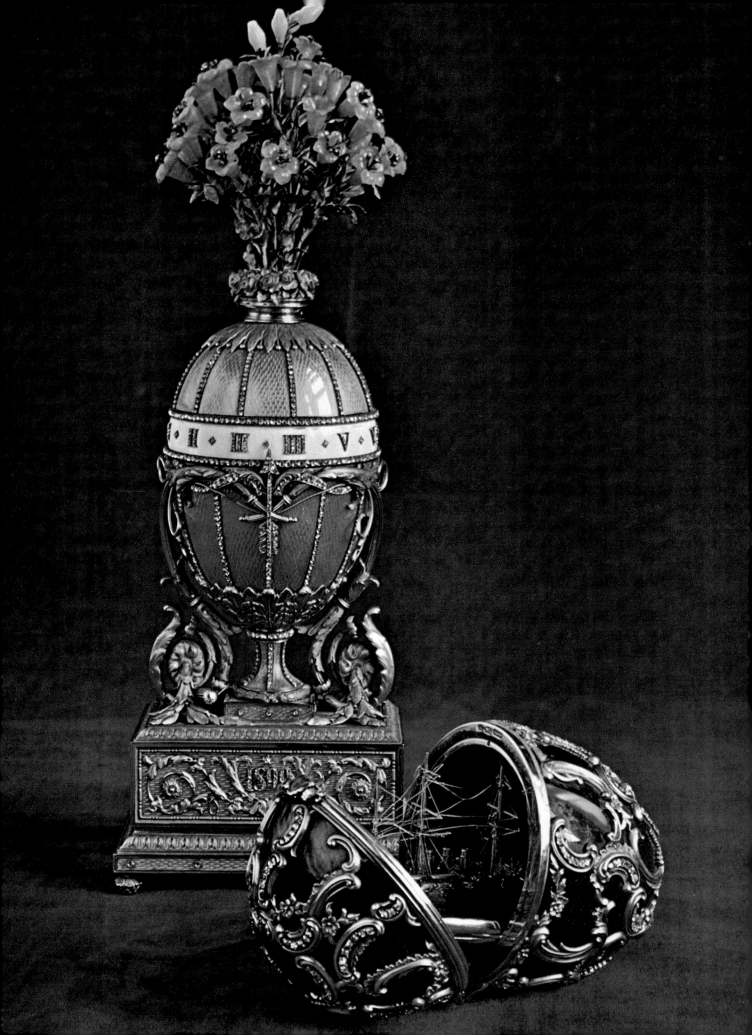

II

The Glory that Easter Celebrates

Two Easter eggs from the hand of Imperial Jeweler Karl Fabergé combine delicate fantasy with the dazzle of jewels and precious metals. The egg on the pedestal, presented by Czar Nicholas II to his Czarina in 1899, supports a vase of diamond-centered lilies and has a rotating clock with diamond numerals. The second egg, opened to display a model of the Imperial Navy cruiser *Pamiat Azova*, was the Easter gift of Czar Alexander III to his consort.

Russians celebrate a full calendar of holidays, public and private, traditional and newly invented, religious and completely secular. On Labor Day (May 1) and Revolution Day (November 7) the streets in every city are festooned with lights and banked with flowers, banners whip in the breeze, endless parades flow past reviewing stands and at night bands play and promenaders watch fireworks that emblazon patriotic slogans across the sky.

New Year's Day is especially dedicated to children, with troika rides through the countryside, trips to the circus, ballet and puppet theater and a visit from Ded Moroz, or Grandfather Frost, who distributes presents and spicy ginger cakes with a lavish hand.

On wedding anniversaries and "name days" (the saints' days that are celebrated as birthdays in Eastern Orthodox lands) friends and families often prepare surprise parties complete with decorated tables, delectable food, icy vodka, toasts, bouquets, gifts, tears, jokes, music, champagne and more toasts. At such parties the note of the past is generally stronger: the traditional drink is hot chocolate served from a copper casserole, and the classic cake obligatory for the occasion is the pretzel-shaped sweet bread called *krendel (Recipe Index)*.

Of all the Russian holidays, the one most deeply rooted in the Slavic past is Easter. On that day Russians around the world share a tradition older than their written history. Emigrés crowd Orthodox churches and cathedrals in alien lands—in Paris, San Francisco, New York, Hong Kong. In the Soviet Union, too, the churches are full, and even people who have abandoned the rituals and beliefs of Eastern Orthodoxy keep the day—from habit, from nostalgia or as a gesture of affection and respect for parents and grandparents.

For Orthodox Russians the preparation for Easter begins in February or early March, seven weeks in advance of the feast itself. It is a bleak season in the north. Short gray days and long cold nights seem to merge into endless wintertime. Ice locks the rivers, and snow falls on snow. The bare trees are black skeletons against the pewter sky. But just when winter seems unendurable and atavistic doubts about spring's return begin to gnaw at even the most rational mind, it is suddenly the week-long Maslenitsa, or "Butter Festival" that precedes the 40 days of Lent.

In pre-Revolutionary Russia Maslenitsa was the occasion for a seven-day carnival. In Moscow and St. Petersburg and in the villages, too, figures in masks and costumes raced through the streets. Men and women, young and old, took turns sliding down elaborately constructed ice hills. The gentry went to balls; traveling troupes entertained the peasants. Every meal was a feast, with mounds of hot *bliny* dripping butter; every mouthful was enhanced in savor and importance by the thought of the long fast ahead.

The last day of the Maslenitsa festivities brought a climax at once gay and melancholy. A straw "Prince Carnival," seated at a bountiful table, was set on a sled and drawn through the streets.

"Stay! Stay!" cried the rollicking crowds as he passed. "Stay with us forever!"

But Prince Carnival's brief reign was over for the year. At the end of his triumphal ride he was enthroned on a bonfire and at sundown he was ceremoniously burned.

In recent times the celebration of Maslenitsa week has been reduced to informal *bliny* parties. We were fortunate enough not long ago to be invited to one in Leningrad by a retired professor, a widower in his eighties, who promised to prepare the *bliny* himself. He was as good as his word. On the appointed night we braved a wind as sharp as a boning knife and walked across a snowy park to his warm, cheerful, flower-filled apartment, fragrant with yeasty dough and hot butter. *Zakuska* was on the table. Vodka stood ready. The other guests had all arrived.

"Please be seated," said our host, "and One—Two—Three! You shall have *bliny*."

Long experience has taught me that in culinary affairs "One—Two —Three!" operations are usually highly skilled performances, well worth watching, and I received permission to stand by and ask questions.

The batter stood ready in a stone crock. It was made, the professor told me, according to his great-grandmother's recipe. A sponge of warm milk, white flour and yeast was allowed to rest and rise overnight. On the morning of the party, buckwheat flour, melted butter, egg yolks, a little salt and sugar were beaten in, and the dough was set in a warm place for a second rising. Just before the guests arrived, stiffly beaten egg whites were folded in.

This Russian kitchen, like many others, had a set of nested *bliny* pans so that several cakes could be fried at once. A lump of butter went into each hot pan to melt and then the professor poured in enough dough to make a very thin, three-inch cake, turned only once. A minute to a side produced a deep golden surface, faintly freckled with brown.

"One—Two—Three!" We were back at the table, eating *bliny* with glis-

Continued on page 49

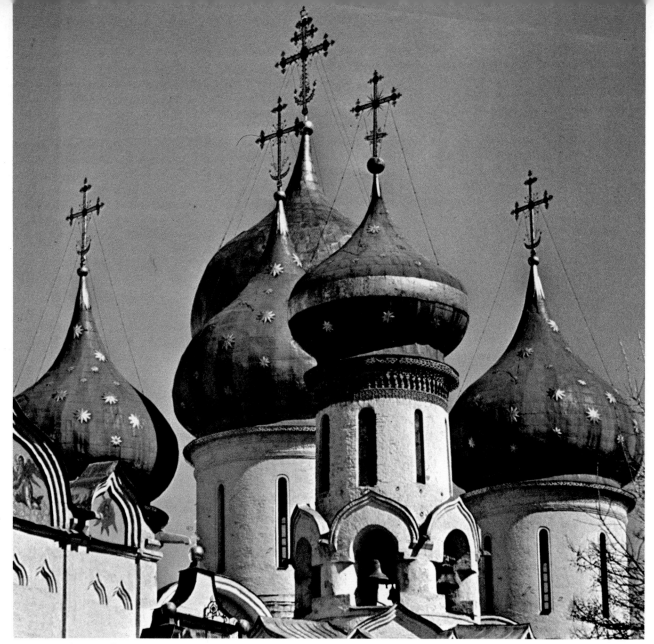

The onion domes of Zagorsk's Troitsky Cathedral, studded with stars and topped by golden crosses, overlook the Troitse-Sergiyeva Monastery, founded in 1340 by the monk Saint Sergius of Radonezh. Here, every spring, food is still brought for Eastertime blessing. The monastery complex of 11 churches and a number of other shrines and buildings is surrounded by a high, thick wall. It often served as a refuge in times of war.

The Unconquerable Feast of Easter

For nearly 1,000 years Easter has been the principal feast day of the Russian calendar, and the Orthodox Easter continues to be celebrated wherever there are Russians to celebrate it, from Smolensk to San Francisco. In churches there is stirring incantation and ritual; at home, equally stirring feasts that progress from appetizers to roasts to rich cakes. In some respects, the rites predate Christianity itself. When Prince Vladimir of Kiev brought Christianity to Russia in the 10th Century, he overlaid Easter upon an older festival that marked the end of bleak winter. "The goodness hidden in the hearts of the holy shall be revealed in their risen bodies just as bare trees put out their leaves in spring," promises an old sermon, and Easter still gains part of its power from this joyful analogy.

41

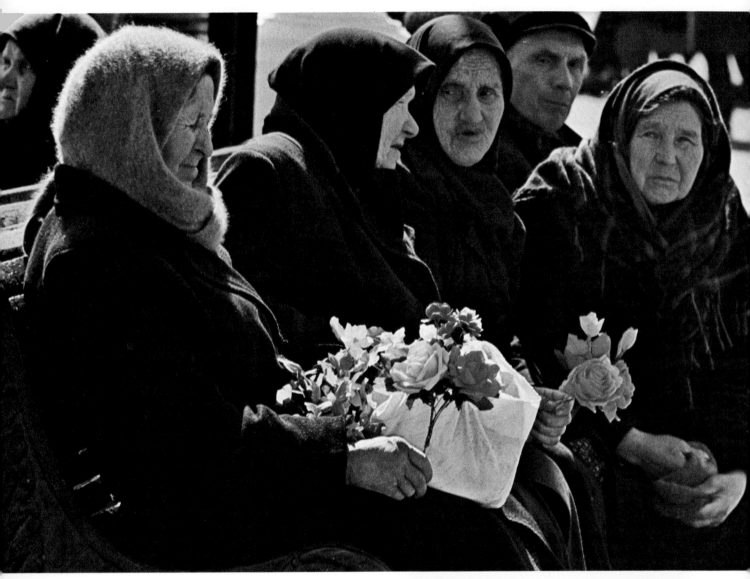

In the courtyard of a 17th century
church, St. Nicholas, in Moscow's
Khamovniki district, women wait for
a priest to bless the Easter cakes they
have wrapped in clean white napkins
(the sprigs of paper flowers will be
used to decorate the cakes). The
special Easter cakes called *kulich* and
paskha, along with the famous dyed
Easter eggs, become an essential part
of the Russian Orthodox celebration.
Particularly important to the day's
ceremonies because it receives a
blessing is the *kulich (right),* a tall
cylindrical yeast cake filled with
raisins and nuts and often iced before
being taken to the church.

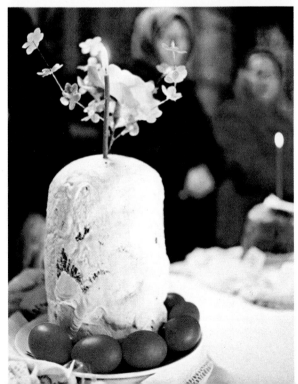

Women unwrap their *kulichi* and set them out for blessing at the Uspenski Cathedral at Zagorsk, one of the many churches in the complex of buildings that make up the Troitse-Sergiyeva Monastery. Depending on the degree of their piety, worshippers may attend only the midnight Resurrection service or stay on through the long Easter mass that follows, ending about 4 a.m. In either case, attendance at church is invariably followed by a feast at home. The classic Russian Easter meal begins with vodka and *zakuska* (appetizers) and ends with *kulich* and *paskha;* in between (for those who can afford it) come cold hams baked in rye dough, the spicy sausage called *kolbase,* cold baked ducks, a chicken-based *salat Olivier,* a cold suckling pig and, of course, Easter eggs.

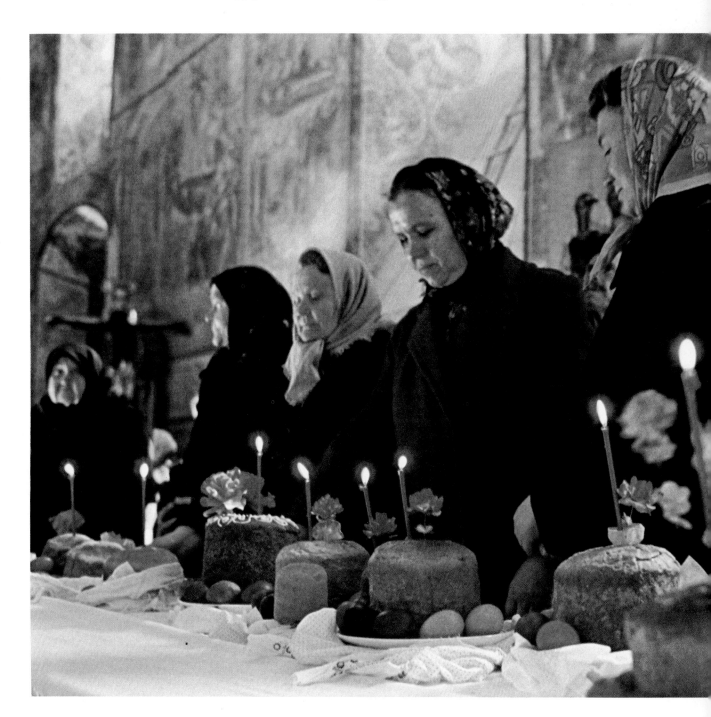

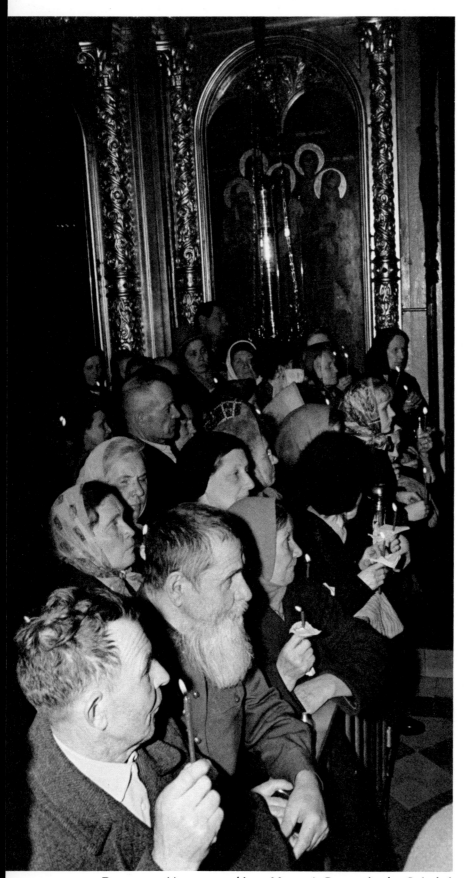

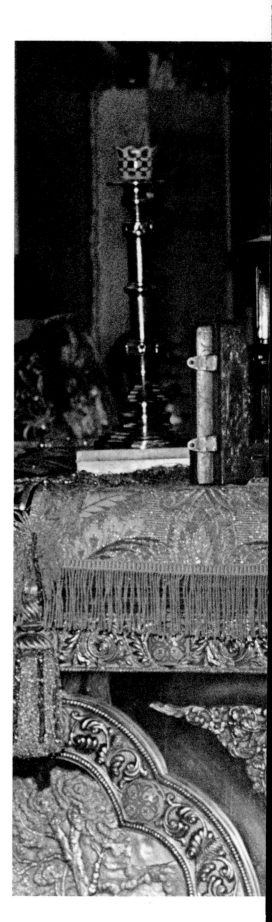

Devout worshippers assemble at Moscow's Bogoyavlensky Cathedral.

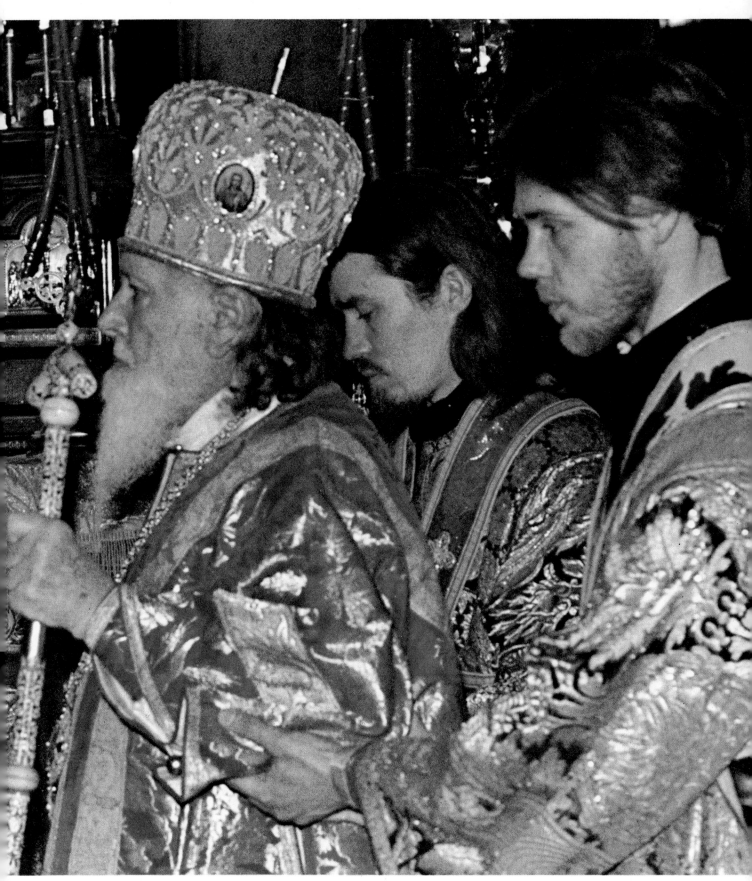

Wearing his miter and followed by attendants, Patriarch Alexis approaches the altar during the Holy Saturday ceremony.

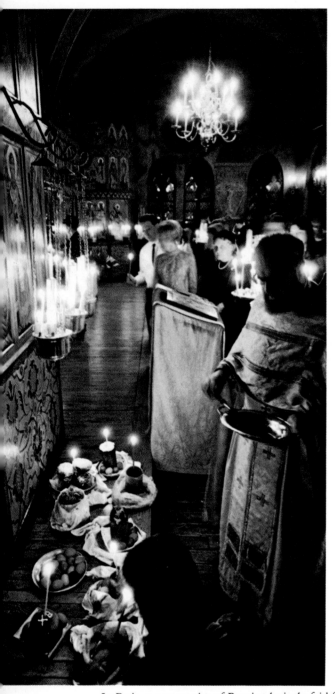

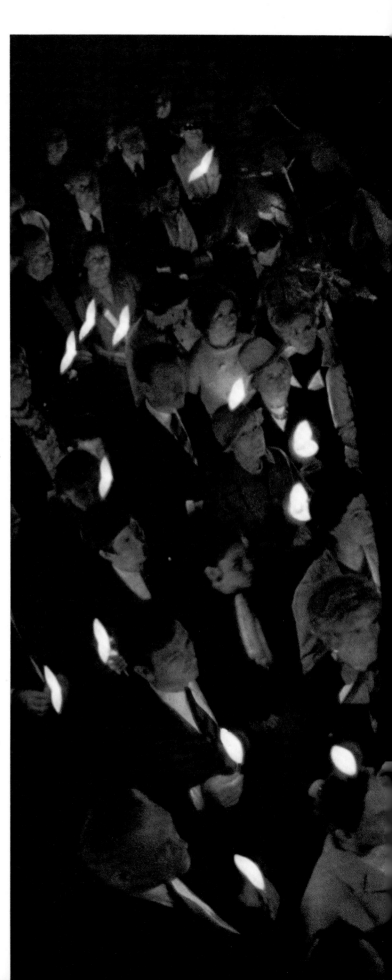

In Paris, a community of Russian émigrés faithfully
observe the ancient Easter of their homeland. Above,
at St. Sergius Russian Orthodox Church, a priest
holds a salver of holy water and a straw whisk to
sprinkle the *kulichi* and eggs arrayed before him. At
right, worshippers leave the church carrying candles.
They will parade around the building three times,
led by the priests and a choir. After the last circuit, a
priest will proclaim "Christos voskres!"—"Christ is
risen!"—and the congregation will respond
"Voistinu voskres!"—"Truly he is risen!"

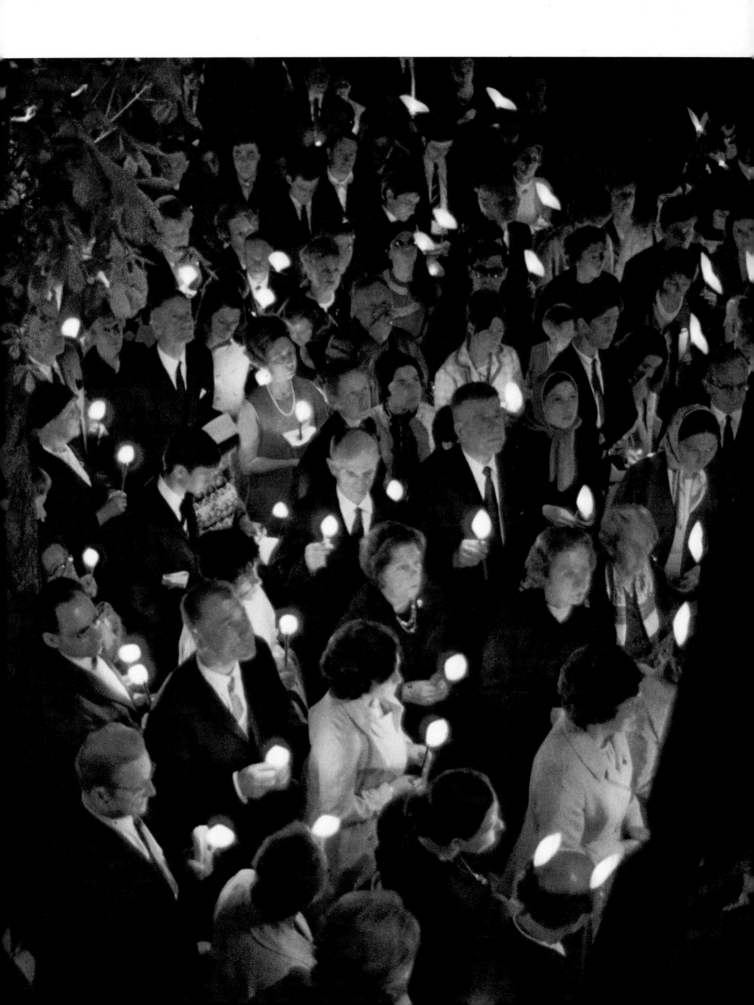

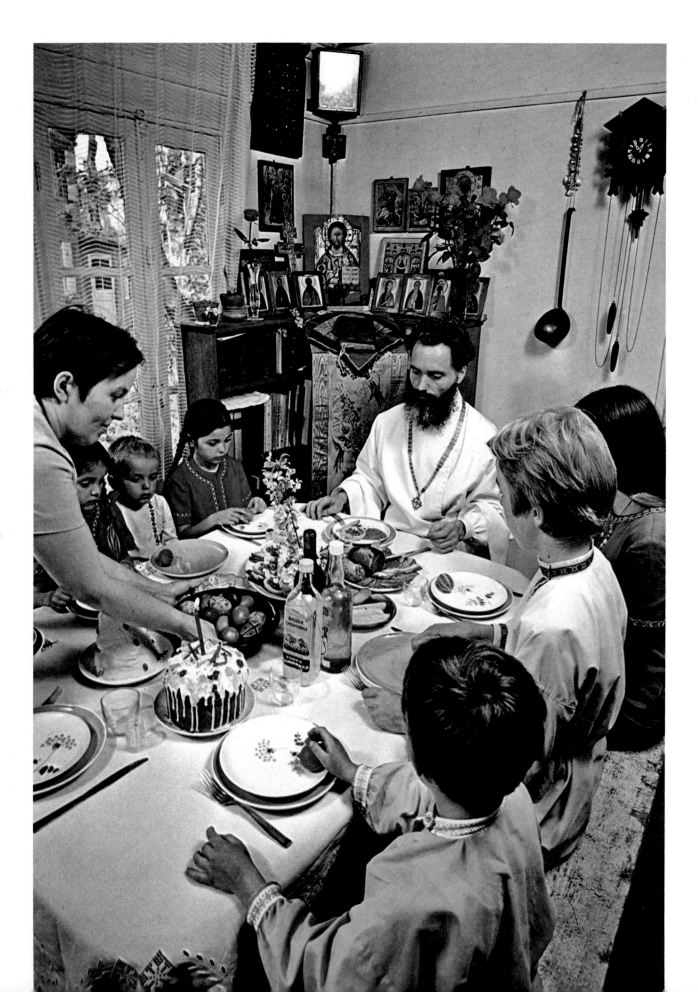

tening sturgeon, pickled herring and heaping mounds of black caviar. After this we had *bliny* laved in melted butter; next came *bliny* stuffed with a mixture of finely chopped mushrooms and onions. When we showed signs of faltering our host reminded us that in the old days *bliny* were served at *every* meal through the whole week of Maslenitsa.

"Often, I remember, my father would eat 30 or 40 at a sitting—and if he were hungry, perhaps 50 or 60. So please, take another."

We all did and between bites we discussed other ways of preparing the batter—with all-wheat flour, with some rye, with baking powder instead of yeast—but no method, we all agreed, could produce better *bliny* than the ones we were eating. It was midnight before we had a final tea and ate the final farewell *bliny*, with black currant jam and sour cream.

Walking home through the silent streets, our boots crunching on fresh dry snow, it seemed warmer, somehow; crossing the park, we were not surprised to see swelling buds on a lilac bush.

Immediately after Maslenitsa week the long Lenten fast began, and few fasts can ever have been more rigorous than those imposed by the Orthodox Church. Today the observance is not so strict, but in the old days neither meat nor animal products of any kind could be eaten; thus eggs, lard, butter, milk and cheese disappeared from the Russian table. For the rich, these restrictions created no real hardship. They made do with pineapples, strawberries, almond "milk," fish disguised as meat—and, not infrequently, meat disguised as fish. (On one occasion a member of the Youssoupoff family served the Metropolitan, or supreme bishop, of Moscow a Lenten fish cutlet made of goose; the culprit was detected and fined half his fortune for the offense). Meanwhile, peasants appeased their hunger by industriously chewing sunflower seeds or pieces of *vobla*, a dried and salted fish whose principal virtue was a tough texture that kept a man's teeth (though certainly not his gastric juices) busy for a long time.

As Lent neared its end, however, the tempo of life speeded up, for the days immediately preceding Easter have always been busy ones for the Russian housewife. She had to clean her house inside and out. In the old days beds, hangings and carpets were taken into the courtyard to be beaten, brushed and aired, while servants in felt boots shuffle-polished the floors to a mirror gloss. Even today, in the Ukraine, farmhouses are replastered and repainted inside and out every spring.

Above all, there is shopping to be done. At one time peasants loaded sleds with carefully hoarded root vegetables such as beets and potatoes, hauled the sleds across the frozen rivers, and set up booths in the city markets. Now the same markets bloom with fresh spring crops—scallions, radishes, salad greens and new peas carried by air freight from the southern republics. The last things to be purchased are the all-important Easter eggs —perfect, fresh, free from the slightest crack or blemish, thick and smooth of shell. Boiled, dyed and decorated, these eggs will adorn the Easter table and be exchanged with friends.

The decorated egg, which predates Christianity itself, surely reached its zenith in Russia at the turn of the 20th Century. In 1884 Czar Alexander III had Karl Fabergé, his court jeweler, make a special Easter present for the Czarina: a white enamel egg that opened to disclose a "yolk" in the form of a

The family of Yuri Drobot, one of the married Russian Orthodox priests living in Paris, sits down to a modest but meaningful Easter feast. Besides the *kulich* and the *paskha* (decorated with the letters XB, the Cyrillic initials of *Christos voskres*), the Drobots' dinner includes vodka, sliced pickles, sausages and Easter eggs that were painted by the children the day before.

golden hen with ruby eyes. The hen bore a replica of the imperial crown, which in turn held a ruby pendant.

The Czarina's pleasure in the gift (a copy of a similar but simpler conceit she had loved as a child in her native Denmark) encouraged the Czar and his successor, Nicholas II, to commission eggs galore. Soon the royal family and the court were exchanging eggs of rock crystal, colored enamels, gold, platinum and ivory—eggs set with rubies, star sapphires, rose diamonds and pearls, eggs containing as "surprises" miniature carvings of people and places, scale models of buildings, yachts and even a train on the Great Siberian Railway (the engine in platinum, the coaches in gold).

Quite different, and for some tastes more beautiful, were the natural eggs decorated by Ukrainian folk artists in designs so complex and minutely detailed that, in the words of one authority, "a painted egg may well be called a miniature mosaic." Archeological evidence indicates that such eggs were made in the Ukraine thousands of years before the beginning of the Christian Era, and that the technique of making them has remained essentially the same through the millennia. That technique is not simply a matter of painting directly upon the egg; instead a design was traced in beeswax on the shell, and this design was slowly elaborated in stages between repeated dippings in baths of vegetable dyes *(see pages 60-61)*. The finished eggs, with their brilliant colors and their intricate geometrical designs based on sun, star, tripod, cross and flower motifs, were true works of art.

Eggs as fanciful as these, of course, were for the few. Most people were satisfied with the small miracles of solid color they could achieve with homely materials—brittle onion skins for an intense saffron, beet juice for red, birch leaves or moss for green, laundry bluing for blue. Decoration, when any was applied, was either painted or scratched on the shell, and took only the simplest forms—a doubled-barred cross, perhaps, or the Cyrillic letters XB, which stands for *Christos voskres* (Christ is risen).

All this egg artistry still goes on before every Easter. After the eggs are dyed, polished with a buttery cloth, arranged on a dish and set aside, the next step of the Easter preparations is to bake the *kulich* or Easter cake *(Recipe Index)*. Like the *bliny* of Maslenitsa week, *kulich* begins with a sponge that rises overnight. In the morning more flour, along with eggs, butter, raisins, almonds, candied fruits, lemon rind and a glass of liqueur, are mixed into the risen dough and the whole is kneaded for 15 or 20 minutes. The mixture then goes into a special *kulich* pan—which looks rather like a length of stove pipe —to rise again. (Theoretically, a *kulich* could be baked in a spring-form pan, but its 12-inch-tall majesty would then be utterly lost and it would be just another cake.)

When the *kulich* has doubled in bulk it goes into the oven. From that moment a special cook's prayer begins. Heaven be merciful to anyone who sets foot in the kitchen, opens the door or speaks above a whisper before the *kulich* is done. There is no good Russian cook who cannot recount a personal horror story of one black day when a passing cart or truck, a ringing telephone, an exhaled breath "killed my *kulich*."

After the *kulich* is safely out of the oven and the pan—and after the cook has quieted her nerves with a glass or two of tea—she covers the top with a sugar glaze and inscribes XB on the side.

A *baba* is sometimes prepared, too, as an extra pastry—and perhaps a few pans of *mazurki,* which are short, rich cakes and *kvhorost,* crisp little buttery twiglets. After the cakes have baked, the meats are roasted, the fowls boiled, the *zakuska* assembled. Last of all comes the *paskha,* a marvel of cottage cheese, rich cream, eggs, raisins, almonds and candied fruit deposited in a four-sided, perforated wood frame in the shape of a truncated pyramid. The mold is lined with cheesecloth and weighed down so that the surplus liquids in the ingredients can seep out. But this mold has more than a purely utilitarian function; it usually has a cross and an XB design carved on its inner sides, so that when the *paskha* emerges it is already decorated.

Very early on the Saturday before Easter Sunday, the festal table is set, always with a white cloth. The Easter eggs are placed at one end, the *kulich* and the *paskha* at the other. Before the family goes to church—usually at 11 o'clock Saturday evening—the *zakuska* and other foods are set out along with the plates, vodkas and glasses.

In the old days a priest used to visit his more aristocratic parishioners and bless their Easter food. Those who could not hope for such an honor brought their holiday fare to the church for the blessing and carried it home again, the *paskha* held carefully in a wicker basket.

The church is full as Easter Sunday approaches. Candles flicker, throwing their light off the golden tracery of the priests' vestments and the jewel-encrusted altar vessels. Just before midnight sonorous voices chant the offices; the swell of the choir rises to fill the vaulted domes. Processions of priests, deacons and the congregation itself move outdoors and circle the church, censers swinging and candles glowing. Then it is midnight. Easter Sunday has come. Families and friends exchange kisses (as they will continue to do, in greeting and farewell, until the official end of the Easter season 50 days later).

"Christos voskres!"—"Christ is risen!"

The answer is returned: "Voistinu voskres!"—"Truly He is risen!"

Now everyone goes home to the waiting tables—to *zakuska,* vodka, ham baked in a crust, a cold turkey in a galantine and a suckling pig roasted to a crackling brown and wreathed in radish roses. Relatives arrive. Friends appear. Greetings are exchanged, again and again. More plates, more chairs, more napkins materialize.

The party rests and naps from time to time, but it never really stops before Sunday night. For three more days, in fact, nothing will be cooked or reheated; the festal table will be sampled again and again. Long before then the *paskha* is tried and pronounced excellent; the *kulich* is cut in rounds across the top, and we hear how it nearly collapsed. And we select an Easter egg with careful attention to the toughness of the pointed end, for we are going to crack eggs together, and by a process of elimination determine who has the strongest one.

The contest is joined; some side bets are made. Accusations are hurled: this egg is not being held straight, that one was struck off center. Finally a victor with an iron-shelled egg and a clever technique emerges—and then, inevitably, he is suddenly defeated by a little boy or girl.

It is Easter. Spring has come again and the world has awakened from its long, dark winter.

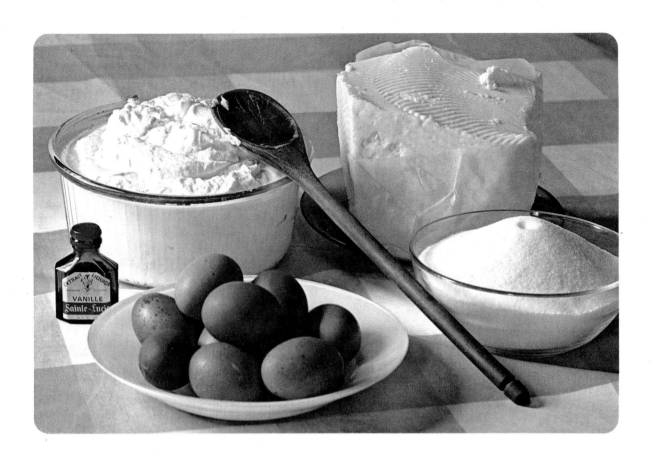

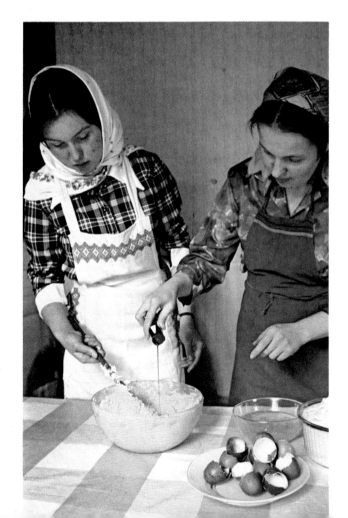

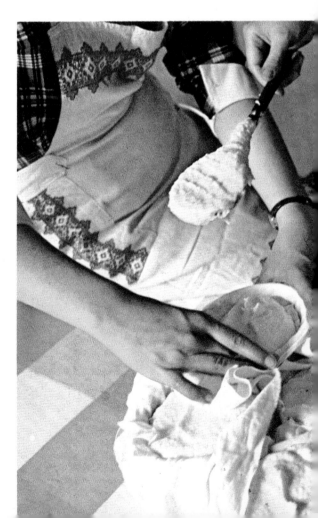

From Pot Cheese and a Few Eggs, a Paskha for the Easter Feast

Priest Yuri Drobot is a man of modest means; the *paskha* that he and his family will share on Easter Sunday in Paris is not nearly so elaborate as the classic nut-and-fruit-filled version made with heavy cream. Nevertheless, the Drobots' *paskha* has the essential ingredients, shown at left: vanilla, puréed pot cheese, unsalted butter, sugar and eggs. The Drobots start work on their *paskha* three days before Easter. Anna Drobot, 15, and her mother *(below, far left)* combine the butter, sugar and eggs and add a dash of vanilla before mixing in the pot cheese. Since the parents and the four oldest Drobot children are all observing a strict Lenten fast, four-year-old André has the job of tasting, a heavy responsibility that he gravely carries out as his mother and sister fill the *paskha* molds *(center)*. The molds will be placed in the refrigerator, weighted down to compress the mixture, for at least eight hours. In the meantime Mme. Drobot undertakes her other Easter duties, such as making and baking the *kulich (right)*.

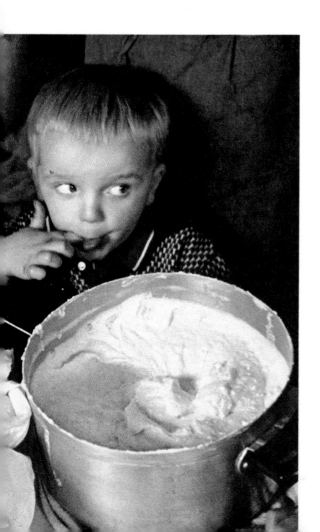

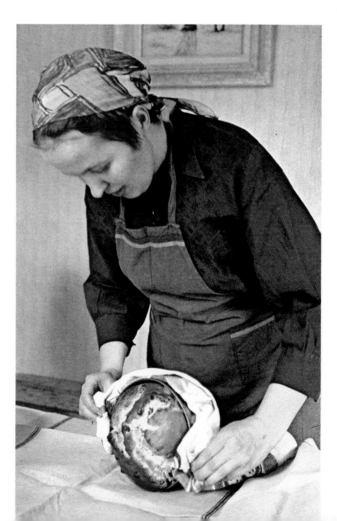

In the Drobot family the children are given—and
joyfully accept—the job of coloring the Easter eggs,
under the supervision of 13-year-old Yuri *(below)*, the
best painter of the group. The children generally color
the eggs with conventional solid dyes, but they also use
oil paints and water colors for more intricate patterns.
At right the four elder Drobot children, all hard at
work, are *(from left)* Maria, nine; Yuri; Alexandra,
seven and Serge, five (four-year-old André must wait
another year for his chance). The association of eggs
and Easter is an ancient one; the egg was a symbol of
the creation of new life even in pre-Christian times.

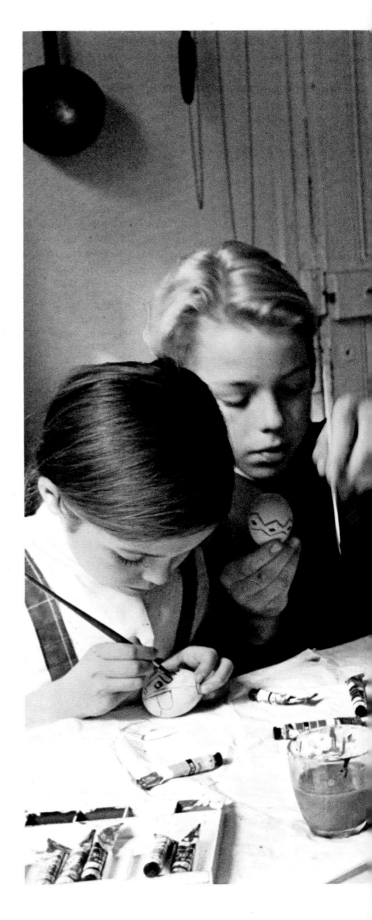

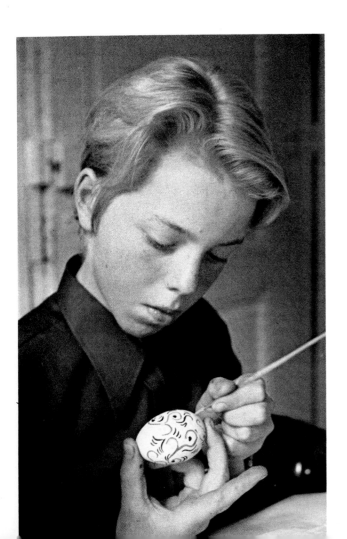

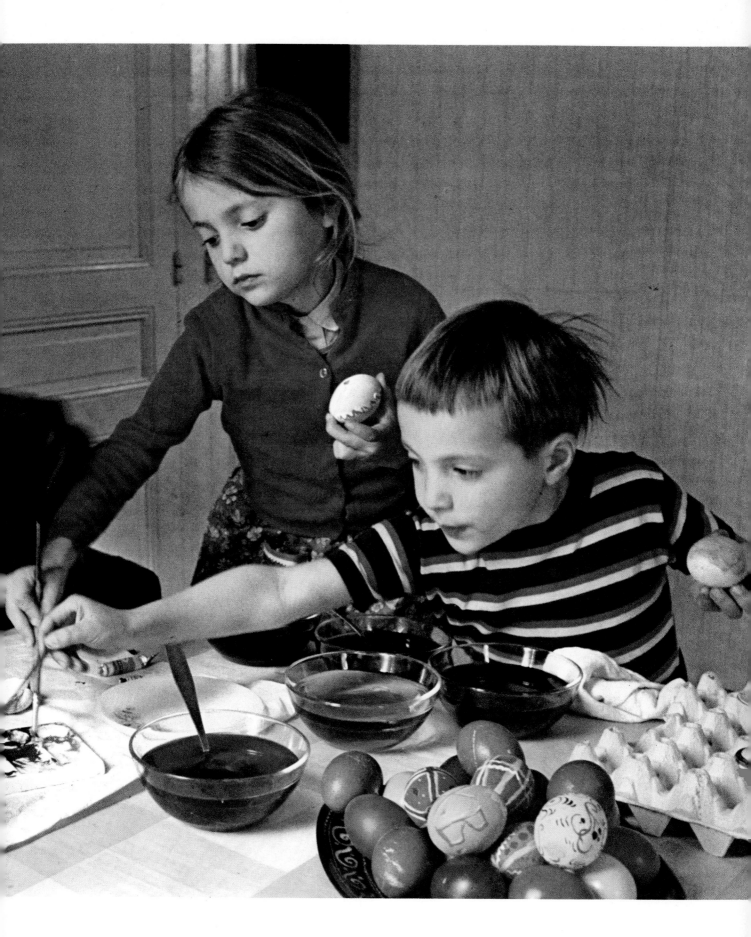

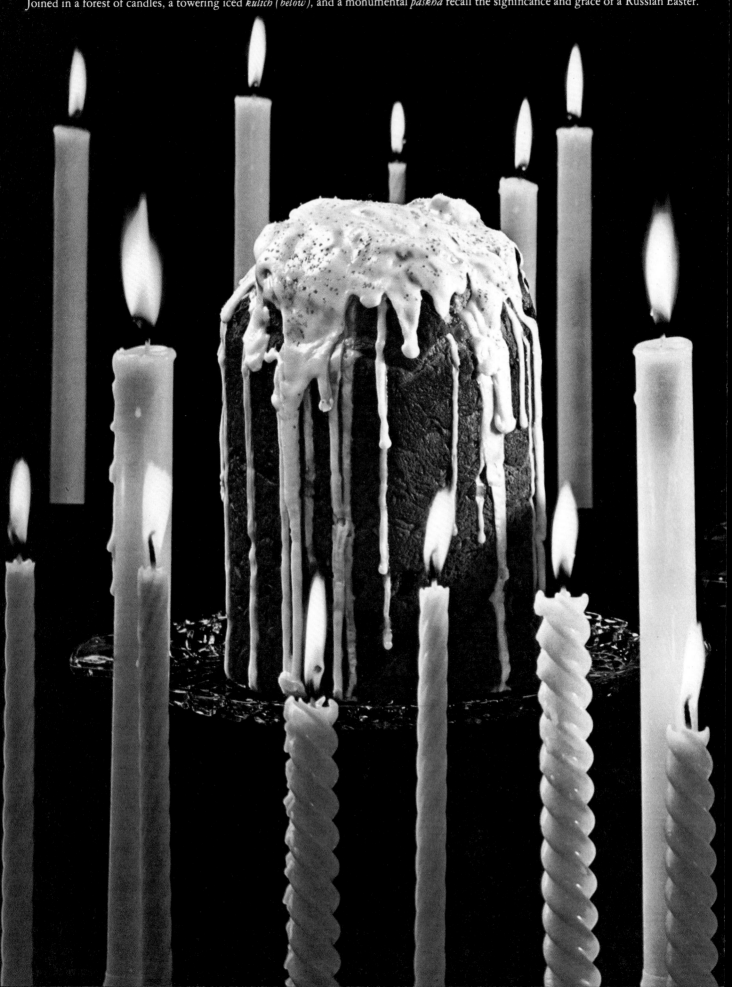

Joined in a forest of candles, a towering iced *kulich* (*below*), and a monumental *paskha* recall the significance and grace of a Russian Easter.

To serve 10 to 12

1 cup lukewarm milk (110° to 115°)
3 packages active dry yeast
½ teaspoon sugar
½ cup sultana raisins
¼ cup rum
2 cups confectioners' sugar
3½ to 5 cups all-purpose flour
1 teaspoon vanilla extract
10 egg yolks
½ teaspoon powdered saffron
½ pound unsalted butter, cut into
    small bits and softened
½ cup slivered or coarsely chopped
    blanched almonds
½ cup mixed candied fruits and
    rinds
3 tablespoons butter, softened

WHITE ICING
2 cups confectioners' sugar
¼ cup cold water
2 teaspoons fresh, strained lemon
    juice

Kulich

EASTER COFFEE CAKE WITH NUTS AND RAISINS

Pour ½ cup of the lukewarm milk into a small, shallow bowl and sprinkle it with the yeast and the ½ teaspoon sugar. Let the mixture stand for 2 or 3 minutes, then stir to dissolve the yeast completely. Set the bowl aside in a warm, draft-free place (such as an unlighted oven) for about 10 minutes, or until the mixture almost doubles in volume.

Soak the sultana raisins in the rum for at least 10 minutes.

Preheat the oven to 400°. Sift the confectioners' sugar and 3½ cups of the flour through a fine sieve set over a large mixing bowl. Slowly pour in the dissolved yeast mixture and the remaining ½ cup of milk, stirring constantly until a stiff batter is formed. Beat in the vanilla and the egg yolks, one at a time. When the mixture becomes too stiff to stir, knead it vigorously with your hands until the dough is smooth and elastic.

With a slotted spoon, remove the raisins from the rum and spread them out on paper towels to drain. Then dissolve the saffron in the rum and pour the saffron and rum over the dough. Knead the dough with your hands until all the liquid is absorbed, and knead or beat in the butter, a few bits at a time, until well combined.

Gather the dough into a compact ball and place it on a lightly floured surface. Knead it by pushing it down with the heels of your hands, pressing it forward, and folding it back on itself. Repeat this process for about 10 minutes. If the dough begins to stick at any point, add as much of the additional flour as you need, ½ cup at a time. Continue to knead until the dough is satiny and elastic, then gather it into a ball again. Place it in a lightly buttered bowl, dust the top lightly with flour and cover the bowl with a kitchen towel. Set aside in the warm, draft-free place for about 1 hour, or until the dough doubles in volume.

Meanwhile, spread the almonds out in a single layer in a cake tin and toast them in the oven for 5 minutes, or until they are lightly and evenly colored, turning them from time to time. In a small bowl, combine the almonds with the candied fruits and raisins. Sprinkle them with a tablespoon of flour and toss them together with your hands.

With a sharp blow of your fist, punch the dough down in the bowl. Add the fruit mixture and knead vigorously until the mixture is more or less evenly distributed throughout the dough.

With a can opener, remove and discard the bottom of an empty can about 6 inches wide and 7 inches high—such as a 3-pound coffee tin. With a pastry brush, coat the sides of the tin with 2 tablespoons of the softened butter. Spread 1 tablespoon of butter on a sheet of heavy brown paper about 22 inches long and use it, unbuttered side in, to line the tin. Let the excess paper hang over the outside of the tin, and tie it around securely with kitchen cord to prevent its rising out of the tin when the cake expands in baking.

Set the tin on a cookie sheet or baking tin and drop in the ball of dough. Cover it loosely with a kitchen towel and set the mold aside in the warm, draft-free spot for another 30 minutes, or until it again doubles in volume and has risen almost to the top of the mold. Bake in the center of the 400°

oven for 15 minutes, then lower the temperature to 350° and bake one hour. The cake will mushroom over the top of the tin and form a cap. Remove the tin from the oven and carefully lift out the cake. Set it upright on a wire cake rack to cool.

ICING: With a wooden spoon, mix together the sugar, water and lemon juice and pour it over the top of the warm cake, allowing it to run down the cake in thin streams.

The Russians prepare *kulich* for serving by first slicing off the mushroom-shaped cap and placing it in the center of a large serving platter. The cake is cut in half lengthwise and finally cut crosswise into 1½- to 2-inch-thick slices. The slices are then arranged around the top of the cake. A traditional accompaniment is *paskha (below)*.

Paskha

EASTER CHEESE PYRAMID WITH CANDIED FRUIT AND NUTS

Drain the pot cheese of all its moisture by setting it in a colander, covering it with cheesecloth or a kitchen towel, and weighting it down with a heavy pot or a small, heavy board. Let the cheese drain for 2 or 3 hours. Meanwhile, combine the candied fruits and the vanilla extract in a small mixing bowl, stir together thoroughly and let the mixture rest for 1 hour. With the back of a wooden spoon, rub the cheese through a fine sieve set over a large bowl. Beat the softened butter thoroughly into the cheese, and set aside.

Over high heat, heat the cream in a small saucepan until small bubbles form around the edge of the pan. Set aside. In a mixing bowl beat the eggs and sugar together with a whisk or a rotary or electric beater until they thicken enough to run sluggishly off the beater when it is lifted out of the bowl. Still beating, slowly add the hot cream in a thin stream, then return the mixture to the pan. Stirring constantly, cook over low heat until the mixture thickens to a custardlike consistency. Do not allow it to boil or it may curdle. Off the heat stir in the candied fruits and set the pan in a large bowl filled with ice cubes covered with 2 inches of water. Stir the custard constantly with a metal spoon until it is completely cooled, then mix it gently but thoroughly into the cheese mixture and stir in the chopped almonds.

Although the Russians use a special *paskha* form in which to shape this Easter dessert a 2-quart clay flower pot with an opening in the bottom is a good substitute. Set the pot in a shallow soup plate and line it with a double thickness of damp cheesecloth, cut long enough so that it hangs at least 2 inches over and around the top of the pot. Pour in the batter and fold the ends of the cheesecloth lightly over the top. Set a weight directly on top of the cheesecloth—perhaps a pan filled with 2 or 3 heavy cans of food—and chill in the refrigerator for at least 8 hours, or overnight, until the dessert is firm.

To unmold, unwrap the cheesecloth from the top, invert a flat serving plate on top of the pot and, grasping the two firmly together, turn them over. The *paskha* will slide out easily. Gently peel off the cheesecloth and decorate the top and sides of the cake as fancifully as you like with the almonds and candied fruits.

The *paskha* may be served alone, or spread in a thick layer on slices of *kulich (left)*, or on sand cake *(Recipe Index)*. Once unmolded, the *paskha* can be safely kept refrigerated for at least a week before serving.

To serve 12 to 16

3 pounds large-curd pot cheese
½ pound unsalted butter, softened
½ cup chopped candied fruits and rinds
1 teaspoon vanilla extract
1 cup heavy cream
4 egg yolks
1 cup sugar
½ cup finely chopped blanched almonds

GARNISH
¼ to ½ cup whole blanched almonds, toasted *(see kulich, opposite)*
¼ to ½ cup candied fruits and rinds

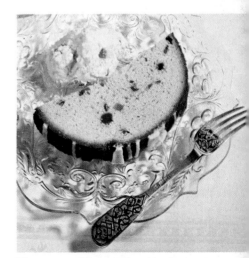

The creamy richness of *paskha*, in which cheese, candied fruits and nuts are blended into an elegant pyramid, is best appreciated when served with slices of its traditional Easter partner, *kulich (recipes on these pages)*. For simpler tastes *paskha* may be complemented by a pound cake.

Decorating Eggs the Ukrainian Way

Easter eggs decorated with intricate and colorful designs have been a Ukrainian art form for centuries. The tools and techniques demonstrated here can be used to produce traditional Ukrainian motifs or your own improvisations. In either case the basic principle is simple: using the equipment shown below (*see page 206*), a raw white egg is dipped into successively darker colors of dye, while areas to be protected against a dye at any stage are covered with beeswax.

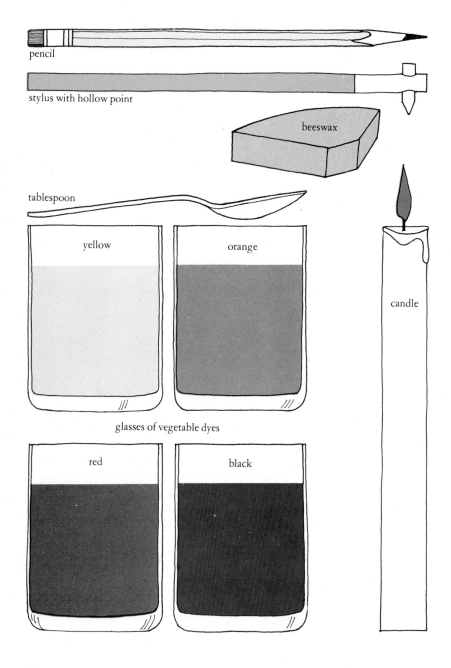

pencil

stylus with hollow point

beeswax

tablespoon

yellow

orange

candle

glasses of vegetable dyes

red

black

1. Holding the pencil steady in one hand and rotating the egg in the other, draw a light pencil line completely around the egg lengthwise.

2. Starting again at the top of the egg, draw another line crossing the first at right angles, thus dividing the egg into quarters.

3. Now draw a third, horizontal line around the middle of the egg.

4. Load the stylus by scraping the open end across the beeswax, and hold the point briefly over a candle flame. Test the flow of wax from the stylus point on a piece of paper, then draw the stylus over the penciled lines on the egg.

5. With the stylus, draw new lines bisecting the open areas and dividing each area into six triangles.

6. Place the egg in a spoon and dip it into the yellow vegetable dye. Gently pat it dry with facial tissue.

7. Draw small circles in alternate triangles with the wax-loaded stylus.

8. The waxed circles will remain yellow when the egg is dipped into orange dye.

9. Pat dry again, then place a dot of wax in the center of each circle.

10. Dip into the red dye, and pat dry.

11. Next draw fine diagonal lines in each of the remaining triangles.

12. Immerse in the black dye.

13. To make the colors gleam on the decorated egg, melt off the protective coats of wax by holding the egg over the flame, rotating and wiping it gently with a facial tissue.

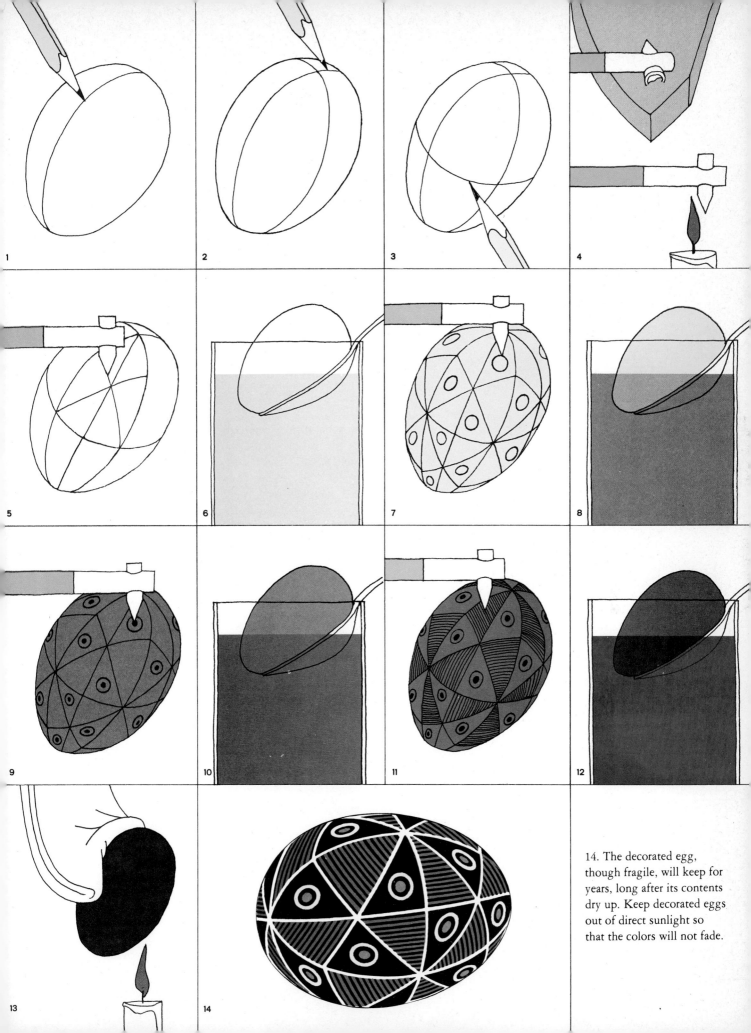

14. The decorated egg, though fragile, will keep for years, long after its contents dry up. Keep decorated eggs out of direct sunlight so that the colors will not fade.

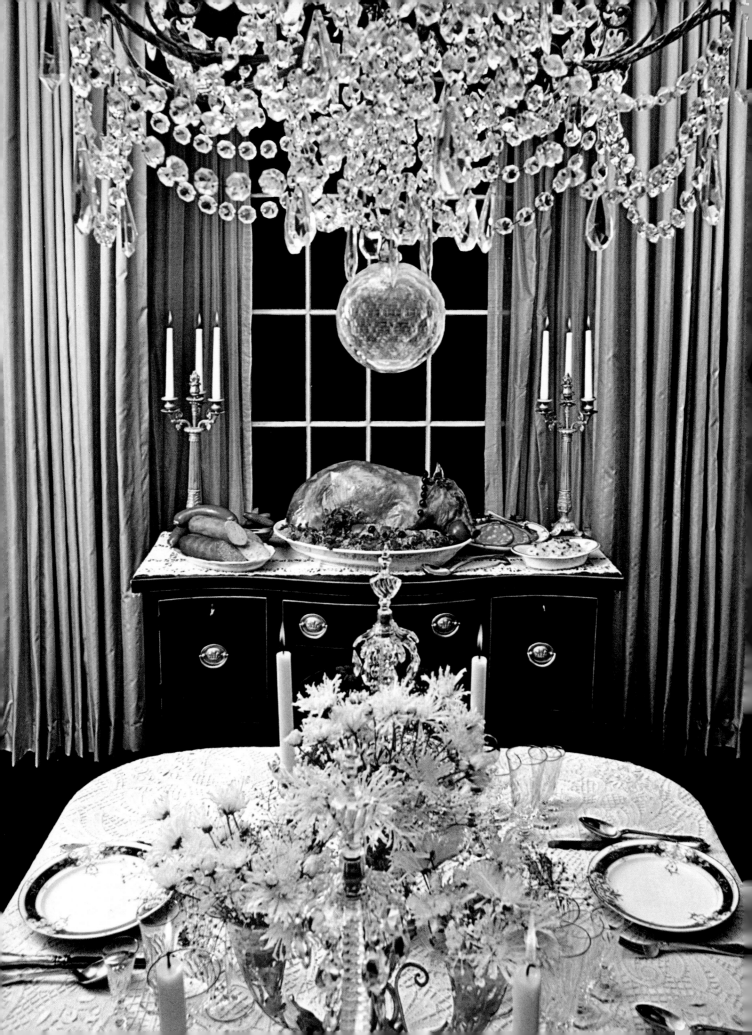

Zharennyı Porosenok
ROAST SUCKLING PIG

Roast suckling pig is a popular main course at Soviet feasts. The smaller the suckling pig the more succulent it usually is. Although usually presented whole, the pig is often more conveniently roasted in quarters as it is here.

To serve 8 to 10

Preheat the oven to 350°. Wash the pig under cold running water and pat it thoroughly dry with paper towels. Sprinkle the flesh liberally with the coarse salt and pepper and rub them into the cavities with your fingers. With a pastry brush, coat the skin and flesh of the quarters and the head of the pig with vegetable oil. Crumple a sheet of aluminum foil into a small ball and insert it into the pig's mouth to keep it open as it roasts. Wrap small sheets of foil around the ears to prevent them from burning.

A 10- to 12-pound suckling pig, the head removed and the body cut into quarters
2 tablespoons coarse salt
2 teaspoons freshly ground black pepper
¼ cup vegetable oil

Place the head in the center of a rack set in a shallow roasting pan and arrange the quarters skin-side up around it. Roast the pig undisturbed for 1¼ to 1½ hours, or until the skin is crisp and the juices run clear when the pig's flesh is pierced with the tip of a sharp knife. Fifteen minutes or so before the pig is done, remove the foil from the ears to brown them slightly.

Serve the pig on a bed of hot *kasha (below),* placing the head in the center with the quarters around it. Replace the foil in the mouth with a fresh apple.

Kasha
BUCKWHEAT GROATS WITH MUSHROOMS AND ONIONS

To serve 6

In a mixing bowl, toss the *kasha* and egg together with a large wooden spoon until the grains are thoroughly coated. Transfer to an ungreased, 10- to 12-inch skillet (preferably one with a nonstick surface) and cook uncovered over moderate heat, stirring constantly, until the *kasha* is lightly toasted and dry. Watch carefully for any sign of burning and regulate the heat accordingly. Add the salt, 3 tablespoons of the butter and 2 cups of boiling water. Stir thoroughly, cover the pan tightly, and reduce the heat to low. Simmer, stirring occasionally, for about 20 minutes. If at this point the *kasha* is not yet tender and seems dry, stir in the additional cup of boiling water and cook covered 10 minutes longer, or until the water is absorbed and the grains of *kasha* are separate and fluffy. Remove the pan from the heat, remove the cover, and let the *kasha* rest undisturbed for about 10 minutes.

1 cup coarse *kasha* (buckwheat groats)
1 egg
1 teaspoon salt
8 tablespoons (¼-pound stick) butter
2 to 3 cups boiling water
2 cups finely chopped onions
½ pound fresh mushrooms, finely chopped

Meanwhile, melt 3 tablespoons of the butter in a heavy 10- to 12-inch skillet over high heat. Add the chopped onions, lower the heat to moderate, and, stirring frequently, fry for 3 or 4 minutes, or until the onions are soft and pale gold. Stir the onions into the *kasha* and melt the remaining 2 tablespoons of butter in the skillet over high heat. Drop in the mushrooms, reduce the heat to moderate, and cook 2 or 3 minutes, stirring frequently. Then raise the heat to high and cook the mushrooms briskly, uncovered, until all the liquid in the pan has evaporated. Add the mushrooms to the *kasha* and onions and toss together. Taste for seasoning.

Kasha may be cooked in advance and reheated, covered, in a preheated 200° oven for 20 minutes or so. Or, it may be steamed by placing the cooked *kasha* in a colander and setting the colander over a deep pot filled with 1 inch of water. Drape the colander with a towel, bring the water to a boil and steam the *kasha* for about 10 minutes, or until it is heated through.

A suckling pig, roasted in quarters and reassembled, rests on a bed of *kasha*.

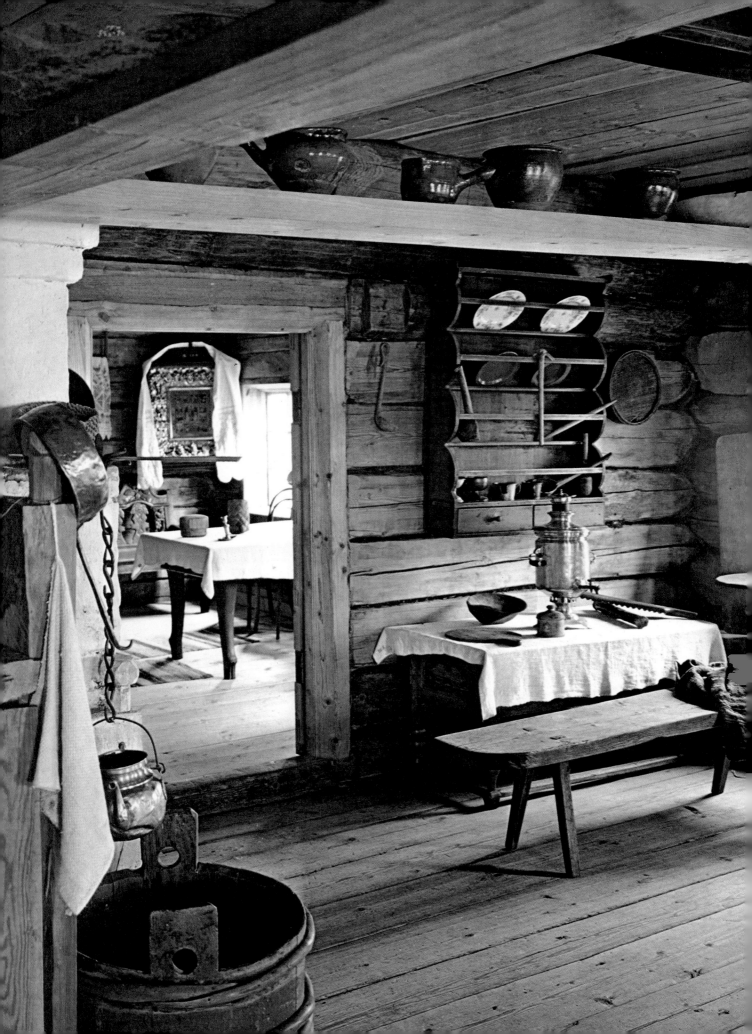

III

The Cuisine
of the People

The Oshevnev peasant house, now part of an outdoor museum at Lake Onega, north of Leningrad, was built only 100 years ago, but its rude warmth is typical of a tradition of craftsmanship in wood many centuries old. Wood is the natural medium of the Russian artisan, and until recent times the endless forests of Russia yielded nearly every object of daily life—furniture, dishes, the house itself.

The high cuisine of Old Russia, with its elaborate service and imported delicacies, existed only for the very few, the great landowning aristocrats and the richest city people. Cities were few and mostly small; the bulk of the people were peasants huddled in and around tiny villages on the great level plain that sweeps eastward through Russia to the Ural Mountains. They were isolated by distance and primitive transportation, and nearly all the foods they ate came from their own small farms and the forests and streams nearby. Most peasants were desperately poor by modern standards, but nevertheless they created out of simple ingredients a very attractive style of cooking which, with additions and elaborations, is the solid base of Russian cooking today. Not until the Russian Revolution of 1917 did this fundamental cuisine begin to undergo significant change.

In the old days, the peasant returning from a long day of labor in the fields joined his family around a crude wooden table in a tiny—sometimes a one-room—wooden cottage. Their repast, illuminated by weak oil lamps or flickering candles, consisted of a single nourishing course. It was simple and cheap, but hearty and flavorful. The head of the house cut the loaf of sour, dark Russian bread into thick slabs and a steaming bowl of *borshch* (beet soup) or *shchi* (cabbage soup) or *ukha* (fish soup) was passed around. When the soup was thin, as it often was, plates heaped high with the coarse cooked grain called *kasha* helped fill the diners' stomachs. The food was lightened—and the spirits of the family lifted—by glass after glass of *kvas*, a thin beer drunk throughout the meal.

The most important pre-revolutionary food was bread, which was taken se-

65

riously, prepared with loving care and much appreciated. Over the centuries, the baking of the Russian peasant's bread developed into a slow, perfect ritual. In the evening the housewife lit a wood fire in her big, brick stove and banked it so it would heat the oven slowly to the right temperature. In the morning she arranged her heavy loaves of dough, which had been rising overnight, on the hearth. There they baked long and slowly and took on a tough crust, a slightly sour, nutty flavor and a wonderful yeasty fragrance.

The traditional loaf was generally made of rye flour, because rye is a dependable crop for the short and fickle Russian growing season. The flour was coarsely ground, and the customary leaven was dough left over from an earlier baking. Other grains such as millet, wheat and barley also were used, but white bread made of refined wheat flour was a rarity. Peasant bread was almost always dark, like pumpernickel, and most Russian bread is dark today. Russians prefer it that way. They do not slice it thin but eat it in thick, man-sized slabs. If they use butter, they may spread it as much as half an inch thick. Bread, they believe, is no petty side dish, it is the very essence of life and should be honored and enjoyed accordingly.

A second basic food that Russian peasants made from their home-grown grain was *kasha (Recipe Index)*. It was customarily made of buckwheat grains or groats (cracked kernels), but could be made of wheat, oats, barley, millet, or any other grain. The housewife fried the grain in a little fat, lard or oil until it was slightly browned and put it in an earthenware pot. She added salted hot water until it covered the grain—according to an old rule, to a depth equal to the first joint of her thumb. Then she set the pot in a moderate oven to heat. After half an hour or so she took it out, added a bit more water and put it back again. The idea was to have the grain absorb as much water as possible without becoming sticky or mushy. If the pot was left in the oven for several hours the *kasha* would be crusty at the bottom but still perfectly good. With proper care to avoid burning on the bottom, *kasha* could also be cooked on top of the stove.

Almost anything could be added to *kasha*. An egg might be stirred into the grain, or fried chopped onions. *Kasha* is excellent by itself, but when fortified with mushrooms or soup stock or chicken it is absolutely delicious. If the family had a piece of meat that was not big enough to serve separately, it was chopped fine and combined with the *kasha* so that each serving would contain a little—a tactful way to divide a scarce delicacy among a large and hungry family.

The third staple of the peasant diet was soup. The commonest kind was *shchi,* which can be called cabbage soup because it always contained fresh cabbage in summer and sauerkraut in winter, although it could include almost anything else the household had on hand. If the family was very poor the *shchi* might be made of nothing but cabbage and other vegetables boiled together and flavored with dill or parsley. The simple dish was not at all bad, and it added invaluable vitamins to a diet that otherwise consisted mostly of cooked grain. More elaborate kinds of *shchi* were simmered with a soup bone or made with soup stock. The most elaborate kinds were thickened with flour browned in butter and cooked with a large chunk of meat that was served separately. But any kind of *shchi* was a hearty dish. The Russians say: "Shchi da kasha, mat nasha." "Shchi and kasha, that's our mother."

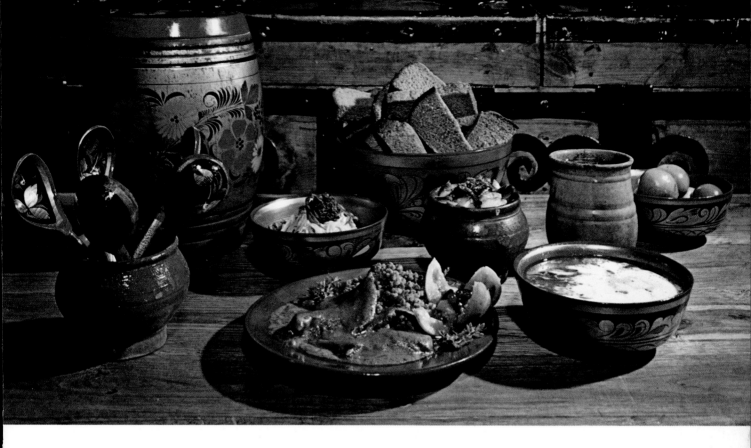

Almost as common as *shchi* and as inexpensive was *borshch (Recipe Index)*, which is based on beets and gets its red color from them. *Borshch*, like *shchi*, might contain nothing but beets, a few other vegetables and flavorings. In prosperous households it took in more and more ingredients, including sausages or a variety of meats, and became an elaborate meal in itself. Often it was hard to tell whether a soup was *borshch* or *shchi*. Some women kept a great pot constantly on the stove and tossed into it anything they happened to have on hand. If cabbage predominated, the soup was *shchi;* if it showed the red of beets, it was *borshch*.

A third basic soup, *ukha*, was made possible by the happy fact that even the bleakest parts of European Russia are thickly laced with slow-flowing, fish-filled streams. No landlord could keep his peasants from fishing. Some of the catch was eaten on the spot, spitted on a peeled willow wand and broiled at the stream bank over a small fire. Others were taken home for *ukha*. The simplest kind was made by simmering cleaned, whole fish in water flavored with herbs and seasonings. If food was in short supply, all parts of the fish were eaten, including the softened bones. In more prosperous times the solid ingredients were strained out to make a clear broth. Sometimes low-quality fish with many troublesome bones were used to make a broth; then they were removed and better fish were added to poach for a few minutes before the soup was served. Russians believe that *ukha* is best when made from several kinds of fish.

For drink the peasant diet had *kvas*, which was much like the "small beer" of Western Europe. It could be made from grain and malt, but was often made from leftover dark bread soaked in hot water and allowed to ferment for a few hours; sugar, fruit or honey customarily was added as a sweetener.

Old-style Russian foods—with a few anachronisms—are set out on wooden vessels in a restaurant at Suzdal, near Moscow. In the foreground is meat boiled in *kvas* (a mild beer), alongside a bowl of the hearty cabbage soup called *shchi*. Behind the meat are *salad zdorovie* (which contains such un-Russian ingredients as squid from the Far East) and stew. The mug holds *pokhlobka*, a potato soup, and at right are pickled tomatoes. Bread and a keg of *medovukha*, a mead made of *kvas* and honey, complete the menu.

67

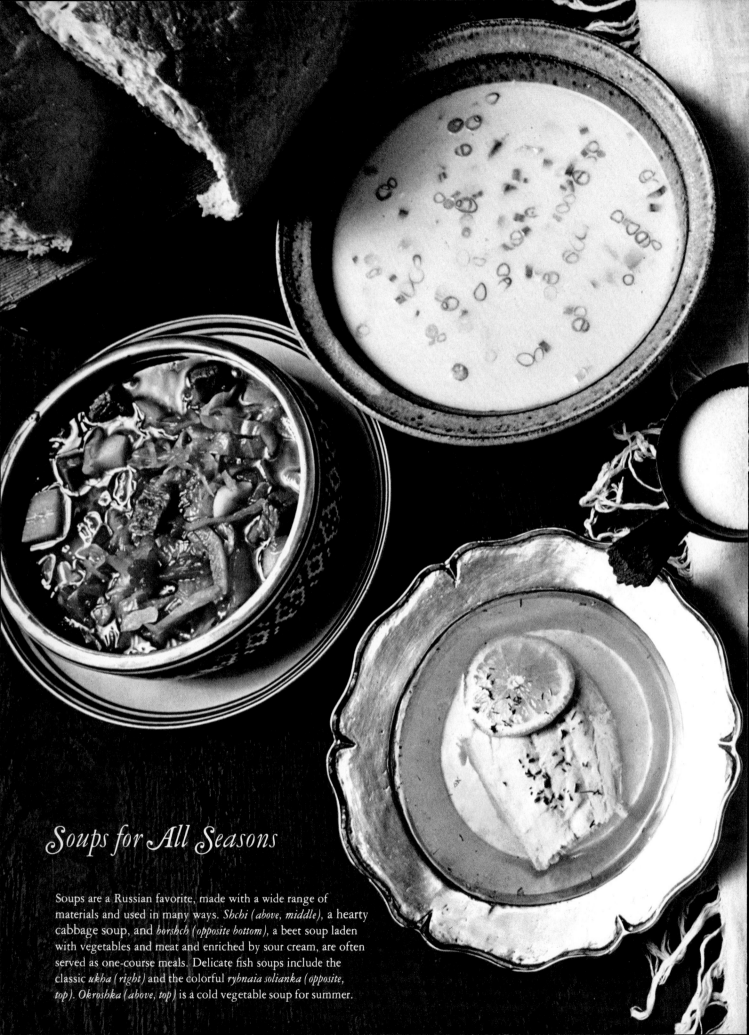

Soups for All Seasons

Soups are a Russian favorite, made with a wide range of materials and used in many ways. *Shchi (above, middle)*, a hearty cabbage soup, and *borshch (opposite bottom)*, a beet soup laden with vegetables and meat and enriched by sour cream, are often served as one-course meals. Delicate fish soups include the classic *ukha (right)* and the colorful *rybnaia solianka (opposite, top)*. *Okroshka (above, top)* is a cold vegetable soup for summer.

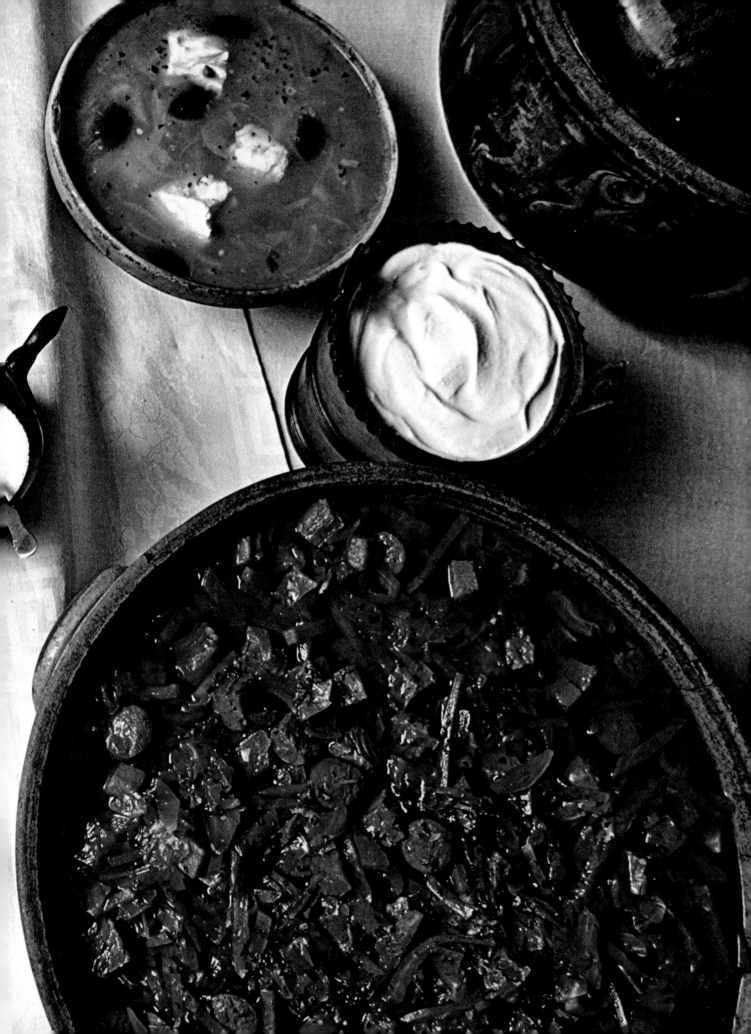

The finished brew could be drunk on the spot or bottled for later use; in some households a part of the brew served as a fermented stock for soups. Homemade *kvas* is somewhat effervescent and only slightly alcoholic. It has never enchanted many non-Russians, but it had an important place in the peasant diet. It was cheap and the yeast suspended in it, like the vegetables in *shchi* or *borshch*, formed a nutritious supplement to a limited diet.

More distinct features of the Russian popular cuisine appeared among people who were prosperous enough to elaborate upon the basic diet. Not all prerevolutionary peasants were poor; some of them had enough good land to produce a surplus of grain for sale and support a few cows, pigs and chickens. There were also townspeople and members of the minor nobility who were not really rich but who still had enough for good living and lavish hospitality. Such households ate very well, and Russians are big eaters. Their enthusiasm is well described in *Oblomov,* a 19th Century novel by Ivan Goncharov that describes the life of Russia's landed gentry. "Food was the first and foremost concern at Oblomovka. What calves were fattened there every year for the festival days! What birds were reared there! What deep understanding, what hard work, what care were needed in looking after them! Turkeys and chickens for name-days and other solemn occasions were fattened on nuts. Geese were deprived of exercise and hung up motionless in a sack a few days before a festival so that they should get covered with fat. What stores of jams, pickles, biscuits! What meads, what *kvases* were brewed, what pies baked at Oblomovka!"

Outside the major cities nearly every prosperous household had a kitchen garden where vegetables flourished during the short growing season. The staples were potatoes, turnips, carrots, beets and cabbages. In the fall root crops were dug and replanted in "sand gardens" in the cellars, where they would keep in reasonably good condition through the long winter. Cabbages and cucumbers, whose vines tangled luxuriantly over the carved fence palings, were eaten fresh or in the form of sauerkraut and pickles. Every garden had tufts of flat-leaf parsley and feathery dill, and currant and gooseberry bushes supplied the makings for preserves. Pickles and preserves were important in Old Russia, and they are important still, for they carry some of the freshness (and the vitamins) of summer into the dead of winter.

A household with a garden, some chickens, a few pigs and a cow or two could command a wide range of the Russian popular cuisine without spending money for commercial commodities. Hams and other pork products were cured for the winter; the parts of the pig that were eaten fresh were generally boiled, sometimes first with a handful of carefully rinsed new hay, then again in *kvas*. Pork chops were cooked with prunes, and the last scraps were folded in cabbage leaves and simmered in tomato sauce.

A cow meant milk, and milk meant an abundance of delicious homemade products; sour cream, clabber, sweet butter for the table, clarified butter for cooking. Cottage cheese was used to make delicacies such as *nalistniki,* which are crisp pancakes stuffed with cheese, and *vatrushki (Recipe Index),* cheese-filled pastry shells. A characteristic Russian trick with milk is to leave a bowl of it in the oven until a brown skin called *penka* forms on its surface. This skin (and the others that form after it is removed) is used, among other things, to separate the layers of elaborate rice- or custard-based desserts.

The final supplements of the basic diet were wild foodstuffs available to almost everyone. Few parts of Old Russia were thickly populated; most villages were near large areas of field or forest or swamp that could provide wild foods for those who knew how to find them. Children were always on the lookout for nettles and other greens for soup; wild garlic to be chopped into sour cream; tiny, aromatic wild strawberries and rose hips for jam. Active men with sufficient skill and courage followed wild bees to their hives and robbed them of their combs of golden honey. Then they and their families could sell the wax, brew heady mead and make crumbly cakes called *medovye prianiki* out of rye meal and strong, dark honey.

Perhaps the best time of year for the hunters of wild food was early autumn, when mushrooms sprout prodigiously in the damp, dark forests of Russia. Many kinds were gathered; Russians have never limited themselves to the common field mushroom that is the only kind widely used in the United States. They enjoy and appreciate white, pink, orange, yellow, bronze, green and black ones, each with its own distinctive flavor. In many places mushrooms are still so plentiful that they are pickled or salted or strung on threads and hung over the stove to dry, and used throughout the year.

From the peasants' simple fare to the varied delights of a wealthy household, the Russian cuisine remained stable until the Russian Revolution of 1917. Then in the space of a few decades, it went through more changes than had occurred in centuries. The Revolution did not immediately abolish poverty nor, to the disappointment of many, did it set all the peasants and workers at the same kind of well-spread table that their former rulers had enjoyed. For a number of years, in fact, their condition was worse rather than better. The socialization and modernization of agriculture was a slow, painful process, but gradually swamps were drained, arid land irrigated, virgin land brought under cultivation and worn-out land improved by better farming practices. High-yielding varieties of grains and vegetables were introduced and scrawny livestock improved by scientific breeding programs. The farmer (officially, there are no more peasants in the Soviet Union) who lived on soup, *kasha* and bread before 1917, eventually came to enjoy a more abundant and better balanced diet, with a chunk of meat in his *borshch*.

While the amount, quality and variety of food increased, it cannot be said that gastronomy flourished during the early years of the Soviet state. The Socialist ethic encouraged asceticism, and popular memory tended to identify the epicure with the exploiter. In any case, people who in less than 40 years had lived through a revolution, two major wars, invasion, enemy occupation and severe famines did not need subtleties of preparation or presentation to make almost any food acceptable.

Paradoxically, it was during this same period of history that Russian cuisine became known and accepted in other parts of the world. Penniless Russian émigrés without professional skills of any kind wisely utilized a lifetime's experience of eating fine food by starting restaurants. In New York, Paris, San Francisco, Shanghai, London and many lesser cities, balalaikas chittered, Cossacks danced and diners discovered the charms of a new cuisine: *botvinia (Recipe Index)*, a sparkling chilled fish soup; *kurnik (Recipe Index)*, a creamy concoction of chicken and rice covered by a puff-pastry crust that shattered at the touch of a fork; and flaming *shashlyk* grilled by a real expatriate

Continued on page 76

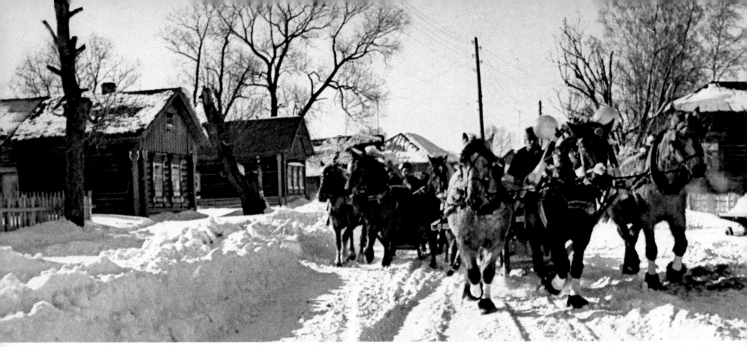

Bundled-up families coming from outlying farms arrive for the Maslenitsa festivities at Stoginskoye in gaily decorated troikas.

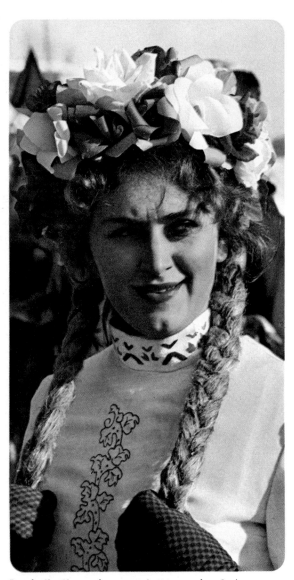

Lyudmila Chervyakova, 19, is costumed as Spring.

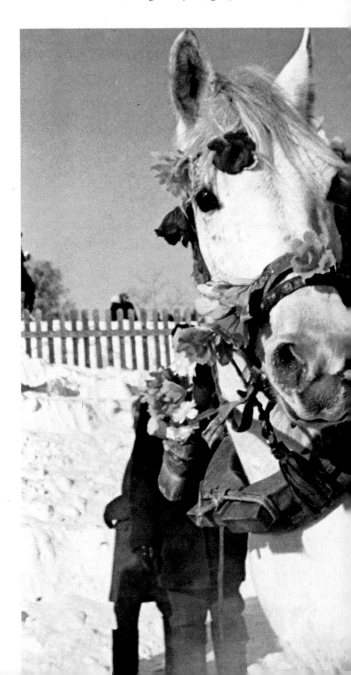

Saying Goodbye to Winter with a Pancake Feast in the Snow

Spring—real spring—comes late to northern Russia; Winter lingers and the nights are freezing cold until well past the equinox. But from time immemorial the people of the northern villages have disdained these uncomfortable realities, saying goodbye to winter with a happy pre-Lenten festival—conducted, if necessary, knee-deep in snow. Like many Russian festivals, Maslenitsa (literally, "Butter Festival") is a blend of Christian and pre-Christian tradition, enhanced by the Russian delight in food—ceremonial bread and salt, buns, bagels, but most delightfully *bliny*, pancakes round like the sun whose coming they celebrate. In the typical northern villages of Stoginskoye and Sereda, it is a time for troika rides and pageants, but also a time for *bliny* eating—*bliny* with butter, with sour cream, caviar, cottage cheese, mushrooms, salt herring or jam.

In the village of Sereda, food vendor Nadezhda Iovleva heaps sour cream on a *blin* for troika driver Pyotr Grigoryev.

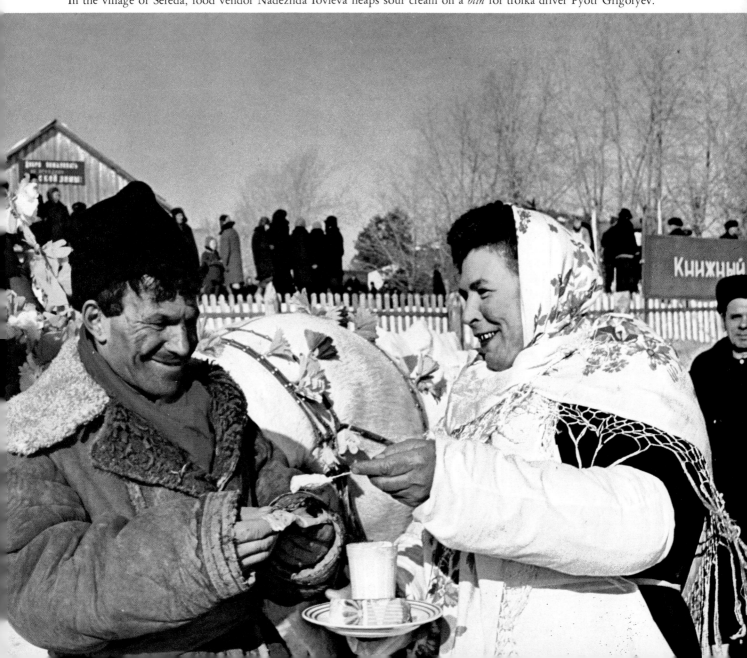

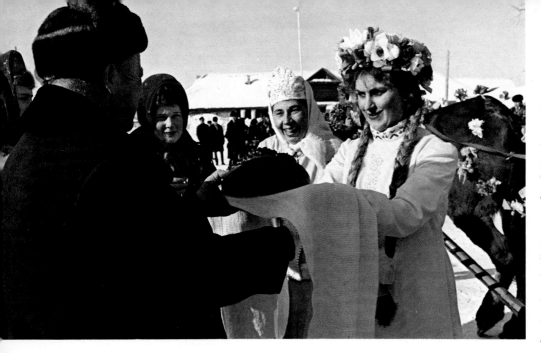

An important Maslenitsa ceremony sees winter out and welcomes spring with an offering of bread and salt. At left, Vladimir Nikitin, chairman of the Krasnaia Niva Collective Farm near Stoginskoye, presents the offering to Lyudmila Chervyakova, gaily costumed as Spring. Behind her, dressed in blue, is Rimma Vasanova, 30, who plays Winter; she will receive a pitcher of wine as a going-away present. Both gifts are shown in the picture at right: Yulia Kononova, 23, holds the bread; Tatiana Solovyeva, a 21-year-old schoolteacher, the wine, now nearly gone after a series of toasts.

In Sereda, vendors preside over bagels, wheat buns and a samovar in front of a banner that reads "Drink hot Russian tea!"

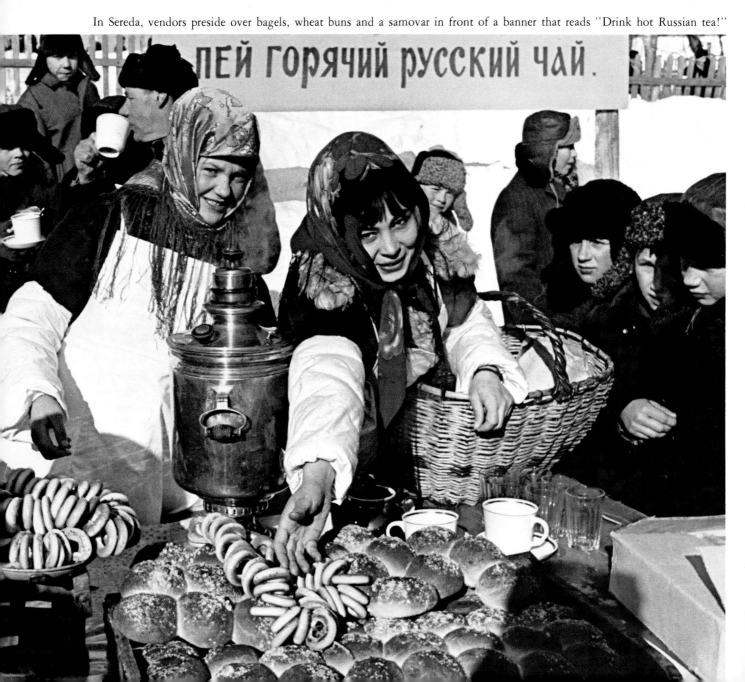

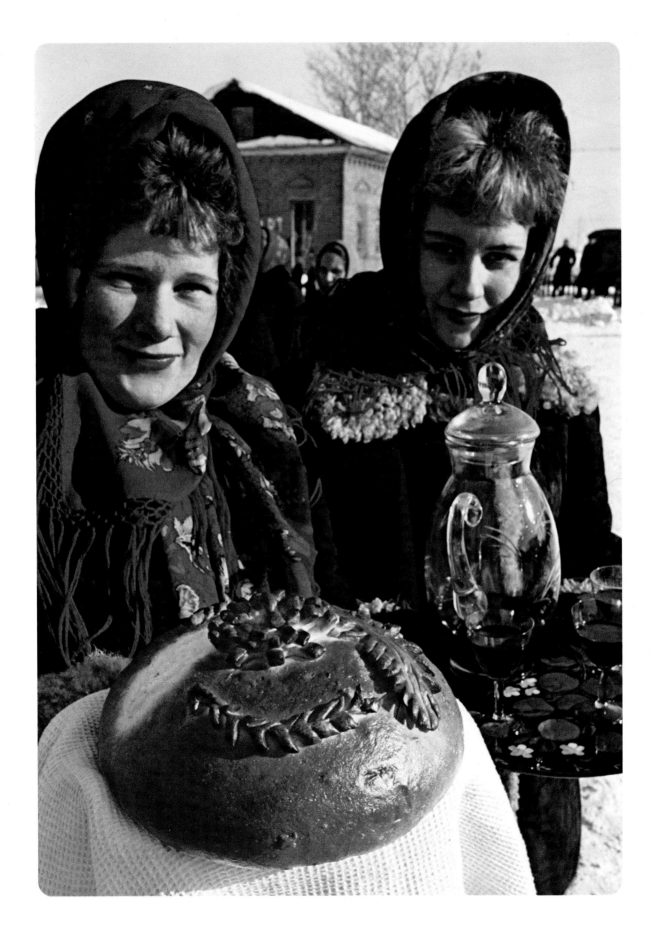

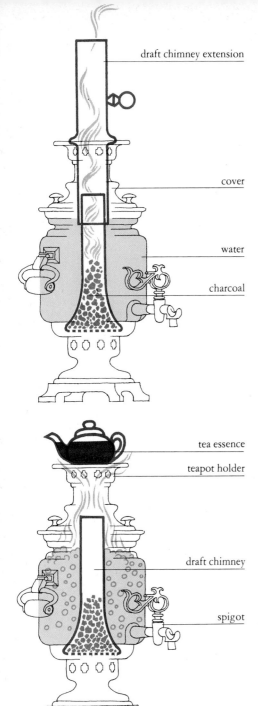

draft chimney extension

cover

water

charcoal

tea essence

teapot holder

draft chimney

spigot

Tea from a samovar is a mixed drink: strong tea from the pot, diluted with hot water. The hostess fills her samovar with cold water and puts burning charcoal in the draft chimney. With the extension fitted on *(top)*, she boils the water. With the extension off and no more smoke coming from the chimney, the samovar is carried to the table. Strong tea essence is poured from the teapot and boiling water is added from the spigot *(bottom)*.

prince and served to the flattered customers by a hand-kissing count.

In Russia itself, when the ravages of World War II were repaired, more and more people had the leisure and money to support an interest in fine cooking. Battered copies of a pre-revolutionary cookbook, Mme. Molokhovets' *A Gift to Young Housewives,* sold for high prices in second-hand bookshops. In 1952, the Ministry of Food Production published *The Book of Tasty and Healthy Food,* a collection of recipes and nutritional instructions. Elderly *ba-bushki* found themselves teaching their modern granddaughters how to make *gogol-mogol,* eggs and sugar beaten to an airy cloud; *smokva,* pastilles of sun-dried fruit, and other delectable dishes of a bygone age.

Even with the best will, however, it takes time to resurrect an almost lost cuisine. For many years tourists found Russia's finest hotels still offering a half-continental, half-Russian menu that was monotonous if not downright bad. By the 1960s decades of slow improvement began to show results. Visitors could enjoy scores of new restaurants offering both Russian and regional food —provided an empty table was available, which was seldom. (One authority estimates that while Paris has a restaurant seat for every 10 inhabitants, Moscow has one for every 30.) A tourist who patronizes the dining room of his hotel faces a different problem. He will find a table marked with his country's flag and permanently reserved for him, a multilingual menu and a choice of seasonal dishes—but the fare is not likely to be exciting and the service will be slow, since most hotel food is cooked to order, and meals there are expected to be protracted social affairs.

For both atmosphere and food, the restaurants operated for Russians, not tourists, are the visitor's best bet, and he will find it worth his while to solve the problem of getting into them. Since reservations are not customarily accepted, he must join the block-long queue waiting outside for a table—or he can follow the advice given to us by a Russian friend: "Walk boldly to the entrance door, knock sharply on the glass with a coin. When the attendant opens the door, talk English at him until in desperation he lets you inside. Then someone will find you a table, because you are foreign guests. But remember, don't speak a word of Russian, for if you do and the queue hears you! . . . I doubt that even your Ambassador could help you."

One night armed with this and other pertinent advice, we selected the Sadko, one of Leningrad's newest and most elegant restaurants, and managed to get a table there. In the spacious, uncluttered interior, panels of opaque glass, beautifully etched, create a soft, diffused light and a showcase background to each party of diners. In one dining room accordions, bass balalaikas and singers provided lively and loud music; in another was a quieter string trio and in the Hall of Banquets (fully reserved, incidentally, for a year ahead) a 50th birthday party danced to an orchestra.

Since we arrived rather late, after an evening at the ballet, we ordered a light supper, leaving the choice of dishes to our waiter. He returned carrying what looked like a brilliantly colored mosaic, big enough to adorn a public building. "A bite of *zakuska,*" he said, "to open your appetite."

The *zakuska* was enough not only to open but also to close our appetites. Slices of cold chicken, turkey, very lean pork and mild cheese ringed the plate, along with beet roses, minced carrot salad, quartered tomatoes, garnet *kliukvy* (miniature cranberries, thin-skinned and juicy). Topping the whole was a pickled mushroom cap, a giant that weighed several pounds and must have been, in its natural state, the throne of the King of the Brownies.

There followed a plate of rosy pink sturgeon, ivory *sevruga* and coral salmon garnished with quartered lemons, the rind of each quarter cut into a neat handle. Tiny glasses were filled with chilled Starka vodka, mildly aromatic and deceptively innocuous. We were ready to leave when a serving cart appeared, bearing a chafing dish of *bliny*. Deftly the waiter rolled the *bliny* with spoon and fork, set them on serving plates, spooned on caviar, rerolled them and stood back to watch our delight and appreciation.

Few Russian restaurants are as good as the Sadko. All are run by a government organization but, just as in non-Communist countries, the skill, enthusiasm and morale of each restaurant's management makes a great difference. In addition, a strict official classification of restaurants largely determines the nature and price of the food. Russian restaurants are of four categories, each plainly identified so a patron will know what to expect to eat and to pay. Those classified as de luxe or ordinary (the Sadko, of course, is de luxe) serve complete meals with most dishes prepared to order. Less expensive is the third category—the *stolovaia*, a sort of luncheonette that offers a limited number of short-order or ready-made dishes and is often self-service. Its *borshch, solianka*, cutlets and similar dishes are hearty popular fare, generally well prepared. The surroundings may be a bit bleak, but are heightened by the good temper and cheerfulness of both customers and attendants.

Cafés, the fourth and final category of restaurants, specialize in snacks and desserts. We dropped in one evening at the Lakomka café in Leningrad, a favorite spot of artists since Pushkin's time. In a little anteroom, a light buffet offered an assortment that included *pirozhki;* tarts filled with garnet-colored berry jam; sponge tortes with mocha frosting; a heap of what looked like golden rubles but proved to be tiny butter cookies; and a special *krendel (Recipe Index)*, a pretzel-shaped, rum-flavored sweet bread sprinkled with almonds and candied angelica. We carried our selections to a table in the main room and watched couples drift in, meet friends, chat, linger on, then go to the buffet for another glass of tea, cup of coffee or glass of white wine —and another ("but only one more") slice of fruit-filled cake.

Russia also has ice-cream parlors, and they are so popular that the lines of people waiting to get into them are unhappily long. Russian ice cream is excellent, and comes in many flavors. It has not yet been "improved" with additions of air, gelatin and unpronounceable chemicals; it is still a blend of pure cream, pure eggs and pure nostalgia.

Like Leningrad, Moscow has elaborate restaurants, though not nearly enough of them. Some are enormous; the Arbat is a huge glass box with tables for 2,000 people and what must be the loudest jazz and the longest menu in the Socialist world. All the big hotels have vast dining rooms and chefs who command a loyal following. But many Russians do not like this mass-produced dining out. The government's Bureau of Public Food Supply is beginning to build restaurants of moderate size that specialize in regional cooking, seafood, game or nostalgic peasant dishes. The best ones go to considerable lengths to create distinctive atmospheres, and the government even promises, in a most unproletarian move, to build "some very, very small places for those people who enjoy most of all just to be quiet."

Continued on page 82

A Delicious Consolation for a Coming Fast

At the heart of the pre-Lenten Maslenitsa festival is the consumption of *bliny*. In Old Russia, seven long weeks of Lenten fasting—during which only vegetables and vegetable oils were allowed on the table—lay in the immediate future, and an orgy of pancake-eating was a consolation for the coming ordeal. Today, Orthodox Russians still observe the old traditions, but for nonbelievers the *bliny* are their own excuse for existence. Made with buckwheat flour, and with yeast, the *bliny* batter must rise for at least six hours. The pancakes themselves can be prepared ahead of time and kept warm, loosely wrapped in a cloth, or they can be served from pan to plate as fast as the cook can operate. Fifteen delicate *bliny* to an eater is a fair allowance —unless, of course, someone is really hungry.

Glafira Fyodorovna Remisova, a Russian *babushka*, or grandmother, lives with her daughter and son-in-law in the village of Sereda in northern Russia. Below, at a *bliny* supper, she serves tea, first pouring into a cup a little of the strong tea essence from the teapot, then drawing hot water from the samovar. Spread on the table in front of her are the parts of the feast that will be eaten along with the *bliny*: portions of a cabbage pie in the foreground; portions of a jam pie next to it; and candy heaped in a compote dish.

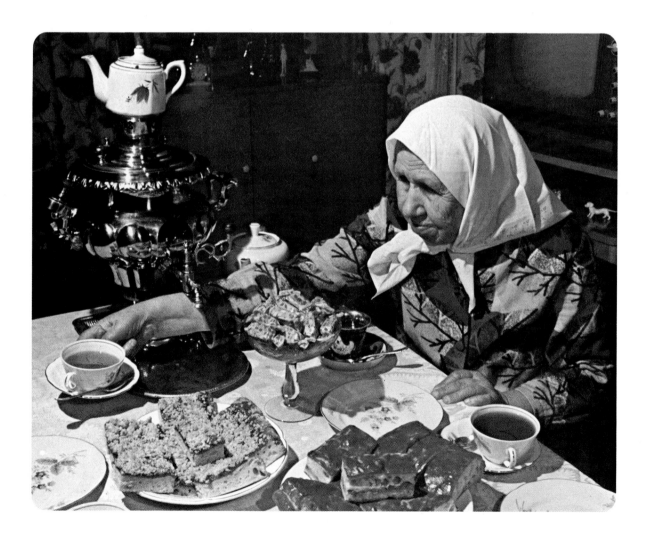

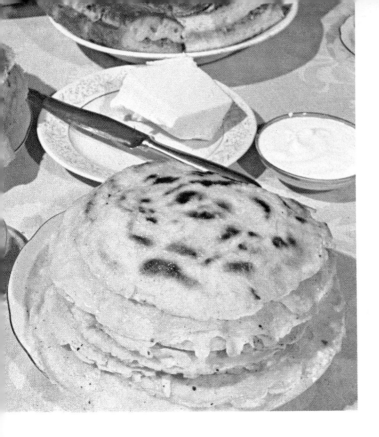

Brought steaming to the table, the *bliny (left)* are flanked by their familiar companions, butter and sour cream. Below, Grandmother Glafira savors a morsel.

Overleaf: Bliny are a rustic invention, but in 1,000 years of eating them the Russians have also made them into an item of haute cuisine. The distinction between the simple and the sophisticated forms of the dish lies mainly in the toppings; but a delicate, well-cooked *blin* can look equally at home on a wooden platter or an imperial plate. From the array shown here, fit for a grand duke or a commissar, the *bliny* may be spread with sour cream or melted butter and then topped with pink sliced salmon, red salmon roe, sliced smoked sturgeon, fresh black caviar or pickled herring.

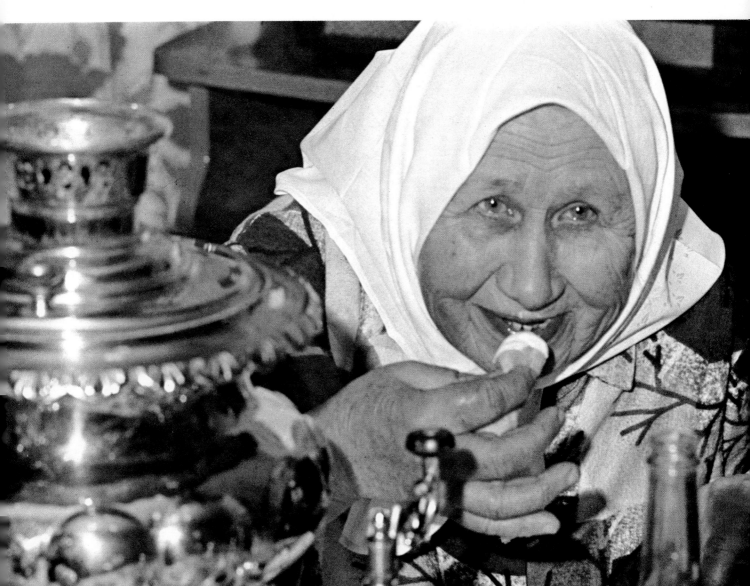

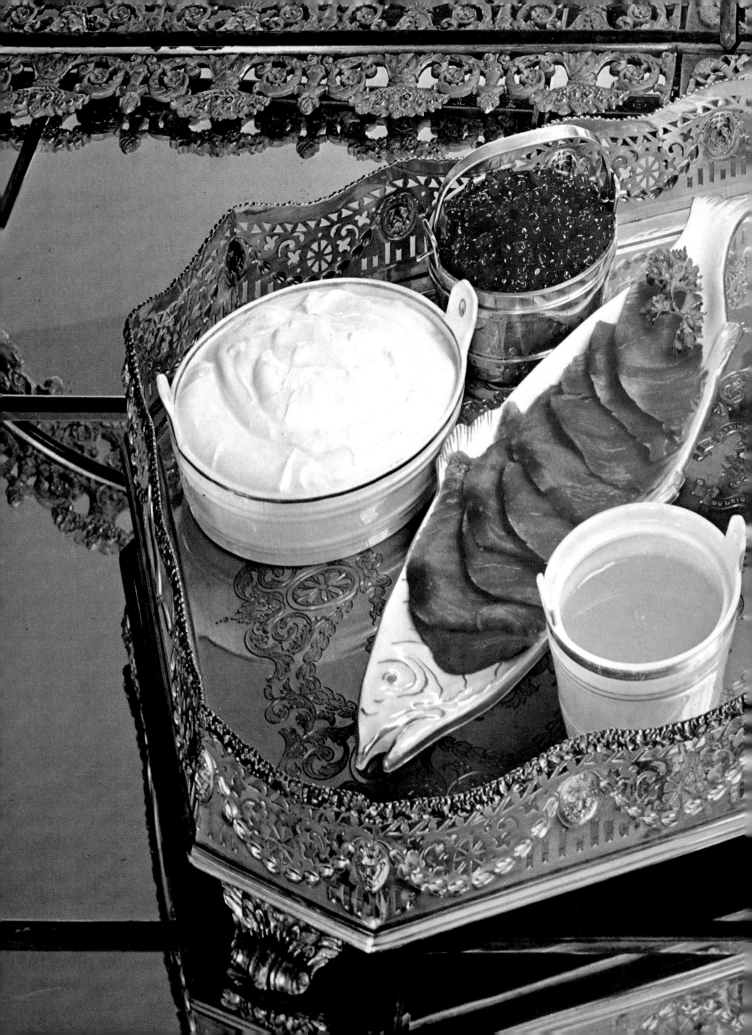

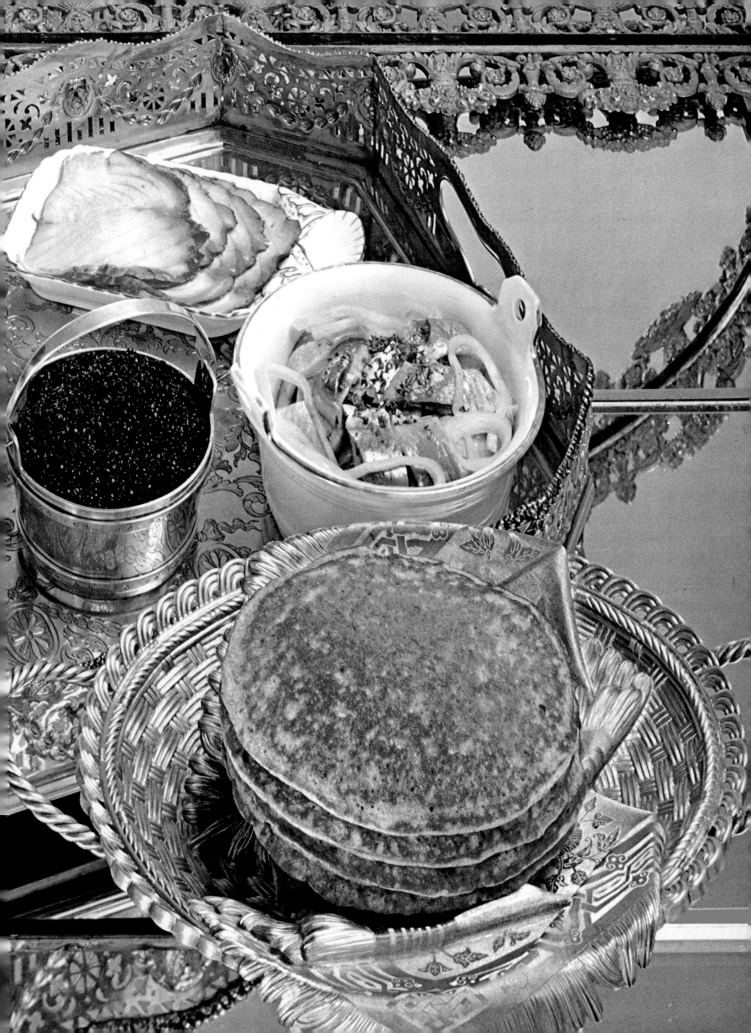

The new restaurants sound promising, but our favorite in Moscow was an old one, the Tsentralnaia on Gorky Street, which flourished as Filippov's in pre-revolutionary days and is still maintained in something close to Czarist splendor. A floor of mellowed tiles, handsome walnut paneling against pale green walls, high ceilings and graceful crystal chandeliers give the room a turn-of-the-century charm. And though the grand dukes and their lovely ballerinas are gone, their places of assignation remain: a row of discreetly curtained booths along one wall.

There, on old fruitwood chairs at a table covered with linen damask we took our places. A waitress brought a pitcher of *kvas* and filled our cut-glass goblets to the brim. She soon returned with vodka and *zakuska:* smoked salmon, red and black caviar, slices of smoky ham, and pickled Antonovka apples, firm-fleshed, almost translucent and with a tartness that lingered on the tongue. There was also a dish of sturgeon salad and small molds of *kholodets:* a mixture of beef, veal and chicken in natural gelatin, served with mustard sauce. For our entrée we had a magnificent beef Stroganov, and our dessert was a *charlottka* that might have been prepared by the great French chef Carême, who for a time was in the service of Czar Alexander I. The great Stroganov family of imperial Russia, which gave its name to beef Stroganov, would not feel too uncomfortable today in the Tsentralnaia.

In theory, of course, there are no social classes in the Soviet Union, but successful artists and writers, scientists, industrial managers and high government officials have enough income to enjoy such restaurants as the Tsentralnaia, often or occasionally. The rest of the time they and people with lower salaries are likely to eat hearty midday meals in canteens attached to the places where they work. These meals vary in price and quality. Some factory workers, in steel mills and chemical plants for instance, get substantial meals at low prices because their work is considered dangerous or unhealthy, while the highest prices are probably those charged by the canteens of research and scientific institutions. A characteristic dish served in the canteens is *kotlety,* a fried patty made of ground meat, onions, eggs and moistened bread and served with potatoes or macaroni.

At 10 o'clock in the morning school children get a hot "second breakfast" such as sausages, *kasha* and milk. Some collective farms have collective eating places; in others, at plowing or harvest time, workers in the fields get hot food carried out to them for the midday meal. Like institutional food everywhere, such meals do not rise to the gourmet level or even to the level of good home cooking, but they are abundant, well balanced nutritionally and far better than the food most Russians got a generation ago.

In Russia as in any country the cuisine can best be judged not in the restaurant but at the family table. Russians are enormously gregarious, and not even the cramped space of older apartments, which makes it necessary to share a kitchen with one or more other families, can keep them from entertaining friends with heaps of food. The quality of the food varies, of course, with the skill and interest of the housewife. Russia has its quota of dedicated cooks, purists who shun short cuts and follow classical methods, and for the benefit of this small but devoted elite, the chefs of de luxe restaurants periodically hold open house to demonstrate fine cookery and introduce new dishes. There are also confirmed non-cooks, but not many.

The great majority of women enjoy cooking, but have only a limited amount of free time (most Soviet women hold full-time jobs) and are eager to take advantage of methods and materials that will ease or shorten their task.

For such women the *gastronom,* or grocery shop, provides increasing help. In most respects they do not match the bewildering lavishness of American supermarkets, but they do offer a good assortment of canned vegetables, fruit, meat and fish as well as raw foodstuffs. There is even canned game, including venison, partridge and *tetereva,* a kind of woodcock; we tried the latter and found it surprisingly fresh in flavor and texture.

Special stores called *kulinaria,* and some of the *gastronoms* as well, sell fully prepared or semi-prepared food for working people to take home with them. That American abomination the TV dinner has not yet appeared in the Soviet Union, but Russians can buy ready-made *borshch* of various kinds; *pirozhki* filled with trout, mushrooms or gelatinous sturgeon spine; tongue in puff-pastry; pork goulash; and stuffed cabbage and peppers. Semi-prepared foods include puff-pastry dough, dumplings ready to be plopped into boiling water, cutlets seasoned and breaded for frying and chunks of marinated meat ready to be grilled as *shashlyk.*

What Russians lack are fresh fruits and vegetables; they have yet to solve the problem of quick transportation for perishable products. In winter Moscow and other northern cities are almost bare of these foodstuffs although the semitropical parts of Central Asia and the Caucasus could supply them the year around. To make up for these deficiencies, many Russian housewives are eager canners and preservers of fresh products in season. When cucumbers are plentiful, they put down great tubs of pickles, and they wait patiently for fresh strawberries, cherries, currants, plums and apples—anything that can carry the cheer and flavor of the growing season into the cold months.

This ample supply enables the Russian family that eats at home to eat very well. There is usually a simple breakfast, of bread and tea, perhaps with an egg. Lunch will start with soup and end with a full course of meat or fish and potatoes or other vegetables. Dinner has the same courses with the addition of a modest *zakuska,* a sweet dessert and a cup of coffee or—more often —tea. The tea is often served with fruit preserves stirred into it.

Much more elaborate than ordinary meals are party meals, and the Russians adore parties. When we arrived in Moscow, we were delighted to find an invitation to dinner from an old friend, Lidia Borisovna. Accepting it, I asked: "May I come early and see exactly how you prepare a dinner, from start to finish?"

"The audience should never be allowed backstage," she said, "but if you really wish, meet me at 8 o'clock sharp at the Nekrasovsky Market."

Exactly to the minute Lidia arrived carrying four of the nylon net shopping bags that are the Russian housewife's badge of office. With her, I walked through wide, immaculate aisles, bordered by stalls of vegetables and fruits from collective farms and from the private plots lovingly cultivated by individuals. We bought a bunch of white icicle radishes, bouquets of parsley and dill, a string of dried mushrooms.

Lidia's next goal was the poultry stand where she bought six plump chickens. By now our bags were bulging, but my hostess was not finished. From the market we took a taxi to a *gastronom.* In size and appearance it resembled

Continued on page 88

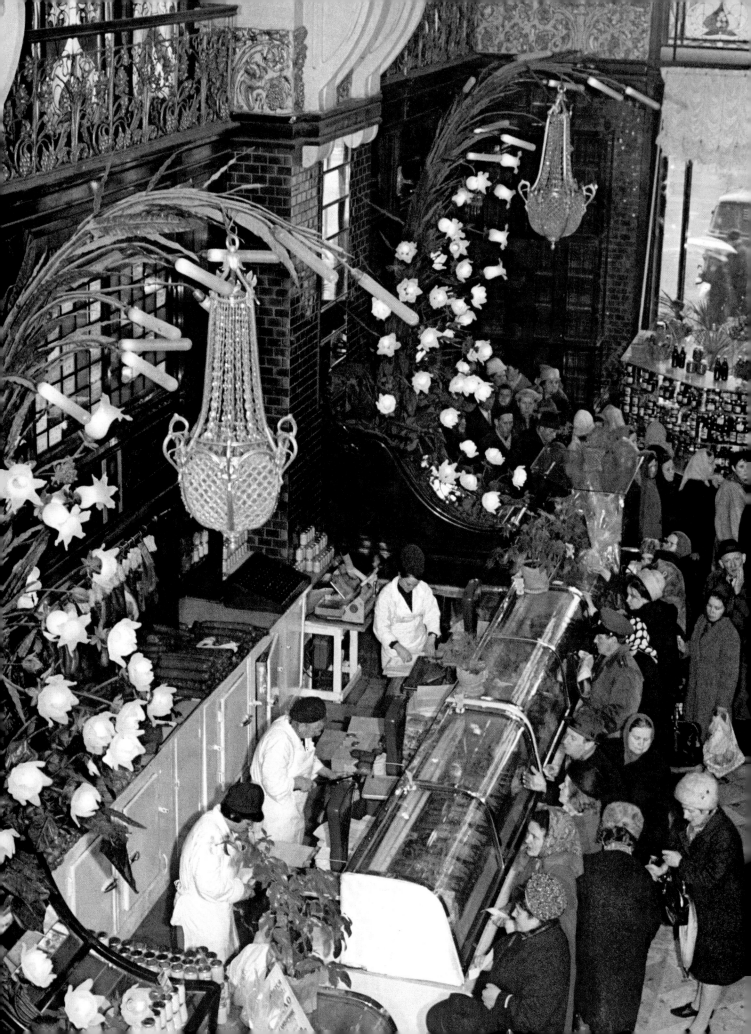

The ornate interior of Tsentralnaia Gastronom in Leningrad is a holdover from Czarist times. Customers wait to be served at the *gastronomia* counter, where ready-to-eat foods like cheese, sausage and meats are sold. A selection of goods from Moscow's Gastronom No. 1 *(below)* is identified by numbers printed on the photograph: spiced pilchard; (2) Rossisky cheese; (3) Swiss cheese; (4) Medynsky hard cheese; (5) unsalted Vologda butter; (6) Pacific herring; (7) Mukuzani No. 4, a dry red Georgian wine; (8) Tsinandali No. 1, a dry white Georgian wine; (9) beef filet sausage; (10) *kolbasa varionaia* (boiled beef sausage); (11) Baltic sprats; (12) fresh caviar; (13) cold smoked whole sturgeon; (14) cold smoked beef sausage; (15) smoked sausage; (16) smoked ham; (17) Moskovskaia vodka; (18) white bread; (19) cold smoked salmon; (20) cold smoked filet of sturgeon; (21) black bread.

Gastronoms to Inspire the Gastronome

About 175 years ago, a food merchant named Yeliseyev made a name for himself in Moscow by purveying quality merchandise to the local gentry. He did so well that in 1802 he was emboldened to expand, opening a handsome shop on St. Petersburg's elegant Nevsky Prospekt. Today, despite the fact that St. Petersburg has become Leningrad and the Yeliseyev signs have long since been taken down, both establishments survive. They bear the savorless names of Moscow Gastronom No. 1 and Tsentralnaia Gastronom *(left)*, but old Yeliseyev probably would approve of the groceries they sell—many varieties of vodka and wine, ready-prepared cuts of meat and fish, cheese and luxury canned goods. Not everyone can shop in the *gastronoms*—the foods there cost too much—but plenty of Russians do. Every day the Tsentralnaia Gastronom sells up to 60,000 customers as much as two-and-a-half tons of sausage alone—not to mention the hundreds of gallons and pounds of Russia's most famous delights, vodka and caviar.

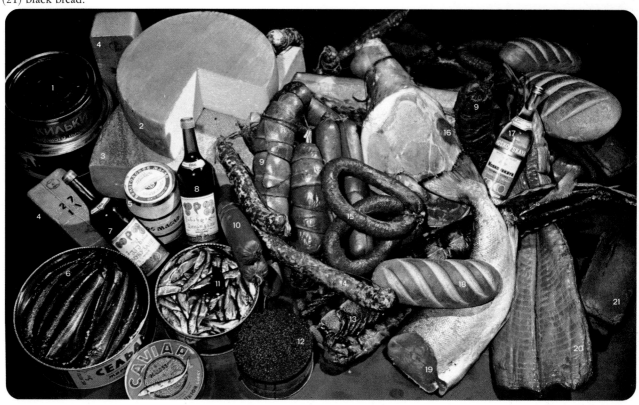

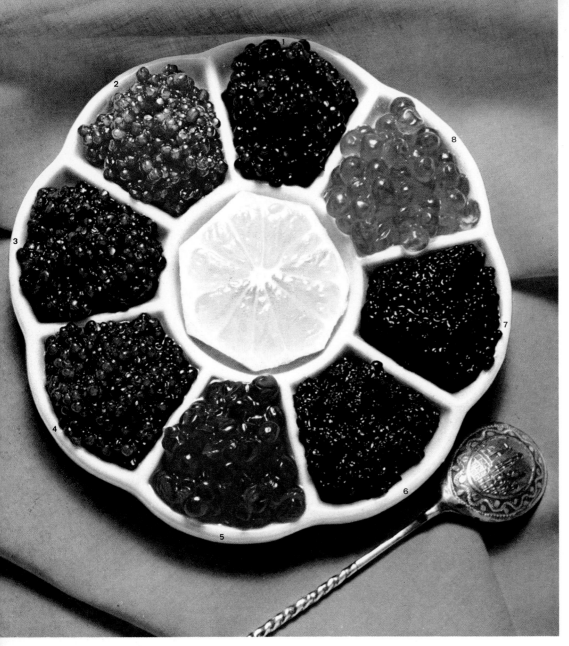

Caviar: From Beluga to Lumpfish

That caviar is known as *caviar* only outside of Russia (the Russians call it *ikra*) is only a minor eccentricity in the mystique surrounding this rare and—to most Westerners—exotic substance. Connoisseurs have developed rules for judging the quality of the best and most expensive caviar (mainly by taste, partly by appearance), for eating it (preferably plain, on unbuttered white or brown bread) and for keeping it (more precisely, not keeping it at all once it has been opened). The rules are good ones, but it would be unfortunate if they discouraged anyone from trying caviar and eating it for enjoyment. Not all types are expensive; some are improved by a squeeze of lemon juice, may be eaten on toast or crackers and are enhanced by an accompaniment of chopped hard-boiled eggs or chopped spring onions. Ringing a lemon slice above are portions of eight different kinds of caviar. The numbered list at right names and describes them.

1 **BLACK BELUGA**
The queen of caviar, beluga comes from sturgeon and is composed of the largest and finest eggs. Beluga sturgeon may reach a length of 14 feet.

2 **GRAY BELUGA**
Gray beluga is distinguished from black by color alone. It is the same high grade of sturgeon caviar, originating mainly in the Caspian Sea.

3 **OSETROVA**
Smaller than beluga eggs, these come from medium-sized sturgeon. It is preferred by many Europeans, but little goes to the United States.

4 **SEVRUGA**
Sevruga is yielded by the smallest sturgeon. Like beluga and osetrova, sevruga may be sold fresh as malossol (lightly salted) caviar.

5 **SALT-WATER SALMON CAVIAR**
Relatively low-priced, red caviar is the roe of salmon caught in the sea. It is produced in Alaska and the Pacific northwest as well as in Russia.

6 **PRESSED CAVIAR**
Pressed caviar is usually a combination of osetrova and sevruga eggs that have been damaged in processing or are too frail to be sold whole.

7 **LUMPFISH CAVIAR**
The roe of lumpfish and whitefish are dyed deep black to produce this inexpensive variety, which is produced mainly in Iceland.

8 **FRESH-WATER SALMON CAVIAR**
Paler in color than the roe of the sea-caught fish, this caviar consists of the eggs of salmon caught during migration to upriver spawning beds.

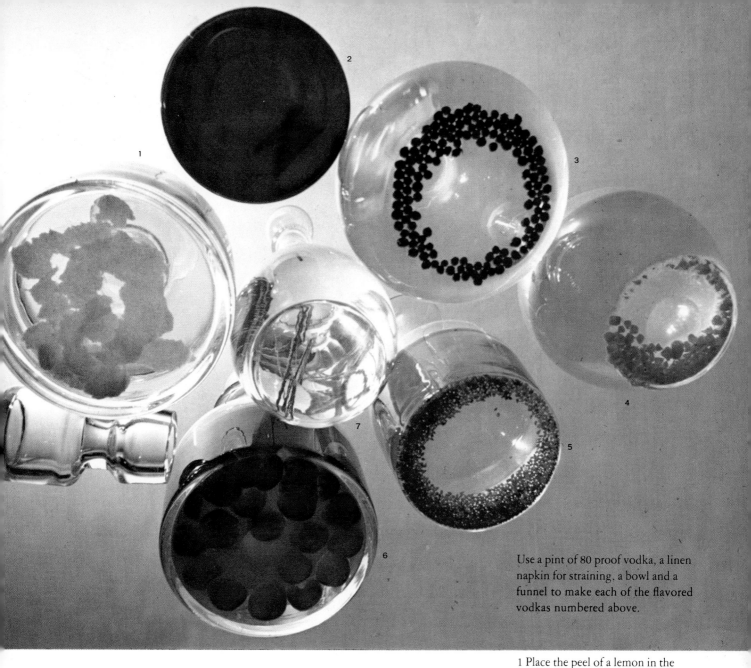

Use a pint of 80 proof vodka, a linen napkin for straining, a bowl and a funnel to make each of the flavored vodkas numbered above.

Vodka: From Cherry Pits to Peppercorns

"The Russian people drink not from need and not from grief," wrote the novelist Andrei Sinyavsky a few years ago, "but from an age-old requirement for the miraculous and extraordinary. . . . Vodka is the [Russian's] White Magic." Ever since it was introduced—as medicine—in the 14th Century, the Russian taste for this powerful alcoholic beverage has never slackened. It is customarily drunk from a small glass in a single gulp, accompanied by appetizers or almost any part of a regular meal, for it goes with any course but the sweet. Vodka should be ice cold, but preferably not served on the rocks, to avoid dilution by the ice. While no Russian would countenance ruining good vodka by making a Bloody Mary out of it, a variety of flavorings can be added to the basic spirits (as seen here, looking up through the bottoms of decanters) to produce an array of subtle liquors fully as interesting as the original.

1 Place the peel of a lemon in the vodka, taking care not to include any white pith; remove after four hours.
2 Place a tea bag and the vodka in a bowl; remove bag after two hours.
3 Add two teaspoons of black or white peppercorns; strain them out after two hours.
4 Wash 20 cherrystones, crush them gently with a hammer and leave them in the vodka for 10 to 12 hours.
5 Place one teaspoon of anise seeds in vodka; strain out after two hours.
6 Put 20 halved, pitted dark sweet cherries in vodka for three hours.
7 Put seven blades of *zubrovka* (buffalo grass) in vodka for four hours, then remove six of them.

an American supermarket, but the system of buying, as in most Russian stores, was far more cumbersome. Before you can purchase anything, you must make a selection and get the attention of a clerk, who tells you the price. Then you go the cashier, pay the sum, get a receipt and claim your purchase. Since each of these steps may involve waiting in a queue, shopping is a time-consuming task even in the newest and most modern *gastronom.*

"Now, one last stop, for the cake" said Lidia. "We'll get that at the Metropole pastry shop." Half the housewives in Moscow seemed to have gotten there before us, crowding in front of a glass case that was filled with works of art executed in several lusciously edible media. We were patient, and at last a superb cream cake was brought out for us, generously admired by all, and boxed, and we were on our way again. "Now I have a problem," said Lidia Borisovna as we settled back in the cab. "When my friends at the apartment house see me coming in with this cake they'll know I'm planning a party, and when they see me with an American friend, they will know why. I could only ask 12 of them. The rest will be hurt."

"I'll carry the cake box," I offered, "and go ahead."

"No, I think you will have to stay in Moscow until I can invite all my friends to meet you—in groups of 12."

I would like to have gone along with her plan, for that dinner party was a great success. Though the day was warm, we had a hot *zakuska:* chopped dried mushrooms simmered in white wine, touched with sour cream, grated cheese and black pepper, then set under the broiler and brought bubbling to the table. Our soup was *okroshka (Recipe Index),* a popular soup for warm weather, made with meat or fish, *kvas* and such greens as scallions and cucumbers, all chilled with ice cubes in the serving plates; it was served with *rastegai,* which are a kind of *pirozhki,* stuffed with gelatinous sturgeon spine. The chickens, split and roasted, had the added tang of a green gooseberry sauce. And, several hours and several toasts later, we came to that rich, beautifully decorated cream cake.

"I have never seen cakes like the ones at the Metropole," I said. "Do they make them there?"

"No, no. This cake comes from the 'Bolshevik' factory."

"Do you suppose I would be allowed to visit it?"

"Why not?" said Lidia. "There are no secrets to making cakes."

A few days later I had an appointment with Anastasia Makarova, director of the "Bolshevik," and visited her cake room, where a score of pretty girls demonstrated their skill. I watched one of them take a pastry tube, fit a nozzle to it, and run off a cream ruffle, squirt out a cluster of tiny mushrooms, set a garden of flowers next to them and finish the whole with a swirl of ribbons. I saw cakes topped with fairy-tale figures, cosmonauts, penguins, a public building, a full-sized bottle of champagne in chocolate cream and a party of bears. But I was still curious about the wonderful quality of the cakes, and I asked Mme. Makarova about that.

"Well," she said, "we use only pure butter, eggs, cream and whipped cream —only the best of ingredients—for to do otherwise is against our rules. And of course, my staff is very proud and very enthusiastic."

Lidia Borisovna was wrong, of course. There certainly *are* some secrets to cake making, and I had just heard them.

The Tsentralnaia restaurant on Gorky Street in Moscow preserves some of the elegance of Russia's Czarist regimes. Founded in 1865 as the Filippov Café, it became part of a hotel-and-restaurant establishment that survived all the upheavals of war and revolution. In the 1930s the Tsentralnaia gained fame as the gathering place for foreign members of the Comintern; today it is one of the city's epicurean landmarks.

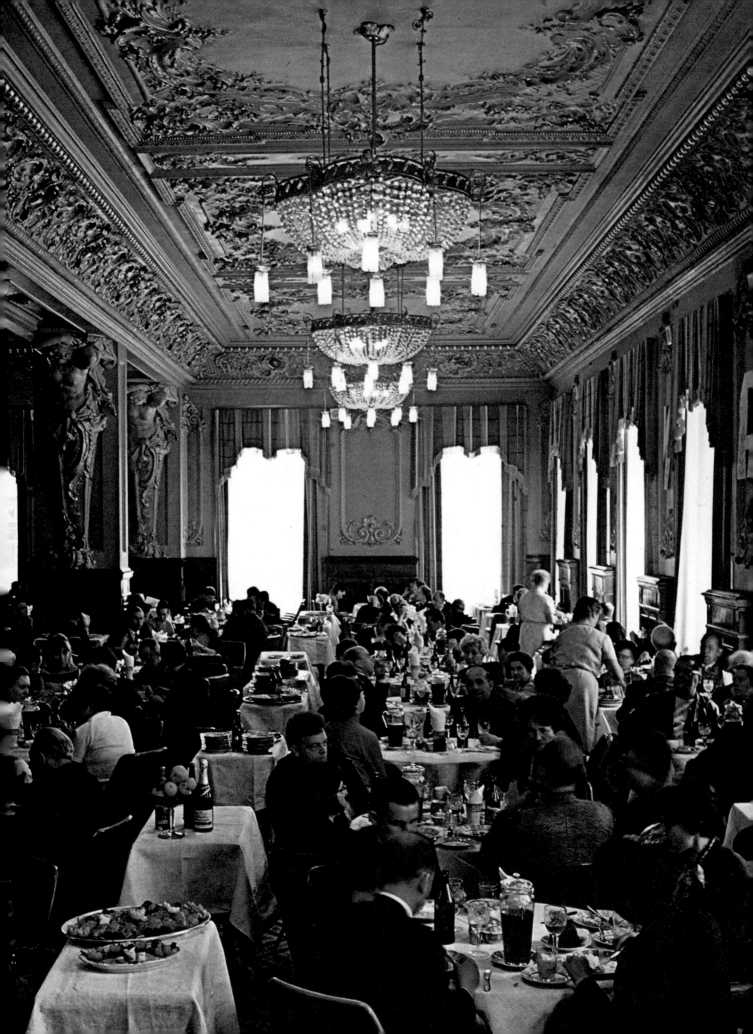

To serve 6 to 8

BEEF STOCK
1 pound fresh lean brisket of beef
5 pounds beef marrow bones, cracked
1 large onion, peeled and quartered
1 large carrot, scraped
2 celery tops, 6 sprigs of parsley
    and 2 bay leaves tied together
1 tablespoon salt

SOUP
4 tablespoons butter
2 cups thinly sliced onions
1½ pounds white cabbage, quartered,
    cored, then coarsely shredded
1 celery root, scraped and cut into
    fine strips
1 parsley root, scraped and cut into
    fine strips
1 pound boiling potatoes, peeled
    and cut into ¼-inch dice (2½ cups)
4 medium tomatoes, peeled, seeded
    and chopped *(see borshch
    ukraïnsky, page 141)*
1 teaspoon salt
Freshly ground black pepper

To serve 6

FISH STOCK
2 cups sliced onions
1 bay leaf
6 whole black peppercorns
3 sprigs parsley
1 teaspoon salt
⅛ teaspoon freshly ground black
    pepper
2½ to 3 pounds fish trimmings: the
    spines, heads, or tails of any
    white-fleshed fish
2 egg whites

FISH
1 pound fish fillets: striped bass,
    sea bass, or any other white-
    fleshed fish
1 lime, thinly sliced
1 tablespoon finely cut fresh dill
    leaves, or finely chopped parsley

Shchi

CABBAGE SOUP

BEEF STOCK: In a heavy 6- to 8-quart pot, bring the pound of beef, beef bones and 4 quarts of water to a boil over high heat, skimming off any foam and scum as they rise to the surface. Add the onion, carrot, tied greens and salt, partially cover the pot and reduce the heat to low. Simmer 1 to 1½ hours, or until the meat is tender but not falling apart. Remove the meat from the pot with a slotted spoon, cut it into small dice and set the dice aside. Continue to simmer the stock partially covered, for about 4 hours longer. Then strain the stock through a fine sieve set over a large bowl, discarding the bones and greens. With a large spoon, skim off and discard as much of the surface fat as you can.

SOUP: Melt the butter in a 3- to 4-quart pot set over high heat. Add the onions, reduce the heat to moderate, and cook 8 to 10 minutes, or until they are soft but not brown. Stir in the shredded cabbage and the celery and parsley roots, cover the pot, and simmer over low heat for 15 minutes.

Pour in the meat stock and add the reserved diced beef. Simmer over moderate heat (partially covered) for 20 minutes, then add the diced potatoes. Cook another 20 minutes and stir in the chopped tomatoes. Cook 10 minutes longer, then add the salt and a few grindings of pepper. Taste for seasoning. Serve hot, accompanied perhaps by *vatrushki (Recipe Index)*.

Ukha

CLEAR FISH SOUP WITH LIME AND DILL

In a 3- to 4-quart enameled or stainless-steel casserole, combine 2 quarts of water with the onions, bay leaf, peppercorns, parsley, salt, pepper and fish trimmings. Bring to a boil over high heat, then reduce the heat to low and partially cover the casserole. Simmer undisturbed for 30 minutes.

Strain the stock through a fine sieve set over a large bowl. Press down hard on the vegetables and trimmings with the back of a large spoon to extract all their juices before discarding them. Return the stock to the casserole.

In a small bowl, beat the egg whites to a froth, add them to the stock, and bring the mixture to a boil over high heat, stirring constantly with a whisk. When the stock begins to froth and threatens to overflow the pan, remove it from the heat and let it rest about 5 minutes. Then slowly pour the entire contents of the pan into a cheesecloth-lined sieve set over a deep bowl. Let the stock drain through the sieve without disturbing it at any point. Discard the contents of the sieve and taste the stock for seasoning. It will doubtless need more salt.

Return the stock to the casserole and bring it to a boil over high heat. Drop in the fish fillets, reduce the heat to low, and simmer the fish uncovered for 3 to 4 minutes, or until it is firm to the touch and opaque. Do not overcook. With a slotted spoon, remove the fish from the casserole to a platter. Pour the soup into a heated tureen or individual soup bowls. Add the slices of the fish and lime, and sprinkle with the cut dill or chopped parsley. Serve at once.

Borshch Moskovskii

MOSCOW-STYLE BEET SOUP

In a 6- to 8-quart pot, melt the butter over moderate heat. Add the onions and, stirring frequently, cook 3 to 5 minutes, or until they are soft but not brown. Stir in the beets, then add the wine vinegar, sugar, chopped tomatoes, 1 teaspoon of the salt and a few grindings of black pepper. Pour in ½ cup of the stock, cover the pan and simmer undisturbed for 50 minutes.

Pour the remaining stock into the pot and add the chopped cabbage. Bring to a boil, then stir in the ham, frankfurters and beef. Submerge the tied parsley and bay leaf in the soup, add another teaspoon of salt, and simmer, partially covered, for ½ hour.

Transfer the *borshch* to a large tureen and sprinkle with fresh dill or parsley. Accompany the soup with a bowl of sour cream, to be added to the *borshch* at the discretion of each diner.

Rassolnik

TART SORREL SOUP WITH KIDNEYS

Cut the pickle in half lengthwise and run a small spoon down its length to remove the seeds and pulp. Place the seeds and pulp in a fine sieve set over a small bowl and press them firmly with the back of a spoon to extract all their juices before throwing them away. Set the juice aside, and chop the pickle as finely as possible.

Melt 4 tablespoons of the butter in a 3- to 4-quart casserole over moderate heat. When the foam has almost subsided, stir in the onions and celery and cover the pan. Reduce the heat to low and simmer gently for at least 10 minutes, or until the onions are soft but not brown. Add the pickle, parsley, sorrel and spinach and stir in the salt and a few grindings of pepper. Pour in the beef stock, stir, and bring to a boil over high heat. Then reduce the heat to low, partially cover the pan, and simmer about 20 minutes.

While the soup is simmering, prepare the kidneys. With a small, sharp knife cut away their knobs of fat and slice the kidneys crosswise into pieces ½ inch thick. Dip the slices in the flour one at a time and shake them vigorously to rid them of any excess flour. Heat the remaining 2 tablespoons of butter and the 2 tablespoons of oil in a heavy 10- to 12-inch skillet set over high heat. When the fat begins to turn light brown, add the kidneys. Stirring frequently, fry them briskly until they are lightly browned (the lamb kidneys will take 2 or 3 minutes on each side, the veal kidneys 4 or 5 minutes). Do not overcook. With a slotted spoon, transfer the kidneys to the simmering soup. Pour off the fat in the skillet and in its place add 1 cup of the soup. Bring the soup to a boil, meanwhile scraping into it any browned bits clinging to the bottom of the pan. Pour the mixture into the soup and stir in the pickle juice.

In a mixing bowl, beat the egg yolk lightly with a fork. Slowly beat in 1 cup of the hot soup, then pour the egg mixture slowly into the casserole, stirring constantly. Simmer a moment or two without letting it come to a boil. Taste for seasoning, then serve the *rassolnik* directly from the casserole or in a large tureen.

You may either stir the sour cream into the soup directly before serving it or present it in a separate bowl to be added to each serving at the table.

To serve 6 to 8

2 tablespoons butter
½ cup finely chopped onions
1½ pounds beets, peeled and cut into strips ⅛ inch wide by 2 inches long (about 5 cups)
¼ cup red wine vinegar
1 teaspoon sugar
2 tomatoes, peeled, seeded and coarsely chopped (*see borshch ukraïnsky, page 141*)
2 teaspoons salt
Freshly ground black pepper
2 quarts beef stock (*see shchi, opposite*)
½ pound white cabbage, quartered, cored and coarsely shredded
¼ pound boiled ham, cut into 1-inch cubes
¼ pound all-beef frankfurters, cut into ½-inch-thick rounds
1 pound boiled brisket from the stock, cut into 1-inch cubes
4 sprigs parsley, tied together with 1 bay leaf

½ cup finely cut fresh dill or chopped parsley
1 cup sour cream

To serve 6

1 medium dill pickle
6 tablespoons butter
1 cup thinly sliced onions
½ cup finely chopped celery
1 cup finely chopped parsley
2 pounds fresh sorrel leaves, stripped from their stems, washed and coarsely chopped
¼ pound fresh spinach leaves, stripped from their stems, washed and coarsely chopped
2 teaspoons salt
Freshly ground black pepper
2 quarts beef stock, fresh (*see shchi, opposite*) or canned
1 pound veal or lamb kidneys, well trimmed of their fat
½ cup flour
2 tablespoons vegetable oil
1 egg yolk
2 cups sour cream (optional)

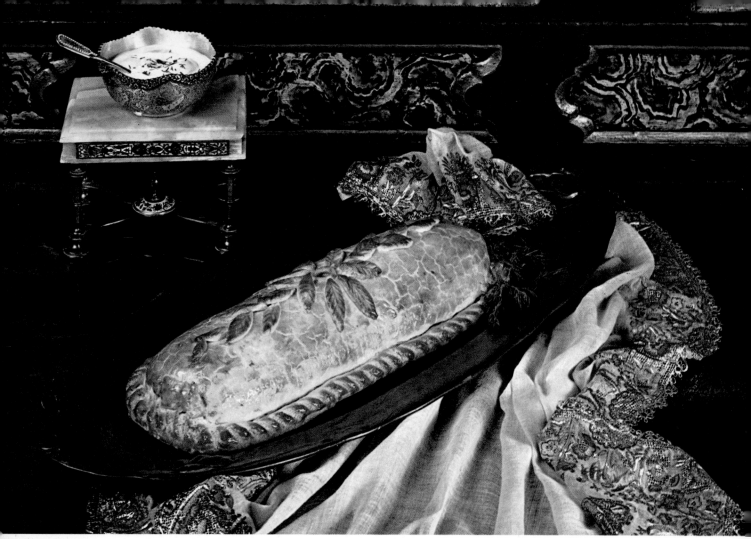

Kulebiaka—flaky pastry enfolding a rich salmon or cabbage filling—is an elegant luncheon or buffet dish served with sour cream.

Kulebiaka

FLAKY SALMON OR CABBAGE LOAF

PASTRY: In a large, chilled bowl, combine the flour, butter, shortening and salt. Working quickly, use your fingertips to rub the flour and fat together until they blend and resemble flakes of coarse meal. Pour 10 tablespoons of the water over the mixture all at once, toss together lightly and gather into a ball. If the dough seems crumbly, add up to 2 tablespoons more ice water by drops. Divide the dough in half, dust each half with flour, and wrap them separately in wax paper. Refrigerate 3 hours, or until firm.

SALMON FILLING: Combine 3 quarts of water, the wine, the coarsely chopped onion, celery, carrots, peppercorns, and 3 teaspoons of the salt in a 4- to 6-quart enameled or stainless-steel casserole. Bring to a boil over high heat, then lower the salmon into the liquid and reduce the heat to low. Simmer 8 to 10 minutes, or until the fish is firm to the touch. With a slotted spatula, transfer the fish to a large bowl and separate it into small flakes with your fingers or a fork.

Melt 2 tablespoons of the butter in a heavy 10- to 12-inch skillet set over high heat. Add the mushrooms, reduce the heat to moderate, and, stirring occasionally, cook for 3 to 5 minutes, or until the mushrooms are soft. With a slotted spoon, transfer the mushrooms to a small bowl and toss them with

To serve 8 to 10

PASTRY
4 cups all-purpose flour
½ pound chilled unsalted butter,
  cut into bits
6 tablespoons chilled vegetable
  shortening
1 teaspoon salt.
10 to 12 tablespoons ice water

92

lemon juice, ½ teaspoon of salt and a few grindings of pepper.

Melt 4 more tablespoons of butter in the skillet over high heat and drop in all but 1 tablespoon of the finely chopped onions. Reduce the heat to moderate and, stirring occasionally, cook 3 to 5 minutes, or until the onions are soft but not brown. Stir in the remaining 1 teaspoon of salt and ¼ teaspoon of pepper and with a rubber spatula, scrape into the mushrooms.

Now melt the remaining 2 tablespoons of butter in the skillet over high heat. Drop in the remaining tablespoon of chopped onion, reduce the heat to moderate and stirring frequently, cook for 2 to 3 minutes, or until soft but not brown. Stir in the rice and cook 2 or 3 minutes, stirring almost constantly, until each grain is coated with butter. Pour in the chicken stock, bring to a boil, and cover the pan tightly. Reduce the heat to low and simmer for 12 minutes, or until the water is completely absorbed and the rice is tender and fluffy. Off the heat, stir in the dill with a fork. Add the cooked mushrooms and onions, rice and chopped, hard-cooked eggs to the bowl of salmon and toss together lightly but thoroughly. Taste for seasoning.

CABBAGE FILLING: Over high heat, bring 4 quarts of lightly salted water to a boil in an 8- to 10-quart pot and drop in the cabbage. Reduce the heat to moderate and cook uncovered for 5 minutes. Then drain the cabbage in a colander and set it aside.

Melt the butter over high heat in a deep skillet or 3- to 4-quart casserole. Add the chopped onions, reduce the heat to moderate, and cook 5 to 8 minutes, or until the onions are soft and lightly colored. Drop in the cabbage and cover the pan. (The pan may be filled to the brim, but the cabbage will shrink as it cooks.) Simmer over low heat for 30 to 40 minutes, or until the cabbage is tender, then uncover the pan, raise the heat to high and boil briskly until almost all of the liquid in the pan has evaporated. Drain the cabbage in a colander and combine it with the chopped eggs, dill and parsley. Stir in the salt, sugar and a few grindings of pepper and taste for seasoning.

TO ASSEMBLE: Preheat the oven to 400°. Place one ball of dough on a floured surface and roll it into a rough rectangle about 1 inch thick. Dust with flour and roll until the dough is about ⅛ inch thick, then trim it to a rectangle 7 inches wide by 16 inches long.

Coat a large cookie sheet with 2 tablespoons of butter, drape the pastry over the rolling pin and unroll it over the cookie sheet. Place the filling along the length of the pastry, leaving a 1-inch border of dough exposed around it. With a pastry brush, brush the exposed rim of dough with the egg-yolk-and-cream mixture. Roll the other half of the dough into a rectangle about 9 inches wide and 18 inches long, drape over the pin and unroll over the filling. Seal the edges by pressing down hard with the back of a fork. Or use your fingertips or a pastry crimper to pinch the edges into narrow pleats. Cut out a 1-inch circle from the center of the dough. If you like you may gather any remaining pastry scraps into a ball, roll them out again, and with a cookie cutter or small, sharp knife, cut out decorative shapes such as leaves or triangles and decorate the top of the loaf. Coat the entire surface of the pastry with the remaining egg-yolk-and-cream mixture, place any pastry shapes on top, and refrigerate for 20 minutes. Pour 1 tablespoon of melted butter into the opening of the loaf and bake the *kulebiaka* in the center of the oven for 1 hour, or until golden brown. Serve at once, accompanied by a pitcher of melted butter or sour cream.

SALMON FILLING

2 cups dry white wine
1 cup coarsely chopped onions
½ cup coarsely chopped celery
1 cup scraped, coarsely chopped carrots
10 whole black peppercorns
4½ teaspoons salt
2½ pounds fresh salmon, in one piece
8 tablespoons unsalted butter (¼-pound stick)
½ pound fresh mushrooms, thinly sliced
3 tablespoons fresh, strained lemon juice
Freshly ground black pepper
3 cups finely chopped onions
½ cup unconverted, long-grain white rice
1 cup chicken stock, fresh or canned
⅓ cup finely cut fresh dill leaves
3 hard-cooked eggs, finely chopped

CABBAGE FILLING

3-pound head of white cabbage, quartered, cored, then coarsely shredded
4 tablespoons butter
2 large onions, coarsely chopped
4 hard-cooked eggs, finely chopped
¼ cup finely cut fresh dill leaves
2 tablespoons finely chopped parsley
1 tablespoon salt
½ teaspoon sugar
Freshly ground black pepper

2 tablespoons butter, softened
1 egg yolk, mixed with 1 tablespoon cream
1 tablespoon butter, melted
1 cup melted butter, hot but not brown, or sour cream

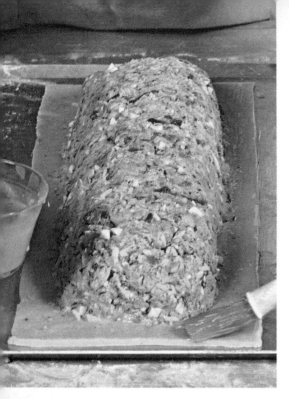

Constructing the Classic "Kulebiaka"

A delicate filling of salmon, mushrooms, onions, rice, eggs and herbs is mounded high on a 7-by-16-inch rectangle of dough that has been set on a buttered cookie sheet *(left)*. With a pastry brush, coat the exposed rim of dough with an egg yolk-and-cream mixture, then drape a 9-by-18-inch rectangle of dough over a rolling pin *(below)* and unroll it over the filling.

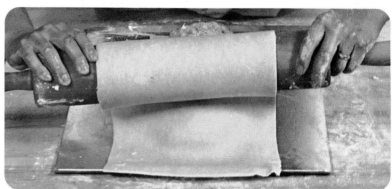

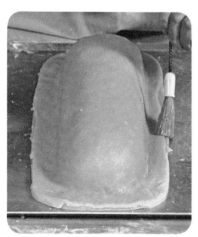

One way of sealing the loaf begins with a gentle brushing of the edges with the yolk-and-cream mixture.

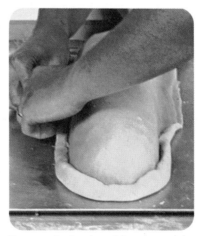

Turn up the border of dough to make a shallow rim around filling. Be careful not to stretch the dough.

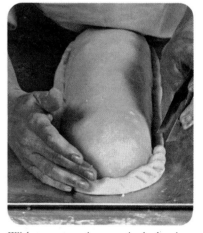

With a pastry crimper, pinch the rim in narrow pleats (or simply make shallow cuts with a small knife).

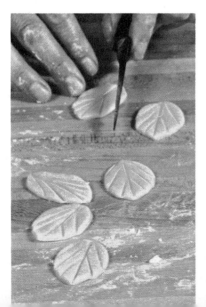

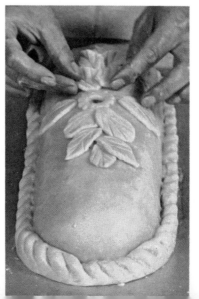

If you like, you may gather any remaining pastry scraps into a ball, roll them out again and, with a cookie cutter, cut out such decorative shapes as leaves *(far left)*. Use a small knife to make leaf veinings on the dough. Cut out a small circle from the center of the loaf and brush the entire surface of the loaf with the egg yolk-and-cream mixture. Then arrange the pastry leaves around the opening *(left)* and refrigerate before baking.

Kvas
MINT-FLAVORED BREAD BEER

Preheat the oven to 200°. Place the bread in the oven for about 1 hour, or until it is thoroughly dry. With a heavy knife, cut and chop it coarsely. Bring 6 quarts of water to a boil in an 8-quart casserole and drop in the bread. Remove from the heat, cover loosely with a kitchen towel, and set it aside for at least 8 hours. Strain the contents of the casserole through a fine sieve set over another large pot or bowl, pressing down hard on the soaked bread with the back of a large spoon before discarding it.

Sprinkle the yeast and ¼ teaspoon of the sugar over the ¼ cup of lukewarm water and stir to dissolve the yeast completely. Set aside in a warm, draft-free spot (such as an unlighted oven) for about 10 minutes, or until the mixture almost doubles in volume. Stir the yeast mixture, the remaining sugar and the mint into the strained bread water, cover with a towel, and set aside for at least 8 hours.

Strain the mixture again through a fine sieve set over a large bowl or casserole, then prepare to bottle it. You will need 2 to 3 quart-sized bottles, or a gallon jug. Pour the liquid through a funnel ⅔ of the way up the sides of the bottle. Then divide the raisins among the bottles and cover the top of each bottle with plastic wrap, secured with a rubber band. Place in a cool —but not cold—spot for 3 to 5 days, or until the raisins have risen to the top and the sediment has sunk to the bottom. Carefully pour off the clear amber liquid and rebottle it in the washed bottles. Refrigerate until ready to use. Although Russians drink *kvas* as a cold beverage, it may also be used as a cold-soup stock. (*See okroshka, below, and botvinia, Recipe Index.*)

Okroshka
CHILLED VEGETABLE SOUP WITH MEAT

With a large spoon, rub the eggs through a fine sieve set over a large bowl. Beat in the sour cream, mustard, salt and sugar, then slowly beat in the *kvas*. Add the scallions, cucumbers and meat, stir, and refrigerate before serving. Taste for seasoning, sprinkle with parsley and serve in chilled soup bowls.

Rybnaia Solianka
FISH SOUP WITH ONIONS, CUCUMBERS AND TOMATOES

In a 3- to 4-quart pot, combine 6½ cups of water, the onions, bay leaf, parsley and 1 teaspoon of the salt. Bring to a boil over high heat, then add the fish, lower the heat, and simmer gently, uncovered, for 6 minutes, until the fish is firm to the touch. Remove the fish and cut it into 1-inch chunks. Strain the fish stock through a fine sieve set over a bowl, pressing down on the onions and herbs with the back of a spoon before discarding them.

In a 2- to 3-quart casserole, melt the butter over high heat. Add the sliced onions, and cook 6 to 8 minutes until the onions are soft but not brown. Stir in the cucumbers and tomatoes and simmer 10 minutes. Pour in the strained fish stock, season with the remaining 2 teaspoons of salt and white pepper, and drop in the fish. Simmer gently a minute or two, until the soup and fish are heated through. Off the heat stir in the capers, lemon, parsley and olives. Taste for seasoning and serve directly from the casserole.

To make 6 cups

1 pound day-old black bread or
   Danish pumpernickel
2 tablespoons active dry yeast
1 cup sugar
¼ cup lukewarm water (110°-115°)
2 tablespoons fresh mint leaves or 1
   tablespoon crumbled dried mint
2 tablespoons raisins

To serve 6 to 8

4 hard-cooked eggs
1 cup sour cream
2 teaspoons Dijon or Düsseldorf
   mustard
1 tablespoon salt
1 teaspoon sugar
6 cups *kvas* (*above*), or less
   traditionally, substitute flat beer
¼ cup thinly sliced scallions,
   including 3 inches of their tops
1 medium cucumber, peeled, halved,
   seeded and cut into ¼-inch dice
½ pound boiled beef, cut into ¼-inch
   dice (*see shchi, page 90*), or substitute
   ½ cup diced boiled ham or veal
3 tablespoons finely chopped parsley

To serve 6 to 8

1 cup coarsely chopped onions
1 bay leaf
2 sprigs parsley
3 teaspoons salt
2½ pounds sturgeon, halibut or
   haddock steaks, cut 1 inch thick
4 tablespoons butter
2 cups thinly sliced onions
1 medium cucumber, peeled, halved,
   seeded and finely chopped
2 tomatoes, peeled, seeded and
   coarsely chopped (*see borshch
   ukraïnsky, page 141*)
⅛ teaspoon white pepper
4 teaspoons capers, drained and
   washed under cold running water
1 lemon, thinly sliced
2 tablespoons finely chopped parsley
12 black olives, pitted

To serve 4 to 6

4 cups large-curd pot cheese or
    cottage cheese (2 pints)
4 egg yolks
⅔ cup all-purpose flour
¼ teaspoon salt
2 tablespoons sugar
8 tablespoons (¼-pound stick)
    melted butter
1 cup sour cream

To make about 40

PASTRY
4 cups all-purpose flour
½ teaspoon salt
16 tablespoons (two ¼-pound sticks)
    unsalted butter, cut into ¼-inch
    bits and chilled
8 tablespoons chilled lard, cut into
    ¼-inch bits
8 to 12 tablespoons ice water

FILLING
4 tablespoons butter
3 cups finely chopped onions
1½ pounds lean ground beef
3 hard-cooked eggs, finely chopped
6 tablespoons finely cut fresh dill
    leaves
2 teaspoons salt
¼ teaspoon freshly ground black
    pepper

Syrniki
SWEET CHEESE FRITTERS

Drain the cheese of all its moisture by setting it in a colander, covering it with a kitchen towel, and weighting it with a heavy casserole. Let the cheese drain undisturbed for 2 or 3 hours, then with the back of a spoon, rub it through a fine sieve set over a bowl. Beat in the egg yolks, one at a time, and gradually beat in the flour, salt and sugar. Shape the mixture into 4 equal balls.

One at a time, place the cheese balls on a lightly floured surface and with your hands, form them into 3- or 4-inch-long sausage-shaped cylinders. Wrap each cylinder separately in wax paper and chill for at least 30 minutes.

With a heavy knife, cut each cylinder into 1-inch-wide rounds. Melt 4 tablespoons of the butter in a heavy 10- to 12-inch skillet. Add 6 to 8 rounds to the skillet, and fry over moderate heat for 3 to 5 minutes on each side, or until golden brown. Transfer the *syrniki* to a heated platter and cover them loosely with foil to keep them warm. Fry the remaining rounds similarly, adding butter to the pan as needed. Serve hot, with a bowl of sour cream.

Pirozhki
SMALL PASTRIES FILLED WITH MEAT

PASTRY: Combine the flour, salt, butter and lard in a deep bowl. With your fingers, rub the flour and fat together until they look like flakes of coarse meal. Pour in 8 tablespoons of ice water all at once and gather the dough into a ball. If it crumbles, add up to 4 tablespoons more ice water, a tablespoon at a time, until the particles adhere. Wrap the ball in wax paper, and chill for about 1 hour. On a lightly floured surface, shape the pastry into a rough rectangle 1 inch thick and roll it into a strip about 21 inches long and 6 inches wide. Fold the strip into thirds to make a 3-layered packet 7 inches long and 6 inches wide. Turn the pastry around and again roll it out lengthwise into a 21-by-6-inch strip. Fold into thirds and roll out the packet as before. Repeat this entire process twice more, ending with the folded packet. Wrap it in wax paper and refrigerate for at least 1 hour.

FILLING: Over high heat, melt the butter in a heavy 10- to 12-inch skillet. Add the onions and, stirring occasionally, cook over moderate heat for 8 to 10 minutes, or until they are soft and transparent but not brown. Stir in the beef and, mashing the meat with a fork to break up any lumps, cook briskly until no traces of pink remain. Grind the meat-and-onion mixture through the finest blade of a meat grinder (or, lacking a grinder, chop the mixture finely). Combine the meat in a large bowl with the eggs, dill, salt and pepper, mix thoroughly and taste for seasoning.

Preheat the oven to 400°. On a lightly floured surface, roll the dough into a circle about ⅛ inch thick. With a 3- to 3½-inch cookie cutter, cut out as many circles as you can. Gather the scraps into a ball and roll out again, cutting additional circles. Drop 2 tablespoons of filling in the center of each round and flatten the filling slightly. Fold one long side of the dough up over the filling, almost covering it. Fold in the two ends of the dough about ½ inch, and lastly, fold over the remaining long side of dough. Place the *pirozhki* side by side, with the seam sides down on a buttered baking sheet. Bake for 30 minutes, or until golden brown. Serve with clear chicken or beef soup, on the *zakuska* table or presented alone as a first course.

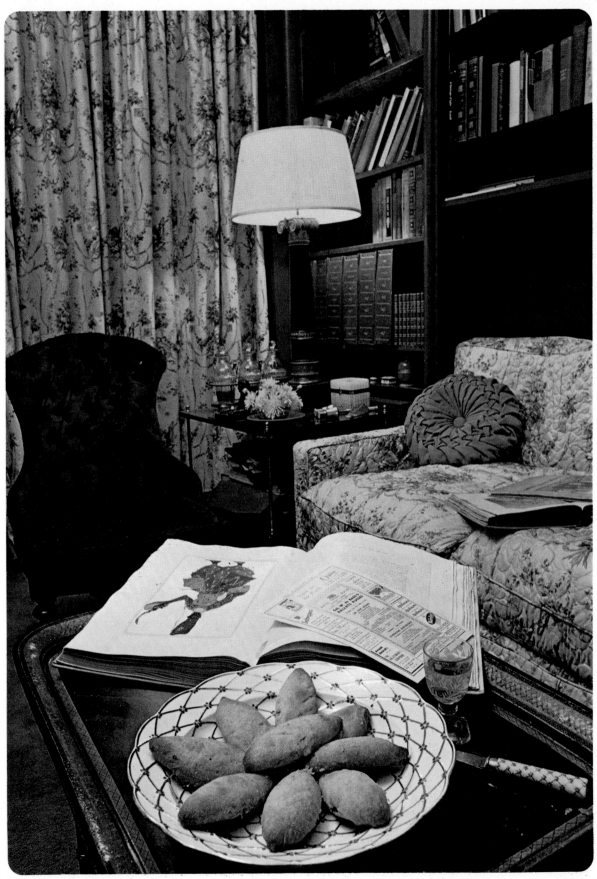

Pirozhki (recipe at left), Russia's famous meat-filled pastries, provide an unusual accompaniment to tea or cocktails.

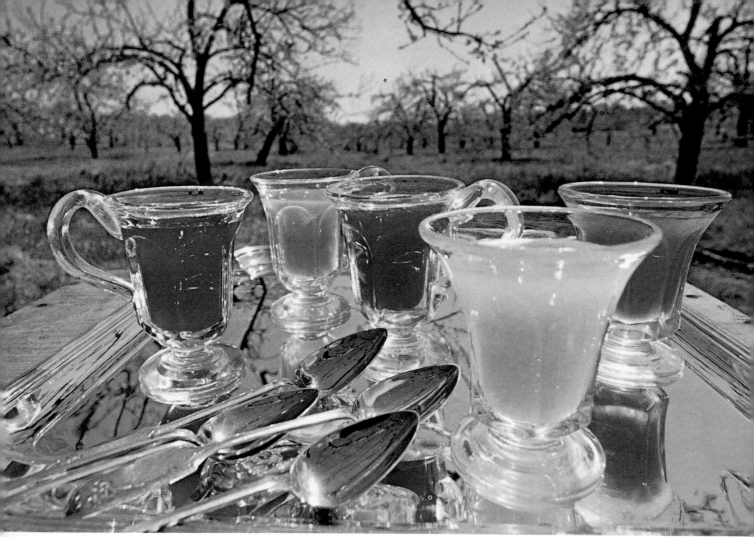

The subtle colors of puréed fruit glow in an array of *kisel,* a summertime dessert popular in the Soviet Union *(recipe opposite).*

Bliny

BUCKWHEAT PANCAKES

"Bliny" have a distinctive taste quite unlike the average griddlecake, mainly because they are made with a yeast batter. Their preparation should start about 6 hours before you plan to serve them. When the batter is complete, the pancakes must be cooked and served at once.

To serve 6 to 8

½ cup lukewarm water (110° to 115°)

1½ packages active dry yeast

½ cup buckwheat flour

2 cups white all-purpose flour

2 cups lukewarm milk (110° to 115°)

3 egg yolks, lightly beaten

½ teaspoon salt

1 teaspoon sugar

½ pound butter, melted and cooled

2 cups sour cream (1 pint)

3 egg whites

16 ounces red or black caviar or substitute 1 pound thinly sliced smoked salmon, sturgeon or herring fillets

Pour the lukewarm water into a small, shallow bowl and sprinkle the yeast over it. Let the yeast stand 2 or 3 minutes, then stir to dissolve it completely. Set in a warm, draft-free spot (such as an unlighted oven) for 3 to 5 minutes, or until the mixture almost doubles in volume.

In a large mixing bowl, combine ¼ cup of the buckwheat flour and the 2 cups of white flour. Make a deep well in the center and pour in 1 cup of the lukewarm milk and the yeast mixture. Slowly stir the flour into the liquid ingredients with a large wooden spoon, then beat vigorously until the mixture is smooth. Cover the bowl loosely with a towel and set it aside in the warm, draft-free spot for 3 hours, or until the mixture doubles in volume.

Stir the batter thoroughly and vigorously beat in the remaining ¼ cup of buckwheat flour. Cover with a towel and let the batter rest in the warm draft-free spot another 2 hours. Again stir the batter and gradually beat in the re-

98

maining cup of lukewarm milk and the 3 egg yolks, salt, sugar, 3 tablespoons of the melted butter and 3 tablespoons of the sour cream.

With a whisk or a rotary or electric beater, beat the egg whites in a large bowl until they form stiff, unwavering peaks on the beater when it is lifted from the bowl. With a rubber spatula, fold the egg whites gently but thoroughly into the batter, cover loosely with a towel, and let the batter rest in the warm, draft-free spot for 30 minutes.

Preheat the oven to 200°. With a pastry brush, lightly coat the bottom of a 10- to 12-inch skillet (preferably with a nonstick surface) with melted butter. Set the pan over high heat until a drop of water flicked across its surface evaporates instantly. Pour in about 3 tablespoons of the batter for each pancake (you will be able to make about 3 at a time, each about 3 or 4 inches wide) and fry 2 or 3 minutes, then brush the top lightly with butter. With a spatula or your fingers, turn the pancake over and cook another 2 minutes, or until golden brown. Transfer the pancakes to an ovenproof dish and keep them warm in the oven while you fry the remaining pancakes similarly, adding additional butter to the pan as needed.

Serve the *bliny* hot, accompanied by bowls of the remaining butter and the sour cream. Traditionally, the *bliny* are spread with melted butter and a mound of red caviar or slice of smoked fish, then topped with a spoonful of sour cream. If you are serving black caviar, omit the sour cream.

Kisel
PURÉED FRUIT DESSERT

Place the apples (or the apricots, strawberries, cranberries or rhubarb) in a 2- to 3-quart enameled or stainless-steel saucepan and pour in the appropriate amount of cold water. Bring to a boil over high heat, then reduce the heat to low and simmer the fruit uncovered for about 10 to 15 minutes, or until the fruit is tender.

With the back of a spoon, rub the fruit mixture through a fine sieve set over a mixing bowl and stir in the appropriate amount of sugar. Return the purée to the pan and bring it to a boil over high heat. Then reduce the heat to moderate, stir in the dissolved potato starch, and, stirring constantly, cook another 2 or 3 minutes, or until the purée just reaches the boil and thickens slightly. Remove from the heat and cool to lukewarm, then pour into individual dessert dishes. Refrigerate for at least 4 hours before serving.

To make 6 servings of each type

APPLE KISEL

2 pounds tart red apples, peeled, cored and cut into 1-inch-thick slices (4 cups)
3 cups cold water
1/2 cup sugar
1 tablespoon potato starch dissolved in 1 tablespoon cold water

APRICOT KISEL

1/2 pound dried apricots (1½ cups)
4½ cups water
4 tablespoons sugar
1 tablespoon potato starch dissolved in 1 tablespoon cold water

STRAWBERRY KISEL

2½ pints fresh strawberries, with hulls removed
2 cups cold water
3/4 cup sugar
1 tablespoon potato starch dissolved in 1 tablespoon cold water

CRANBERRY KISEL

3 cups uncooked whole cranberries (1½ pints)
2 cups cold water
3/4 cup sugar
1 tablespoon potato starch dissolved in 1 tablespoon cold water

RHUBARB KISEL

1½ pounds rhubarb, cut into 2-inch lengths (4½ cups)
3 cups cold water
3/4 cup sugar
1 tablespoon potato starch dissolved in 1 tablespoon cold water

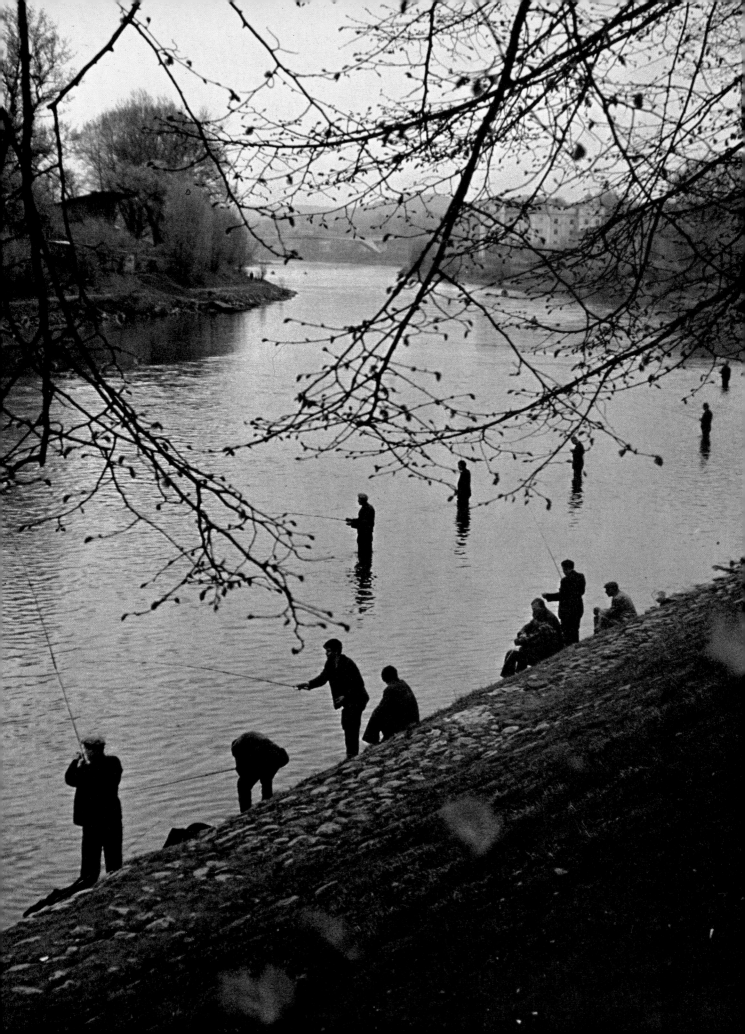

IV

The Baltic States: A Fertile Seacoast

As dusk falls across the Neris River in Vilnius, Lithuanian men patiently angle for perch and pike. This kind of fishing is a favorite sport all over the Soviet Union; the playwright Anton Chekhov maintained that a perch caught on a hook satisfied him "much more palpably than reviews and an applauding gallery."

Green is the dominant color of the Baltic Republics. As I flew from city to city in the Baltic Republics of Estonia, Latvia and Lithuania, everywhere I looked I saw green. There is the rich green of fertile pasture land, the dark green of pine and spruce, the lovely silver green of birch. In summer the sun shines late into the evening, setting afire the orange tips of the northern pines, and the dawn breaks so early that people sleep through the morning hours under a blanket of bird song. Approached by air or driven through by car, the rolling land presents a picture of utter tranquillity, with well-kept fields and innumerable blue-green lakes that reflect the sky.

The three Baltic states lie some 400 miles west of Moscow, in a northern spur of the great Russian Plain. Covering an area about the size of New England and including a population of a little over six million people, they fan out into the waters of the Baltic Sea in a gentle crescent. But the apparent peacefulness of the region is deceptive: It belies the history of three countries where, until fairly recent times, the inhabitants lived "as on a darkling plain swept with confused alarms of struggle and flight." The relative flatness of the land encouraged good farming, but it favored invasion as well. Countless soldiers of fortune from East and West have stormed across this vulnerable terrain. Among the first to come, as early as the Ninth Century, were Viking raiders; they were repulsed. So, in turn, were the Slavs and Mongols, pushing up from the south and halted in part by the barrier of dense forest. But as more and more trees were felled to accommodate the spread of agriculture, the Baltic peoples found themselves victimized by others who coveted their fertile land, their ice-free ports and their rich fisheries.

101

For centuries they had lived apart. They were pagans up to the 13th Century, worshippers of "springs and trees, mounds and hills, steep stones and mountain slopes." Their one major contact with the outside world had been through the amber trade (amber still washes up on their beaches). But when an occasional traveler came their way, they welcomed him into their midst with warm hospitality. In the First Century A.D. the Roman historian Tacitus described them as excellent farmers, and rated them above their "indolent" German neighbors. An 11th-Century German missionary bishop found them "a most humane people"—although it greatly puzzled him how they could have such high moral standards when they insisted upon worshipping trees. This aberration was forcibly remedied in the 13th Century when German missionaries and the military and religious order called the Teutonic Knights, motivated as much by greed as by pious zeal, undertook to make them Christians—and to take over their land. The "stubborn pagans" resisted fiercely, and when at last they were conquered, they subjected themselves to their masters in law and religion only. No matter who dominated them thereafter—Danes, Swedes, Germans, Poles, Russians—the Baltic peoples remained free in spirit, preserving their ancient languages and cultures right up to the present time.

I have known Estonians, Latvians and Lithuanians almost all of my married life. I had heard about their countries and sampled their family recipes for years; I detected not only nostalgia in their voices when they spoke of their fatherlands, but pride as well. Almost none of my friends have been back; war and changes in regime have made it difficult for them to return for a visit. But their homelands, I discovered, lived inside them—and in their kitchens. If few had been able to take their possessions with them, they had come away with their folk songs and recipes, ready to resume life elsewhere and to go on being themselves.

The Baltic peoples are singing peoples; all their national consciousness and all their love of nature is expressed in a huge body of folk songs (no fewer than 500,000 of these songs have been collected in Latvia and Lithuania alone, and the folk-music archives at Estonia's University of Tartu contain 250,000 *pages* of songs). And they are also eating peoples, whose big-boned bodies carry flesh and muscle well, reflecting the hard work they do. "We Latvians," a friend of mine said to me shortly before my husband and I left for the Soviet Union, "we like to eat, and good and plenty." She paused, and I could tell by her expression that she was home again in Latvia. "I still remember hot bread from the oven, a big slice. Mother put a piece of herring on it and on top—sour cream. It tasted better than cake!"

Even before visiting the region for myself, I knew from dishes I had eaten in the homes of my Baltic-American friends that Baltic cooking had a sturdy plainness to it. I thought of it as direct and touchingly honest, as my friends are—and every bit as warming. It was always prepared with feeling, and served in heaping mounds with all the pleasure that goes with giving. Heavy emphasis was placed on bread and potatoes, pork and fish, and such dairy products as milk, sour cream and cottage cheese—the last utilized in a spectrum of dishes ranging from caraway-sprinkled casseroles to dumplings and pancakes. And though such down-to-earth ingredients do not generally produce subtle results, I detected a delicate flavor of the past in what I ate, a

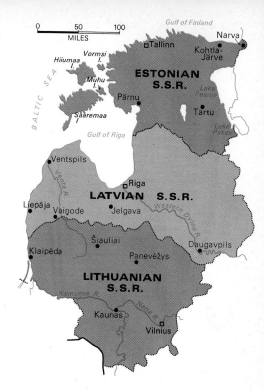

taste perhaps of the Middle Ages when rye, not wheat, was the basic grain and honey, not sugar, was everybody's sweetener.

Honey fresh from the comb is still used by the Baltic peoples in a variety of time-honored ways. It is essential to the production of the mildly fermented *krupnikas*, the Lithuanian national drink, into which goes a veritable spice chest of flavors—cloves, allspice, cinnamon, ginger, caraway, cardamom, nutmeg and saffron. It is beaten into cake batter, dribbled onto tortes and spread atop slices of farmers' cheese or raw, crisp cucumber. It is combined with tart apples and spices to produce "apple cheese"—a Lithuanian specialty that involves baking the fruit, sieving it, simmering it, and finally pressing the pulp between two boards and drying it in the oven.

I have come across recipes for unleavened buckwheat bread, which must be as old as the earth itself, and for *skaba putra*, a venerable sour-milk and barley soup that is allowed to ferment for 6 to 12 hours, then is chilled for the same length of time. It is served cold with sour cream, and customarily eaten in Latvia with herring or bread and butter. In Lithuania the traditional Christmas Eve dish, *ăvižinē košē*, or oatmeal porridge, is also fermented—but after standing 24 hours, it is boiled and then served with poppy-seed milk, a boiled syrup containing pounded poppy seeds, chopped almonds, milk and sugar. The survival of such dishes says much about the tenacity with which Baltic peoples cling to the old things they consider their own.

While dishes like these reach deep into the past of the Baltic lands, many others are Russian, or at least have Russian prototypes. But I have always been very careful not to say so. When people have been eating a dish for as long as they can remember and make it as their mothers and grandmothers made it, they like to claim ownership. And the variant is often as delicious as the original, in an entirely different way. Estonian stuffed cabbage (*Recipe Index*) is a good example. Its filling consists of three kinds of meat—veal, pork and beef—rather than the beef alone that is usual in the Russian version; it is bigger and juicier; and it is traditionally served with lingonberries.

I went to the Baltic Republics in search of what I already knew to be there, and I found it; but I also discovered a great deal more. The countryside was as green as I expected; in the forests the moss lay ankle deep. The cities were ancient as I had been told, with copper church towers that rise in needle-sharp steeples to lofty weather vanes and crosses, and red tile roofs so slanted that they look like two playing cards leaning together. In the markets sat rosy-cheeked old women selling baskets of mushrooms and bunches of herbs. But somehow I was not prepared for the differences I observed, many of them subtle to be sure, but all of them significant, separating Estonians from Latvians and Latvians from Lithuanians in kitchen as well as outlook. Though my Baltic-American friends spoke with dissimilar accents, I had made the mistake of lumping them and their cooking styles together. And there was something else I was not prepared for: the newness of so much that we saw. Had I taken into account the industriousness of my friends, perhaps I would not have been surprised by the industriousness of the peoples they left behind them along the Baltic.

Estonia, the first Baltic Republic we visited, reminded me of Scandinavia, as indeed it should have. Tallinn, the city where we stayed, was founded over 750 years ago by the Danes (Tallinn means "Danish City" in Estonian)

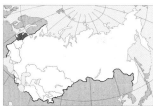

The Baltic Republics of Estonia, Latvia and Lithuania, occupying the eastern coast of the Baltic Sea, are among the smallest in the Soviet Union. But their economic importance is out of proportion to their size because of the fertility of the coastal plain and the value of its offshore fisheries. The Republics produce 13 per cent of the nation's fish and seafood products, and about a twentieth of its milk and eggs.

and the Danes were replaced by the Swedes. Both left an indelible mark upon the architecture of the city; some of the medieval buildings would look as much at home in Stockholm's old town as they do in Tallinn's —and so for that matter would some of Tallinn's new buildings in modern Stockholm. Even the shop signs suggest Scandinavia. One day, following the scent of fresh bread down a winding cobblestone street, we came to a bakery and found hanging over the door a gold, pretzel-shaped pastry exactly like the ones identifying similar shops in Denmark, Norway and Sweden.

The influence of Scandinavia can be tasted in Estonia no less than seen and heard. A Swede would not find himself out of place—or out of sorts —at an Estonian table. The assortment of cold foods that often begins a meal includes many of the same salty smoked fish dishes and herring specialties that the *smörgåsbord* does in Sweden, and the drink that goes best with it is, I think, icy vodka infused with caraway—the flavoring in aquavit.

Even when Estonian foods resemble those of Scandinavia, however, they can be charmingly different. Swedish meatballs and Estonian meatballs *(Recipe Index)* have in common the meats that go into them, veal, pork and beef; but there the resemblance ends. Estonian meatballs are, in fact, hamburgers —large patties that are flattened and fried in a pan. A similar difference of size occurs in the case of pancakes. We rose one morning to find pancakes on the breakfast menu of our hotel, and we ordered them, expecting to be served something like the characteristically small Swedish pancakes. Instead, we got one pancake each. My *pannkook (Recipe Index)* was as golden as a Swedish pancake and as buttery crisp around the edges, and I spread rubies of lingonberry preserves on top; but it was completely set apart from the Swedish kind by its diameter. It was almost as big and as round as the plate on which it was served. Later I discovered the batter for an Estonian pancake is allowed to stand for hours, overnight sometimes, which somehow blends flour, eggs and sugar in a pancake of omeletlike consistency. George and I ate pancakes for breakfast—but Estonians usually eat them for dessert.

Something else the Estonians share with the Scandinavians is a sweet tooth —and its indulgence in a cozy atmosphere. Down the dark, narrow alleys of Tallinn can be found many inconspicuous café doors. Push one open, and inside you enter a mellow world of relaxation, with people reading newspapers or talking in low voices while sipping coffee and eating butter-rich pastries and cream cakes. The tradition is an old one, going back to the early 18th Century, when coffee first became popular in Northern Europe and inspired a slew of baked goods to go with it. Nowhere in the Soviet Union is coffee so good or fortifying as it is in Estonia and Latvia. It is sometimes served with a heaping spoonful of whipped cream melting on top—a luxury in Moscow, but not in the Baltic Republics, where dairying is a major occupation.

One of the most enchanting places we saw in all the Soviet Union was a café on the outskirts of Tallinn. It is called the Flower Pavilion—and it is exactly that. My husband and I had been touring the city all day, and I was tired. When our guide suggested that we visit the pavilion, an inviting-looking glass-and-brick structure on a hillside, I begged off, but George decided to take one quick look. He came back moments later, filled with excitement. "You must come," he said. I got out of the car somewhat reluctantly. There were wide flights of glass-enclosed stairs to climb, but George took my arm

Spread on a table in an old-fashioned Latvian kitchen are the makings of a porridge called *skaba putra,* a classic Baltic dish consisting of sour milk *(in the large bowl),* barley *(in smaller bowl),* potatoes and salt pork. The typical accompaniments shown here are black bread and fresh radishes. The kitchen, equipped with a cast-iron, wood-fueled cooking stove and a brick oven, is now a museum piece. The house containing it, built in 1859, was moved from its original site to an open-air museum on the outskirts of Riga, Latvia, along with other old country buildings.

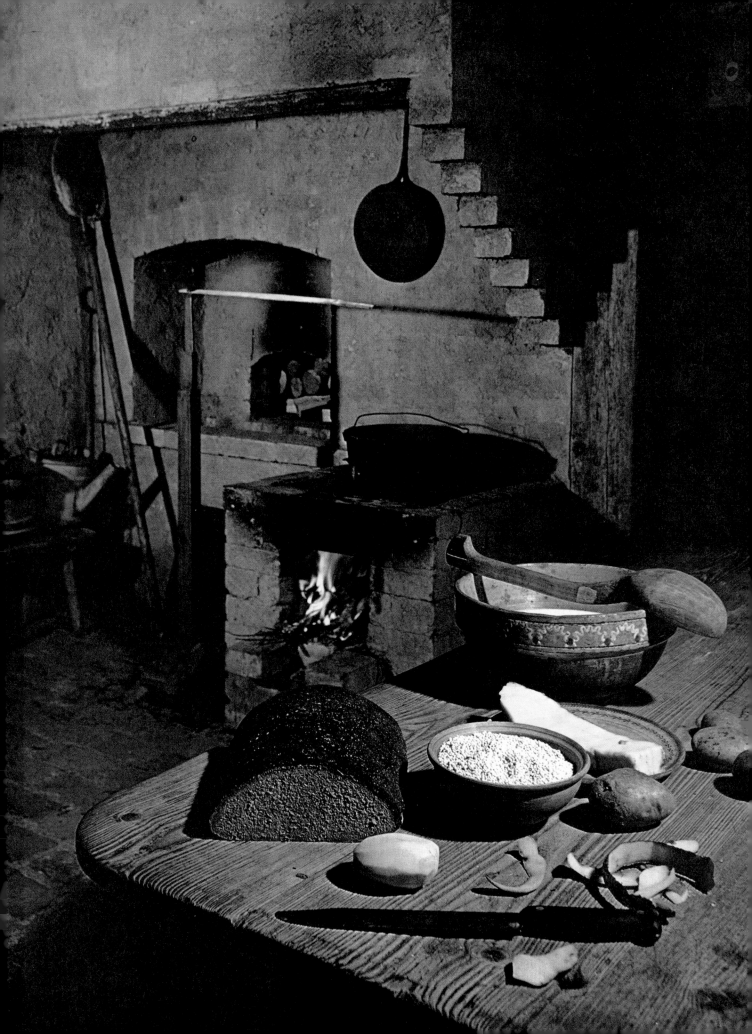

and led me on. Along either side of the steps were banks of flowers—on that day, they were chrysanthemums. At the top, we found ourselves in a sun-filled room, with huge windows and masses of brilliantly colored chrysanthemums banked up against the walls and around pillars. We were the only people there. Several tables spaced wide apart were covered with glowing white tablecloths; on one, the food for a tea party had been laid out, with a plate of open-faced sandwiches at each place, almost exactly like Danish *smørrebrød,* at the side a platter jammed with little cakes spread with thick frosting and whipped cream. We sat down at one of the unoccupied tables, near a tier of yellow chrysanthemums that reflected a golden light into our faces. What better place to rest than here, I thought.

A black-clad waitress with curly blond hair came to our table and asked if we cared for something to eat and drink. Suddenly, it seemed that we did. We ordered sandwiches, dessert and coffee. The sandwiches were special: the bread was, as it might be in Denmark, thinly sliced white bread, well buttered, and the ham and cheese had been placed on top with exquisite care—the edges of both had been delicately ruffled. We had two of these apiece and then settled back in the warm sunshine to wait for dessert. The waitress returned bearing an enormous tray. We were expected, her smile informed us, to sample all the sweets it bore. But that was plainly impossible. From an array that included rich gooseberry tarts, apple cake with whipped cream, and a variety of rum *babas,* I chose a simple bun. It had a baked sweet-sour topping of cottage cheese mixed with sugar and raisins. The cottage cheese, the waitress told us, is always heaped on thickly in Estonia—so thickly, according to one saying, that when the first bite is taken, your nose should dip into it. One bun was all I had room for; George sampled more widely, taking a slice of the apple cake and a piece of yellow, grainy-textured *liiva kook,* or sand cake *(Recipe Index).* The speed with which they disappeared convinced me that they must have been very good too.

We felt as comfortable as cats in the warm sunshine, overcome by an inertia that might have kept us at the Flower Pavilion the rest of the day had we not been lured to investigate the grounds behind the café. There we found a sculpture garden, and to our amazement, the works were not the heroic, monumental figures of official Socialist Realism, but modern pieces made of stone, metal and ceramic and displaying style—even wit. I fell in love with one enchanting conceit that exhibited an appealing Soviet practicality. It was a ceramic grill for roasting meat—but a grill with the head of a ram at one end and a curled metal tail at the other for shaking the grate.

The next day we flew to Latvia, Estonia's sister republic. As we dipped for a landing at Riga, the capital, I remembered that I had a special mission in Latvia, and vowed to accomplish it as soon as I could. Before leaving the United States, I had visited a Latvian friend in New York. Over the long years of our friendship we had talked often about going to Latvia together one day —and now I was going without her. I wanted to find a gift for her that would be special, something that would not merely remind her of home but actually *be* a piece of home. "Would you like me to bring you some amber?" I had asked her. She shook her head. "No," she said solemnly, "I want you, if you please, to bring me two pieces of bread, one piece of black bread and one piece of light bread. I want, before I die, to taste that bread again, I want to feel it in my teeth. I just want to taste it once more.''

After settling in our hotel in Riga, we went out to dinner and ordered as typical a Latvian meal as we could find. I asked for *kurzemes* pork, named after the town where my friend's mother had been born; George had *ligzdinas,* a large, moist patty with a surprise. As he cut into it, the meat—beef mixed with a little pork and bread—broke open to reveal a whole peeled hard-boiled egg. My *kurzemes* pork was fresh ham, pounded until thin, floured, browned and then simmered with onions in bouillon to which sour cream and mushrooms were added. It was extremely tender and not at all fatty. With our main courses came potatoes in several guises, including a potato basket for each of us, a crisp shell about the size of a cupcake, filled with canned peas, the prestige vegetable bar none in the Soviet Union. (We even saw people eating peas for breakfast, and with as much gusto as they ate caviar.) In addition to the pea-filled baskets, there was something that I will call a potato sundae—French fries topped with shoestring potatoes. We got the distinct impression that Latvians really liked potatoes.

With our meal came a large stack of bread, an almost black, tangy, sourish pumpernickel type and an oatmeal-colored, rich, whole-grain light bread. Tasting it I understood why Latvian bread was so lovingly remembered. I slipped a slice of each type into a plastic bag I had waiting in my pock-

Estonian herring salad, or *rossolye,* is a satisfying dish of the Soviet Union's northern seaboard. Besides herring it contains meat—ham, beef, veal or lamb (the version below has ham)—and at least five other ingredients: hard-cooked eggs, beets, potatoes, dill pickles and apples. Dressed with a sour-cream-and-mustard mixture, the salad refreshingly combines sweet and sour, tart and bland.

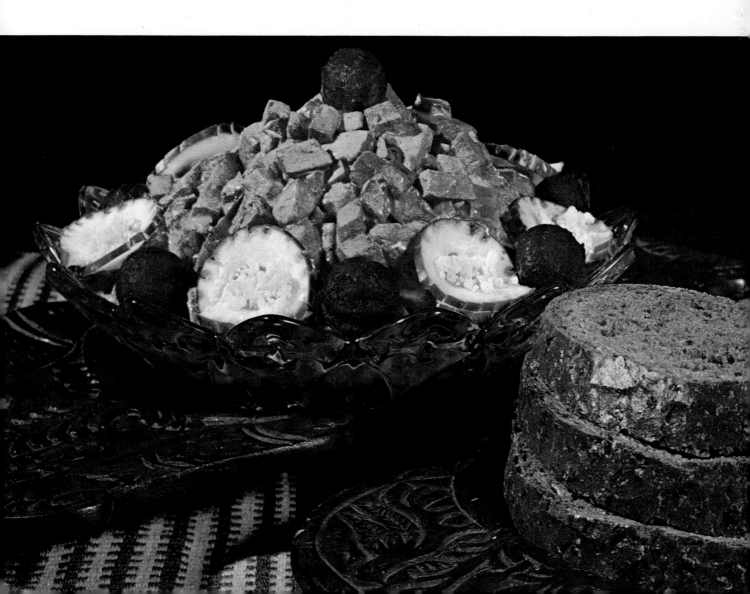

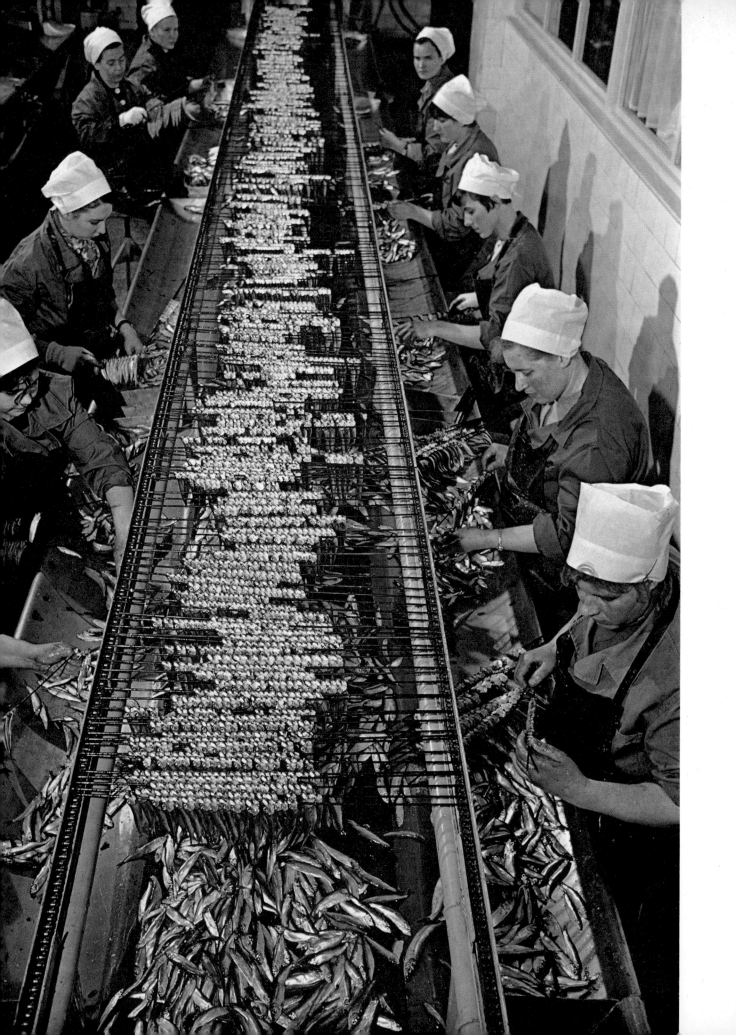

etbook, and later that night I took the bread out and put it on the radiator to dry; by midmorning it was ready to be packed carefully in my suitcase and taken back to my Latvian friend in America.

The next day we breakfasted early and went off to market, the biggest market in the Soviet Union. It occupies several converted Zeppelin hangars, originally built at Vaiņode by the Germans during World War I, then moved 80 miles to Riga in the 1920s; and it overflows onto several acres outside. At first we thought that we had come to the wrong place, for all we saw were flowers—tubs of flowers, pots of flowers, baskets of flowers, jars with flowers jammed down into them, paper cornucopias with flowers bunched inside. There were dahlias, flame red and bright orange; chrysanthemums, yellow, white and rust; Michaelmas daisies; purple asters and pink cyclamen. And all the green string bags dangling from the fingers of the shoppers had bouquets bobbing out their tops. The flower explosion, we soon realized, had been brought on by the threat of frost in the air; the growers had stripped their gardens in the hope of earning a little money before the winter set in and there would be no more flowers to sell.

At Soviet markets two types of vendors are to be seen: those from a collective or state farm, and private individuals who sell produce grown in their own farming plots or gardens. Some of the latter are entrepreneurs who hope to make a quick profit with a particularly scarce item. At the Riga market we saw a group of men who had flown in from Azerbaijan, 3,000 miles to the southeast, with 10 bags of melons. They were charging eight rubles (about nine dollars) for a melon and they were getting it.

We strolled around outside before entering the old hangars sheltering the meat and fish stalls. Long wooden tables held piles of vegetables and fruit, carefully arranged to look as attractive and appetizing as possible. At one stall, four plump potatoes had been laid out on a plastic doily. Carrots and radishes had been scrubbed until they glowed. Bunches of dill provided a note of fresh green and, in the midst of so many flowers, looked somewhat like the asparagus fern that florists insert into bouquets in America.

Inside, we came to the area where fish is sold. If I lived in Latvia, I would want to eat fish all the time. The variety was enormous, and I could see from the cold glitter in the eyes of the specimens I examined that they had been caught only recently. Freshness is a serious concern of the Soviet shopper —and especially so when it comes to fish. Indeed, some women prefer to buy their fish alive. I have seen fishmongers throughout the Soviet Union make a cone of old newspapers, scoop a flouncing fish from a tank, pop it into the cone, ladle in some water, fold the cone over at the top and hand the package to the shopper who then puts it into her green string shopping bag and nonchalantly carries her squirming purchase home.

The Latvians are the great fishermen of the Soviet Union. Before World War II, they concentrated on the Baltic coast, supplying the eels, sprats and herring that are still a major part of the diet of the country. But with the development of fishing cooperatives and the introduction of new equipment after the war, they took to ranging far afield, into the Norwegian Sea, the North Sea, the Atlantic, and even the Caribbean Sea. Their trawlers—and the factory ships that follow along behind to process the catch—now turn up off the coasts of Africa, Iceland and Newfoundland.

Preparing sprats for passage through an automated 40-minute smoking process, Latvian women thread the fresh fish on long metal rods. Their factory on the Gulf of Riga is part of the 12,000-member Ninth of May Fishing Collective. Trawlers belonging to the collective range as far as the Grand Banks off Newfoundland, while smaller Ninth of May craft work the Baltic's coastal waters.

The sight of so much fresh fish in the market made us hungry for fish, and we went off to lunch. The restaurant we picked, the Pearl of the Sea, lies in a seaside resort not far from Riga. It is a cantilevered, glassed-in structure jutting over the white sand beach and offering an uninterrupted view of sea and sky. We decided to have a fish *solianka (Recipe Index)*, a savory dish that could be called either a thin stew or a thick soup, depending on how you chose to look at it.

After *solianka*, dessert seemed an impossibility; if I had not been so anxious to try a cake called Alexander torte *(Recipe Index)*, I might have settled for a cup of coffee. I had heard my Latvian and Estonian friends talk about it, and though they had promised to bake me one, somehow they had never gotten around to it. Alexander torte, I was happy to discover, is more cookie-like than cakelike in consistency. It consists of two thin, crisp layers mortared with raspberry conserve and iced with a lemon-and-sugar glaze.

After lunch we decided to pay a visit to an ethnological museum located in a large park at the edge of the city. Following the example of the Swedes, who were the first in Europe to set up open-air museums, the Latvians have brought together farmers' and fishermen's homes from all over the country and re-erected them in clearings among the pines and ancient oaks. It is an enchanting place, representing the Latvia of the past—the Latvia that is still alive in the memory of my friends. The houses, dating from the 18th and 19th Centuries, generally were built with no more than three rooms, and the kitchen was easily the most important of the three. Each house was furnished as though a family still lived in it; the utensils were worn with use, and beautiful for being so. In the kitchen of one was an ingenious churn made from a hollowed-out log and mounted on a pair of rockers. To make butter, the housewife had only to rock the log.

Behind one gray wooden house, its thatched roof covered with emerald moss, we paused in front of a giant rosebush. Dangling from its branches were orange rose hips, almost as big as plums. George picked one and broke it open to reveal the fuzzy choke inside. Rose hips are still sold in Baltic markets, to be made into jams and purées. They are a particularly rich source of Vitamin C and are much used during the winter. Close by the rosebush was a windmill, its blades motionless in the soft autumn air. Latvia was once known for its windmills, and with brown Latvian cows grazing in front of them (cows of a special breed that produce especially rich milk), the low, flat landscape must have had a Dutch look.

Only a day after visiting the ethnological museum, with its pervasive atmosphere of the peasant past, we found ourselves at the very forefront of the Soviet Union's 20th Century in the bustling industrial city of Vilnius, the capital of Lithuania. We came by plane, and the initial impression we had from the air was of an old city, its skyline jagged with church spires. But on the ground the city proved to be anything but old-fashioned. Savagely shelled and bombed during the war, Vilnius had rebuilt itself. The modern architecture is graceful and human in scale, blending with the traditional —or even with the very old, of which a great deal still remains.

In its way, the new architecture can be taken as a manifestation of the Lithuanian spirit of independence. Plainly rejected in the planning of the city was the wedding-cake style of architecture that marred post-war Moscow.

The Lithuanians possess a deep sense of their own nationhood. During the Middle Ages, their country stretched from the Baltic to the Black Sea, and was one of the most powerful duchies in Europe until it merged with neighboring Poland in 1569. Though Lithuanians thereafter had a number of masters, they kept their ancient tongue and their strong spirit of independence.

Their cooking displays a similar individuality. (Some of it, I think, only a Lithuanian could care passionately about. A favorite dish is pig's stomach, stuffed with potatoes and herring, and baked; another is fried black bread, heavily flavored with garlic.) But there are many other foods to rouse the appetite and roundly satisfy it. The most delicious sausages I ate in the Soviet Union I had in Lithuania. One, called *sviežià dėsrà*, contained ground beef and pork and was flavored with garlic, black pepper, chopped parsley and nutmeg. The sausage was served hot, and the tomato sauce that went with it also had a touch of nutmeg.

Before World War II, many Jews lived in Lithuania, and they adapted or developed their own special dishes. Vilnius was once a center of Jewish learning and culture; more than half its citizens were Jews. After the Nazi holocaust, only a handful remained, but among these a few still cook as of old. In their homes—and in the homes of many gentile Lithuanians—can be found the melt-in-the-mouth honey cake called *lekakh*, and crunchy-edged *kugelis*, grated potato puddings baked with eggs and onions *(Recipe Index)*. *Kugelis* can seem a simple thing to make, but only the true cook knows that old potatoes give the best results, and that the grated potatoes should stand exactly two and a half inches high in the baking dish.

Since World War II, Lithuanian cooking has acquired a much broader base, at least in Vilnius, a city that in recent years has attracted skilled workers and technicians from all over the U.S.S.R. A Russification of the kitchen is taking place, partly as a result of communal dining halls in factories, where the dishes reflect the standardized training of Soviet cooking schools.

There are scores of cooking schools scattered throughout the Soviet Union. One of the best is in Vilnius, and it proved to be not only a place where young people learn to cook, but also a canteen servicing Vilnius' 400-year-old university. We got a behind-the-scenes look at mass-feeding operations —and, as it turned out, found ourselves being mass fed.

It was 12 o'clock and the students were streaming into the university dining hall. Making selections from the cafeteria counter, a line moved past the tables, each attractively set with flower-patterned restaurant china and a small bouquet of fresh flowers. George and I donned white uniforms, complete with a chef's hat for him and a kerchief for me, and were taken back into the kitchen where the white-clad pupils of the culinary school were at work in an atmosphere of hushed concentration. Instructors passed from group to group, commenting on the dishes in progress. Several girls were making *virtiniai* (called *pelmeni* in Russia)—a boiled dumpling made of noodle dough and stuffed with mashed potatoes, although meat, cheese or almost any vegetable is also used. To make first-class *pelmeni* takes a certain skill: The dough must be rolled thin, but not so thin that it bursts when dropped in the bubbling water. A pretty young instructor was carefully inspecting the *pelmeni* made by the girls. Whenever she came upon any that had burst or were badly shaped, she would point out to the student cook her mistake; she man-

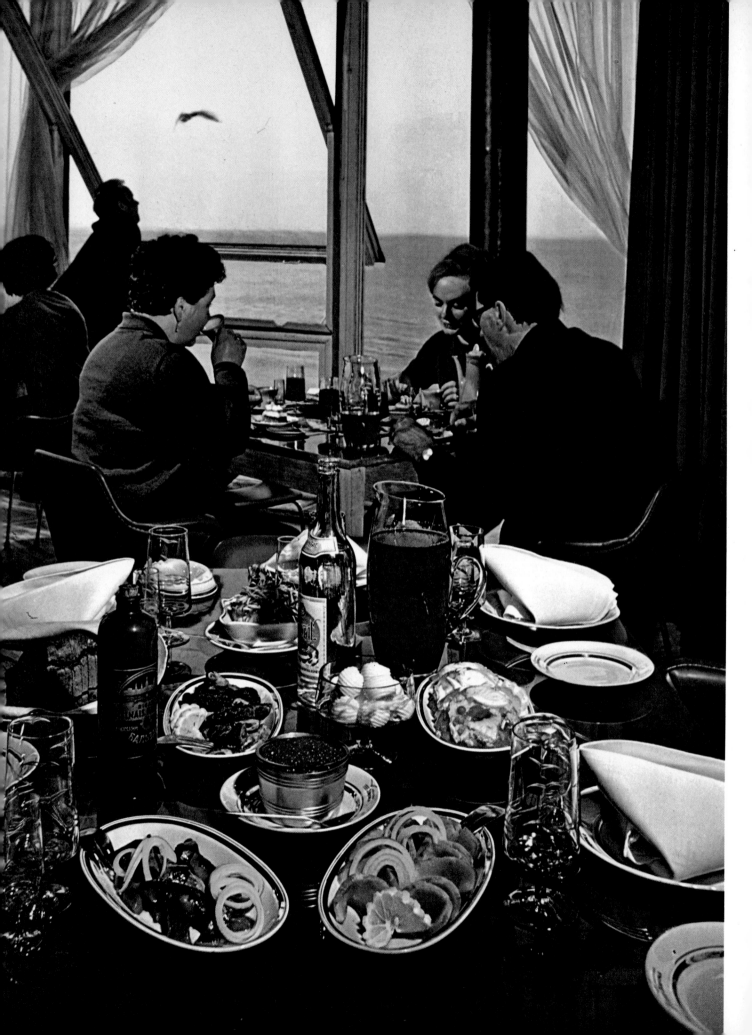

aged to do this with great dignity and concern, almost as though she were correcting a faulty premise in logic or a mistake in a geometry lesson. The student, in turn, would listen carefully, apply herself to rectifying her error and —lo!—produce perfect *pelmeni.* Smiles on both sides.

At a stove, pupils were frying another Russian dish, *kotlety,* ground meat mixed with moistened bread crumbs, finely chopped raw onion and a little milk. Close by, others were deep-frying the little oblong meat pies called *pirozhki.* Another group was making potato pancakes. "You have wonderful potatoes," I said to the instructor in charge. "Yes, we think we do," she said. "Lithuanians eat lots of potatoes. In fact, we eat so many potatoes we have a central potato peeling plant here, and peeled potatoes are delivered all over the city every morning."

Now came the time to try some of the food. The first thing brought to our table in the student dining room was a platter of *pelmeni,* the boiled dumplings, with a touch of melted butter and a topping of sour cream. I expected them to be as heavy as lead, but they were light—and almost as surprising was the agreeable taste and texture of noodles and mashed potatoes combined. Next came the potato pancakes, delicious, too. After that the *kotlety* arrived, brown on the outside, very moist and tender inside. We could eat no more, not even one of the crisp, finger-length *pirozhki,* and we made an attempt to get up. "Oh, no, wait," said one of the girls, "you haven't had your dessert yet!" And on came the final course—not one dessert but three: a delicate fruit gelatin; a thickened pudding with apples, pears and cherries cut into it; and a rich-looking dish that, as far as I could ascertain, was scarcely more than a mountain of whipped cream.

After a meal like that, there was only one thing to do—walk. And we found plenty of opportunity for that at the "apple fair." An exhibition of apples did not strike us as the most exciting thing to attend, but people kept insisting that we visit it—and how glad I am that we did. I found out that the Lithuanians, for all their progress, are tree worshippers still.

The apple fair was being held in a pavilion located in a park. Similar pavilions can be found throughout the Soviet Union; they serve as permanent exhibition centers for displays of the workers' achievements and resemble nothing so much as a perpetual American county fair—minus the midway. The apple fair had attracted a great throng. A queue of at least 1,000 apple lovers ran completely around the pavilion waiting to get in. As tourists—which, in Lithuania, means welcome guests—we were accorded the privilege of entering the pavilion without having to queue up. The moment we stepped inside, we were enveloped in the sweet perfume of apples. Every kind of apple raised in Lithuania seemed to be on display, ranging from pale ivory to brilliant crimson. All the state and collective farms had sent their apples, and so had a great number of individual growers. The bakers and other food processors had cooperated with the apple growers, using the fruit as the basis for innumerable desserts and treats. There were ginger cookies made with ground apples, tarts with sliced apples on top, puffs with apples inside, tortes, apple-cream cakes (including one surmounted by a pineapple cornucopia stuffed with jellied crab apples), candies made of apple paste, apple juice, apple syrup, even apple wine. And passing to and fro were apple-cheeked Lithuanians, oohing and aahing over everything they saw.

The Juras Perle Restaurant (Pearl of the Sea) on the beach at Bulduri, near Riga, is famous for its seafood and the beauty of its view over the Baltic. The table in the foreground is set in typical Latvian style with smoked salmon, herring with onion, red caviar, fried lamprey, sturgeon in jelly and straw potatoes. A pitcher of cranberry juice accompanies the feast, along with bottles of vodka and an herb liqueur called Balsam.

To serve 4 (8 to 10 pancakes)

1 cup all-purpose flour
2 cups milk
2 egg yolks
2 tablespoons sugar
¼ teaspoon salt
2 egg whites
3 tablespoons butter
½ cup lingonberry preserves, or
substitute any berry preserves

Pannkoogid
DESSERT PANCAKES

Place the flour in a large mixing bowl and, with a large spoon, slowly beat in the milk a half cup at a time. Then beat in the egg yolks, sugar and salt. When the ingredients are thoroughly combined, set the batter aside in a cool —not cold—place for at least 3 hours or even overnight.

Just before making the pancakes, beat the egg whites in a large bowl with a whisk or a rotary or electric beater until they form stiff peaks on the beater when it is lifted out of the bowl. With a rubber spatula, gently but thoroughly fold them into the batter.

Preheat the oven to 250°. With a pastry brush, lightly coat a 5- to 6-inch crêpe pan or skillet with 1 teaspoon of the butter. Pour in ½ cup of the batter, tilting the pan to spread it evenly. Fry over moderate heat for about 3 minutes on each side, until the pancake is golden, turning it over with a spatula. Slide the pancake onto an ovenproof platter and keep it warm in the low oven while you fry the remaining pancakes in similar amounts. Serve the *pannkoogid* on heated dessert plates, accompanied by a bowl of berry preserves.

To make about 4 dozen

½ pound unsalted butter, chilled
and cut into bits
3 to 3½ cups all-purpose flour
3 tablespoons sugar
1 egg
1½ cups (12 ounces) raspberry
preserves
2 tablespoons softened butter

WHITE ICING
2 cups confectioners' sugar
¼ cup cold water
2 teaspoons lemon juice

Aleksander Torte
RASPBERRY-FILLED PASTRY STRIPS

In a large mixing bowl, combine the chilled butter, 3 cups of the flour and the sugar and, with your fingertips, rub until the mixture resembles flakes of coarse meal. Beat in the egg and continue to mix until the pastry is smooth. Shape it into a ball, wrap it in wax paper, and refrigerate 1 hour, or until the dough is firm.

With the back of a spoon, rub the preserves through a fine sieve set over a 1-quart saucepan, then cook over moderate heat, stirring constantly, for 3 to 5 minutes, or until they thicken into a thin purée. Set aside off the heat.

Preheat the oven to 250°. Cut the chilled pastry in half and shape each half into a rectangle. One half at a time, roll the pastry between two sheets of lightly floured wax paper into a rectangle approximately 10 inches wide and 15 inches long. With a pastry brush, coat each of 2 cookie sheets with 1 tablespoon of butter and sprinkle them with flour, tipping the sheets from side to side to coat them evenly. Then invert the sheets and tap them against a hard surface to dislodge any excess flour. Following the pictures opposite, use the wax paper to lift the pastry onto the sheets. Bake 40 minutes, or until the pastry begins to turn a pale gold. Watch carefully for any sign of burning and regulate the heat accordingly.

With a metal spatula, spread the raspberry purée evenly over one sheet of the pastry, covering it completely and smoothly. Slide the second sheet of pastry gently onto the first.

With a spoon stir the sugar, water and lemon juice together in a large mixing bowl to form a thin paste. Spread the icing smoothly over the top layer of pastry with the spatula, and set the cake aside to cool to room temperature. With a small, sharp knife or pastry wheel, slice the *Aleksander torte* into strips 1 inch wide and 2 inches long.

Bulvių Maltiniai
FRIED POTATO PATTIES

To serve 8 to 10

3 pounds baking potatoes, peeled and quartered
1 egg
½ to ¾ cup flour
2 teaspoons salt

4 tablespoons butter for frying

Bring 4 quarts of water to a boil in a 6- to 8-quart pot and drop in the potatoes. Boil briskly, uncovered, until they are soft enough to be easily pierced with a fork. Drain them thoroughly in a large sieve and force them through a ricer or mash them in a bowl with a fork. Beat in the egg, ½ cup of flour and the salt, and continue to beat vigorously until the mixture is smooth and dense enough to hold its shape almost solidly in a spoon. (If the mixture seems too fluid, beat in the remaining flour, a tablespoon at a time.)

Gather the potato dough into a ball, place it on a heavily floured surface and pat it into a thick rectangle. With a floured rolling pin, roll it into a large rectangle about 1 inch thick, dusting it frequently with a little flour to prevent it from sticking to the pin or board. With a sharp knife or pastry wheel, cut 2-inch-wide strips down the length of the dough, then slice diagonally into 2½-inch-wide lengths. Gently score the top of each diamond-shaped patty by making shallow lines down its length.

Melt 2 tablespoons of the butter in a heavy 10- to 12-inch skillet set over high heat. When the foam has almost subsided add 6 or 8 of the patties and brown them 3 to 5 minutes on each side, turning them over carefully with a large spatula. Transfer the patties to a serving platter and cover them loosely with foil to keep them warm while you fry the remaining patties, adding more butter to the pan as needed.

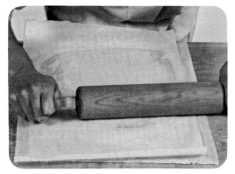

Roll half of the delicate *Aleksander torte* pastry between two sheets of lightly floured wax paper.

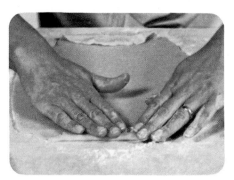

To make a 10-by-15-inch rectangle, fold in any excess edges, cover with wax paper again and roll smooth.

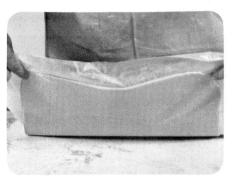

Peel off the top sheet of wax paper and use the bottom one to lift the pastry onto a cookie sheet.

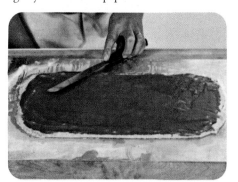

Similarly roll the remaining dough and bake each separately. Spread one layer evenly with raspberry purée.

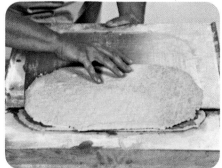

Gently slide the second layer of pastry off its cookie sheet onto the raspberry-covered layer.

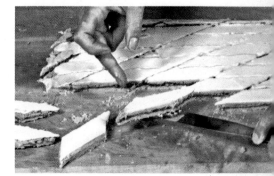

Cover the top layer of pastry with lemon-flavored sugar icing, cool, then slice into 1-by-2-inch strips.

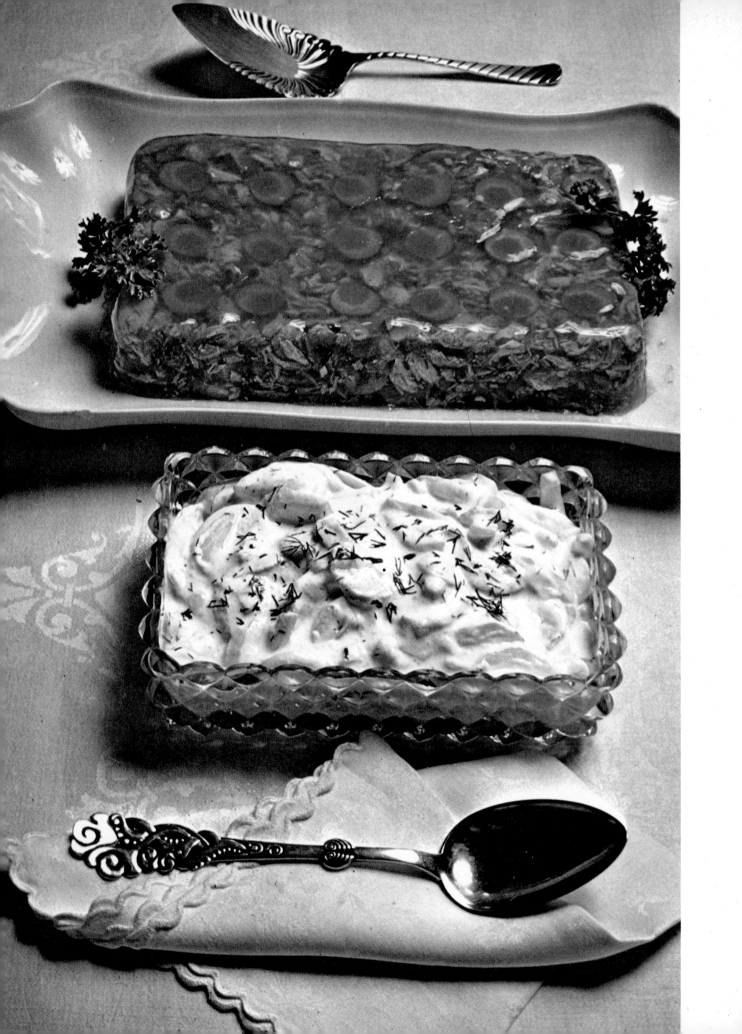

Agurkai su Rukcscia Grietne

CUCUMBER-AND-SOUR-CREAM SALAD

In a mixing bowl, combine the cucumber slices, salt and vinegar and toss them about with a large spoon until the cucumber is well moistened. Marinate at room temperature for 30 minutes, then drain the cucumbers through a sieve and pat them thoroughly dry with paper towels. Place them in a large mixing bowl.

Separate the yolks from the whites of the hard-cooked eggs. Cut the whites into strips ⅛ inch wide and 1 to 2 inches long and stir the egg whites into the cucumber.

With the back of a large spoon, rub the egg yolks through a fine sieve set over a small bowl. Slowly beat in the mustard, sour cream, white wine vinegar, sugar and white pepper. When the dressing is smooth, pour it over the cucumbers and toss together gently but thoroughly. Taste for seasoning.

To serve, arrange the lettuce leaves on a large flat serving plate or on small individual plates and mound the salad on top of them. Sprinkle with dill and refrigerate until ready to serve.

Sult

JELLIED VEAL

In a heavy 4- to 6-quart casserole, combine the veal, pig's knuckles, onion, carrot, and water and bring to a boil over high heat, meanwhile skimming the foam and scum from the surface as they rise to the top. Then add the whole peppercorns and bay leaves, reduce the heat to low, and simmer partially covered for about 3 hours, or until the veal is tender enough to be easily pierced with a fork.

With a slotted spatula, transfer the veal and pig's knuckle to a plate. Strain the cooking stock in the casserole through a fine sieve set over a large bowl and let it rest for about 10 minutes. Then with a large spoon, skim off and discard all the surface fat. Pour the stock into a small pan and boil it briskly, uncovered, until it has cooked down to 4 cups.

When the veal and pig's knuckle are cool enough to handle, trim off the fat with a small knife and cut the meat away from the bones. Discard the bones and cut the meat into ¼-inch-wide shreds.

Arrange the carrot slices in concentric circles in the bottom of a 2-quart charlotte or a similar mold at least 3 inches deep. A teaspoon at a time, sprinkle the carrots evenly with the stock, and continue adding the stock by teaspoons until the carrots are half submerged but not floating in the liquid. Carefully place the mold in the refrigerator without dislodging the design and chill for at least 1 hour, or until the stock has firmly jelled.

By this time the remaining stock should be cool. Stir in the meat, salt and garlic and taste for seasoning. Then pour the entire mixture into the chilled mold. Refrigerate for at least 4 hours, or until the stock is firm.

To unmold, run a knife around the inside edges of the jellied veal. Dip the bottom of the mold briefly in hot water, then invert a flat serving dish on top. Holding mold and plate firmly together, turn them over. The jellied veal should slide out easily. Traditionally, *sult* is served as a first course or on the *zakuska* table.

To serve 4 to 6

4 medium cucumbers, peeled, halved, seeded, and cut crosswise into ½-inch-thick slices
1 tablespoon coarse salt, or substitute 2 tablespoons table salt
½ teaspoon white distilled vinegar

DRESSING

3 hard-cooked eggs
1 teaspoon prepared mustard, preferably Dijon or Düsseldorf
⅓ cup sour cream
2 teaspoons white wine vinegar
¼ teaspoon sugar
⅛ teaspoon white pepper

4 to 6 large lettuce leaves, well washed and dried
1 tablespoon finely cut fresh dill leaves

To serve 6 to 8

1½ pounds shoulder of veal cut into 2-inch pieces
1½ pounds fresh pig's knuckles, cracked with a cleaver
1 large onion (about 1 pound), unpeeled
1 large carrot, scraped and cut crosswise into ⅛-inch-thick rounds
2 quarts cold water
6 whole black peppercorns
3 bay leaves
1 tablespoon salt
1 teaspoon finely chopped garlic

Sult, an Estonian specialty of jellied veal, accompanied here by a cucumber-and-sour-cream salad, makes a refreshing first course or light summer meal.

To serve 8 to 10

½ pound ground lean veal
½ pound ground lean pork
½ pound ground lean beef
½ cup fresh bread crumbs, made
  from homemade-style white bread,
  pulverized in a blender or finely
  shredded with a fork
1 cup finely chopped onions
2 eggs
Salt
Freshly ground black pepper
A 5-pound boned shoulder of veal
4 hard-cooked eggs, peeled
1½-2 cups cold water, or 1½-2 cups
  chicken stock, fresh or canned
½ cup sour cream

To serve 6 to 8

DRESSING
3 teaspoons powdered mustard
1¼ teaspoons sugar
1 to 2 tablespoons warm water
1 cup sour cream

SALAD
2 hard-cooked eggs, finely chopped
2 large or 4 small boiled and peeled
  fresh beets, or 4 canned beets,
  cut into ¼-inch dice
1 pound (about 3 medium) boiled
  potatoes, peeled and cut into ¼-
  inch dice
1 pound (about 2) sour dill pickles,
  cut lengthwise into narrow strips,
  then crosswise into ⅛-inch-wide
  bits
1 fillet of pickled or *matjes* herring,
  drained and cut into ¼-inch dice
1 pound boiled beef, or cooked ham,
  veal or lamb, trimmed of fat and
  cut into ½-inch dice
1 large, tart red apple, cored, peeled
  and cut into ¼-inch dice
3 hard-cooked eggs, cut into quarters

Täidetud Vasikarind
ROAST STUFFED SHOULDER OF VEAL

To make the stuffing, combine the ground veal, pork and beef in a large mixing bowl, and add the bread crumbs, onions, water, eggs, 1 tablespoon of salt and 1 teaspoon of pepper. Mix with your hands or a large spoon until all the ingredients are well combined. Then vigorously knead the mixture for 3 to 5 minutes, or until smooth.

Preheat the oven to 350°. Skin-side down, spread the veal shoulder flat on a table and, with a small, sharp knife, make small cuts in the thickest areas of the meat so that it lies even flatter. Lay a sheet of wax paper over the veal and with the side of a cleaver or meat pounder, pound the meat to a fairly uniform thickness. Remove the paper and sprinkle the veal liberally with salt and somewhat more discreetly with pepper.

Spread half the stuffing on the veal, leaving a 2-inch border of the veal exposed all around the sides. Lay the hard-cooked eggs in a row down the length of the stuffing and spread the remaining stuffing in a layer over them. Bring one long side of the veal over the filling to the middle, and tuck in the two ends. Now bring the other side over the filling, enclosing it snugly. With strong kitchen cord, tie the rolled veal crosswise at 2-inch intervals, then with more cord tie it lengthwise.

Place the rolled veal seam-side down in a shallow roasting pan just large enough to hold it comfortably. Pour in 1½ cups of cold water or chicken stock and roast for 2 hours, undisturbed, basting the veal from time to time with the pan juices. When the meat is a deep golden brown, carefully transfer it to a serving platter and cut off and discard the strings.

Bring the juices remaining in the pan to a boil over high heat. If most of the liquid has cooked away, add the remaining ½ cup of water or chicken stock to the pan, meanwhile scraping into it any brown bits that may be clinging to the pan. Off the heat, stir the sour cream into the sauce, a tablespoon at a time. Taste for seasoning and pour into a sauceboat.

Slice the roll crosswise into 1-inch rounds and arrange them slightly overlapping down the center of a large heated platter. Moisten them with a few tablespoons of sauce and serve the remaining sauce separately.

Rossolye
ESTONIAN VINAIGRETTE WITH HERRING AND BEETS

DRESSING: In a small bowl, combine the dry mustard with ¼ teaspoon of the sugar and stir in 1 to 2 tablespoons of warm water, or enough to make a thick paste. Set aside for 15 minutes. Then stir in the sour cream and the remaining teaspoon of sugar.

SALAD: In a large mixing bowl, combine the finely chopped eggs, diced beets, potatoes, pickles, herring, meat and apple. Add the sour cream dressing and toss together lightly but thoroughly until all the ingredients are well moistened with the dressing.

Traditionally, *rossolye* is mounded high on a square or round serving plate, garnished with sliced hard-cooked eggs, and chilled. Serve as a first course or as part of a *zakuska* table.

A surprise stuffing of chopped meat and hard-cooked eggs enriches an Estonian specialty, *täidetud vasikarind,* or rolled shoulder of veal. Accompanying the dish are crisply fried potato patties.

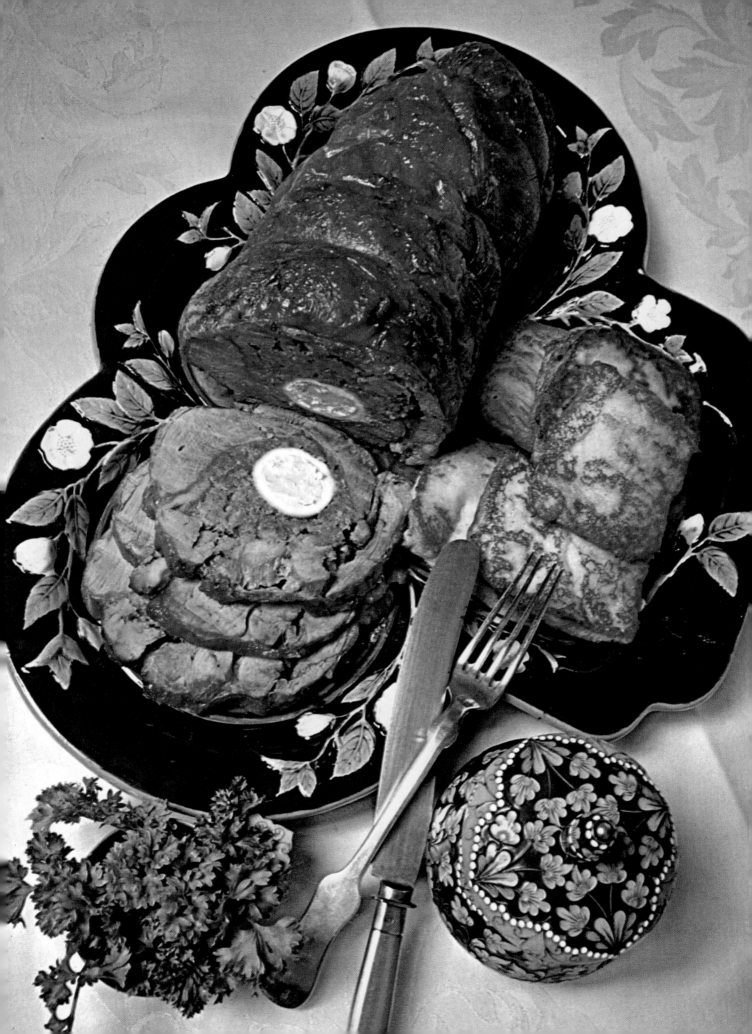

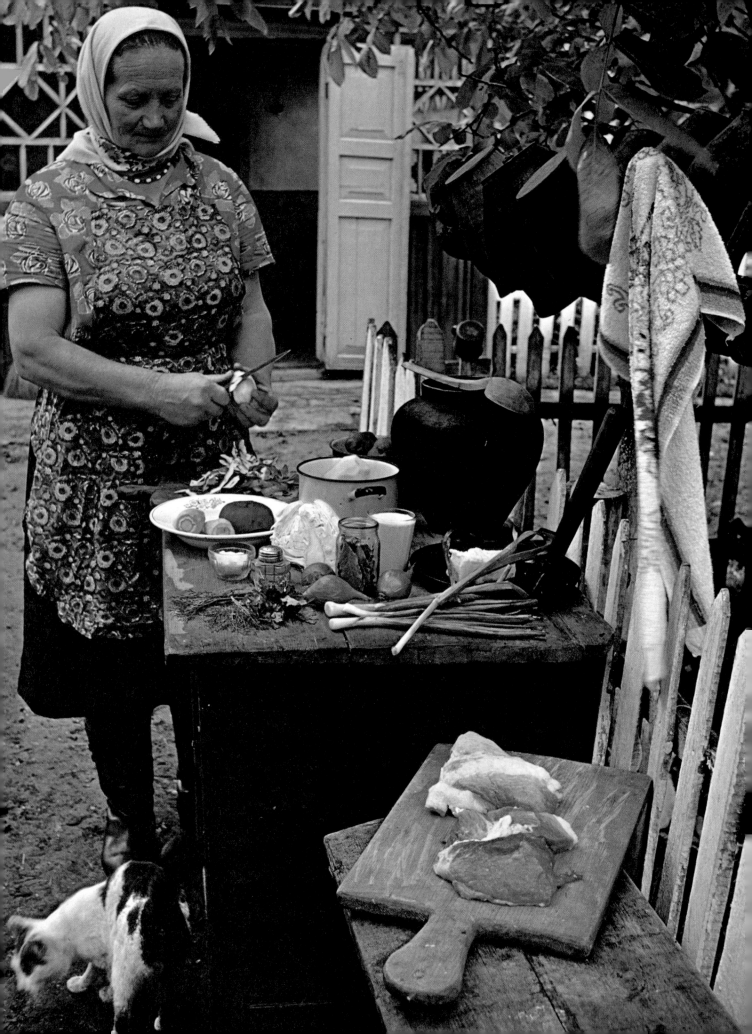

V

Ukraine: Breadbasket and Sugar Bowl

Peeling potatoes, Khristina Djima of the Ilyich Collective Farm near Kiev, begins the preparation of Ukrainian *borshch* for a dinner *(page 128)*. Among the other ingredients in her version of the soup are beets, cabbage, carrots, onions, garlic, pork fat, bay leaves and sour cream. Meat for the soup, a cut of boned pork, lies on the cutting board in the foreground.

As a traveler moves southwest from the Baltic States and the Russian Republic, the land around him changes. The rolling green plains, which in the north grew monotonous, become a magnificent sweep of beauty. Under a brilliant sky, flower-edged fields roll on and on in limitless swells to meet the horizon that rises far to the west in the distant peaks of the Carpathian Mountains. This is the Ukraine, the second largest (after Russia itself) of the 15 Soviet republics in population and production, the third largest (after Russia and Kazakhstan) in sheer size.

Like the Russians, the Ukrainians are Slavs, but Slavs with a language, a literature, a culture and a cuisine very distinctly and proudly their own. Despite repeated occupations of their land—by Mongols, Poles, Lithuanians, Turks and Germans—the Ukrainians have kept their independence of spirit and their national traditions. And they have been blessed by nature. Rich and deep and black, the Ukrainian soil—the famous *chornozem,* or "black earth" —fills the air with a loamy fragrance; abundant rain and mild climate make this soil one of the most fertile croplands in all the world. For centuries the Ukraine was called "the breadbasket of Europe," and plowing, sowing and reaping set the rhythm of life there. In time, golden grain and all that comes from it became a symbol of the Ukraine as well as its basic food.

The Frenchman Honoré de Balzac, who visited the Ukraine in the 1840s, noted, with proper French respect: "I counted 77 ways of making bread" —and a Ukrainian added, with proper pride, "No one has ever counted all our cakes." The range of these baked goods is no less awesome than their number. Among the "plain" breads (if any example of Ukrainian baking

121

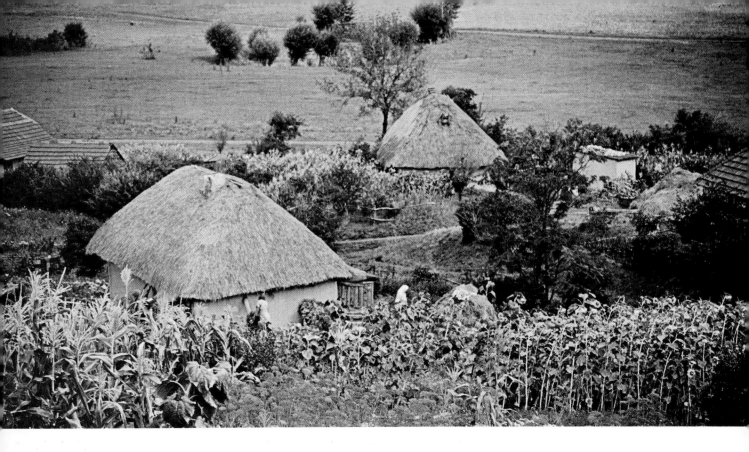

The rich, warm countryside of Poltava is typical of the Ukraine —gently rolling land, deep black soil, cottages and copses. This region, one of the world's most fertile, is still the Soviet breadbasket, although the Soviet government has been opening the so-called "virgin lands" of its eastern steppes to large-scale grain production. Here in Poltava nearly everything that springs from the earth means wealth: even the sunflowers are valued for oil and for their edible seeds.

can be called plain) are such everyday fare as *agnautka*, a flat, whole-grained loaf; *polianitsa*, a white mound of bread two feet around, topped with a crusty cap; and *ukrainka*, a heavy, dark, rough-textured product that comes in three-pound loaves shaped like cartwheels. Then there are special breads for almost every important occasion in Ukrainian life. Honored guests are greeted with a fresh loaf bearing a shaped mound of salt. A bride and groom are blessed, the dead are remembered and Christmas is celebrated with an intricate, triple-braided ring of especially rich bread called *kalach*, which symbolizes both good fortune and eternity. On New Year's Eve unmarried girls foretell their futures with small sour-dough rolls called *balabushky;* according to tradition, a girl who finds a coin baked into her *balabushka* will be married before the year is out. And for the wedding itself, seven bridesmaids will grind flour from wheat grown in seven different fields to bake a *korovai*—a good-luck loaf ornamented with such emblems as rosettes, nesting doves and hearts and flowers of dough.

Along with these plain and ritual breads there is a profusion of sweet rolls and other sweet-dough delights. Their very names, linked together, make a kind of poem—*pampushky, rohalyky, zavyvanets, bulochky, palochky, perekladanets*. These translate, respectively, into doughnut puffs, either plain or filled with rose petals; almond horns; sweet dough filled with fruit and nuts and shaped in a roll, coil or ring; crumb-sprinkled buns; soft, sweet "sticks," and layered coffee cake. And these are but a prelude to the true cakes, which include tarts and tortes, sponge cakes and wafers, strudels and fritters, meringues and thin pancakes. There are loaf cakes and cakes shaped into roses, balls, knots, shells, horns or crowns; there are plain cakes and cakes filled with poppy seed, cream, nuts, fruits, honey or cheese.

"How do you ever learn to bake them all?" I asked a Ukrainian friend.

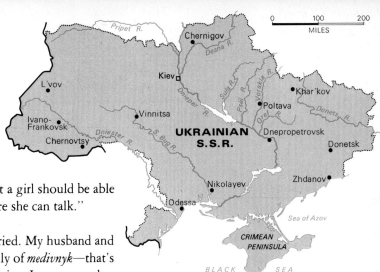

"By starting early. My grandmother always said that a girl should be able to sift flour before she can walk and knead bread before she can talk."

"Did you?"

"No. On the contrary, I learned nothing until I married. My husband and I were living in Moscow then, and he talked so longingly of *medivnyk*—that's a honey cake—that I wrote my grandmother for the recipe. I soon got a letter from her explaining just how to boil the honey and beat in the eggs and listing all the ingredients—but not giving the quantities of any of them. I asked her, 'How much of each ingredient?' Back came her answer: 'How can I tell you? It depends on whether you want enough for a wedding, a medium-sized party or a present.' I worked it out, but it took time."

For all their profusion and richness, breads and cakes represent only a part of the culinary wealth of the Ukraine. Early travelers in the region marveled at the abundance they saw on every side. One visitor described "smiling cottages" surrounded by gardens full of melons, eggplants, cucumbers, and pumpkins "of a size that would need but wheels to be a coach." Michael the Lithuanian, who went to the Ukraine on a diplomatic mission in the mid-16th Century, noted in his diary that "the rivers are filled with an immense quantity of sturgeon and other big fish. Therefore, many rivers are called 'golden,' especially the Pripet, which . . . at the beginning of March is filled with such a great quantity of fish that a spear thrown into the water stands upright, as if pushed into the ground. I would not have believed this, had I not seen for myself how the people fished. . . ." Elsewhere, a chronicler of the 17th Century saw a single cast of a net at the mouth of the Orel River bring in no less than 2,000 fish, the smallest of them a foot long.

Modern visitors find the same rich plenty, and on an even vaster scale. Grain is still important but other crops have become more prominent. Driving through the countryside George and I saw sugar beets in mile-long rows (the Ukrainian "breadbasket" is now sometimes called the "Soviet sugar bowl"), sweeps of orchards with heavily laden fruit and nut trees, potato fields that stretched beyond the eye's pursuit, and vast tracts of mammoth-headed sunflowers. The sunflowers are grown for their seeds, which are either pressed into oil or cracked and roasted to make a snack that is a favorite in every part of the Soviet Union. The foothills of the Carpathian Mountains, blue and purple shadows on the western horizon of the Ukrainian plain, provide pasturage for beef and dairy cattle breeds, such as the Simmental, Red Steppes and Grey Ukrainians.

With such a brimming cornucopia spilling its bounty, Ukrainian cookery has always displayed a greater variety of raw materials than that of the Russian Republic. More meats are used. Beef round is often sliced into steaks, spread with seasoned bread crumbs, rolled up and either oven or pot roasted, then served with a savory sauce of the stock and sour cream. A liberal addition of bread crumbs also goes into *sichenyky* and *kotlety;* Ukrainian cooks

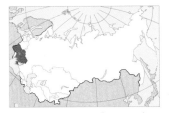

Among the 15 republics making up the Union of Soviet Socialist Republics, the Ukrainian S.S.R. is second only to the Russian S.F.S.R. in population and production and is surpassed only by Russia and Kazakh in area. The rich black soil of the Ukraine produces such abundant crops of grain that the region was formerly known as "the breadbasket of Europe." In recent times it has become the producer of more than half the Soviet Union's sugar (all derived from sugar beets) and has earned the new nickname of "the Soviet sugar bowl."

argue that the crumbs are the secret of keeping these patties juicy, for the ground meat or vegetables will not otherwise retain the moisture of egg and milk. Pork from big white Mirgorod pigs is well finished and carefully cut. We sampled a crackling pork roast glazed with tart applesauce and touched with spices, and a dish of pork chops baked with pungent caraway seeds.

Fish are still plentiful. Sturgeon from the Sea of Azov is common everywhere and—for that reason, perhaps—is treated more casually than in the north; sometimes it is simply boiled, without seasonings or condiments to dispute its quiet authority. Herring are smoked or pickled, and eaten the year around. River fish, such as pike, perch and carp, are often stuffed with crumbs and baked; alternatively, they may be fried in a batter or simmered in sour cream. A pike in glistening jelly is a traditional dish for Christmas Eve.

The long Ukrainian growing season, now further extended by the wide use of greenhouses, makes vegetables abundant throughout the year. Corn, which flourishes in the Ukraine, is eaten on the cob, and the meal is used for a porridge and a soft spoon bread. Beets, potatoes and cabbage are year-round staples. The beets are often shredded and baked in butter and vinegar, but the ways of preparing cabbage are limited only by the ingenuity of the cook. Sometimes a cabbage is wilted, a meat-and-crumb mixture is tucked between each leaf, and the whole head, tied with string, is simmered in tomato sauce. Single cabbage leaves are filled with cooked rice, either alone or combined with meat or mushrooms, then rolled into packets called *holubtsi* ("little pigeons") and simmered (*Recipe Index*). As a variation, beet leaves may make the wrapper and bits of raised yeast dough, the filling; spinach, the outside leaves of lettuce, and even grape leaves are also used for the same dish. The crown of cabbage cookery, and the "proof-piece" of a good Ukrainian cook, is *nakypliak*, a steamed cabbage soufflé. A first-rate *nakypliak* takes a good two hours to concoct, but it is worth every minute of the time, for the first bite reveals hitherto unsuspected qualities in a homely old friend.

As might be expected, the versatility of grain is utilized to the utmost. Wheat, millet, pearl barley and buckwheat are baked or steamed as *kasha*, to be eaten with milk at breakfast and with meat at other meals. More elaborately, wheat grains are combined with honey, poppy seeds and stewed, dried fruit to make *kutia*, a traditional meatless dish for Christmas Eve. Flour not only goes into breads and cakes but is converted into rich egg noodles called *lokshyna*, eaten alone or with meat, vegetables or soft curd cheese (*Recipe Index*). Boiled, drained and fried, *lokshyna* has the luminosity of new straw, the flavor of unthreshed grain. Utterly different in texture and taste is the popular dish called *halushky*—bits of dough made from wheat flour, milk and egg yolks, boiled in water or broth and served with sour cream or onions that have been browned in sunflower-seed oil (*Recipe Index*).

The most typically Ukrainian flour-based dish, however, is probably the dumplings called *varenyky* (*Recipe Index*). The dish is permanently listed on all restaurant menus, there are cafés that serve nothing else, and in most households it is made once or twice a week. Everyone in the Ukraine knows that good *varenyky* must be made with a dough that is tender and thin, yet has enough strength and elasticity to encase the filling without bursting when it boils. The number of "right" ways to achieve this ideal, however, must very nearly equal the number of good cooks in the republic.

124

Continued on page 129

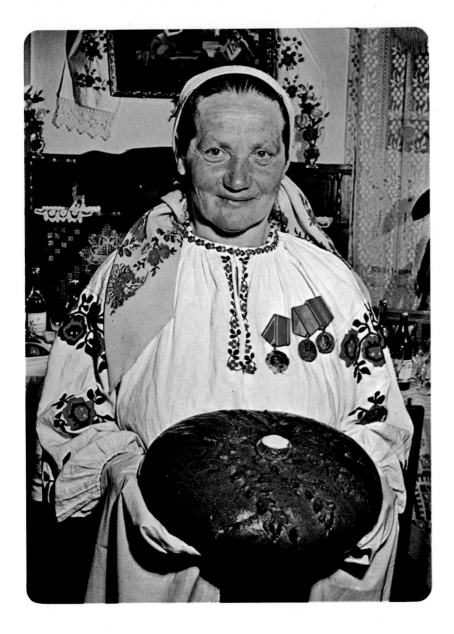

Dressed in her best embroidered blouse, Khristina Djima welcomes guests with the traditional loaf and mound of salt. She wears the Order of Lenin and medals for labor achievements and for service in World War II.

Overleaf: Scores of different breads are baked at a single Ukrainian shop on Kreshchatik Street in Kiev. The assortment shown, keyed by numerals printed on the picture, consists of three major kinds: black breads, sweetened white breads and unsweetened white breads. Perhaps the most renowned of Ukrainian breads are *chernyi khlib,* or the dark rye or black breads (10, 20, 24, 25). Most of the white breads have more or less sweetening and are commonly served with tea or coffee. Among these are *khala* (28, 15), braided twists baked with and without poppy seeds; *zdoba* (2, 3, 5, 7, 16, 17, 18, 19), which are sweet buns; *perepychka* (1, 12); a sweetened version of *kalach* (8), a popular white bread; *kruchenyk* (9, 14, 21), a twisted bun; and *rizhok* (23), a little horn. Sweetened specialty breads include *solomka* (4), which is a bread straw, and *bublyky* (26, 30), bagel-like hard rolls. Most popular unsweetened white bread is probably *korzh* (6). Others include unsweetened *kalach* (11, 13, 29); *frantsuzski kalach* (22), a French-influenced *kalach;* and *polianitsa* (27).

Bread and Salt, Edible Symbols of Ukrainian Hospitality

In the Ukraine—as in most of the Soviet Union—the symbolic *khlib i sil* (the Ukrainian words for bread and salt), offered on a folded white cloth, is hospitality made tangible. Bowing, the host and hostess declare Prosymo zavitaty (welcome, with good will) and present the loaf to the guest. He is expected to cut a slice of bread, dip it in the salt and eat it. This age-old custom is often interpreted to mean that, even in a house too poor to offer more than bread and salt, the guest is welcome to share. But however poor the house, there is nothing poor about the splendid variety of Ukrainian breads.

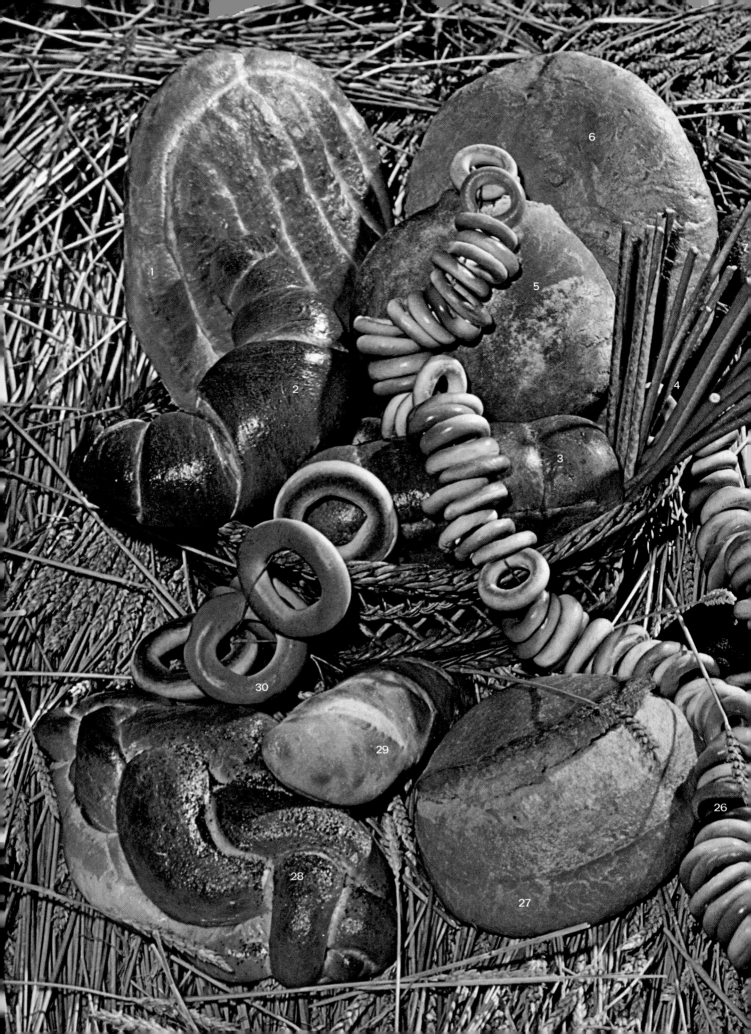

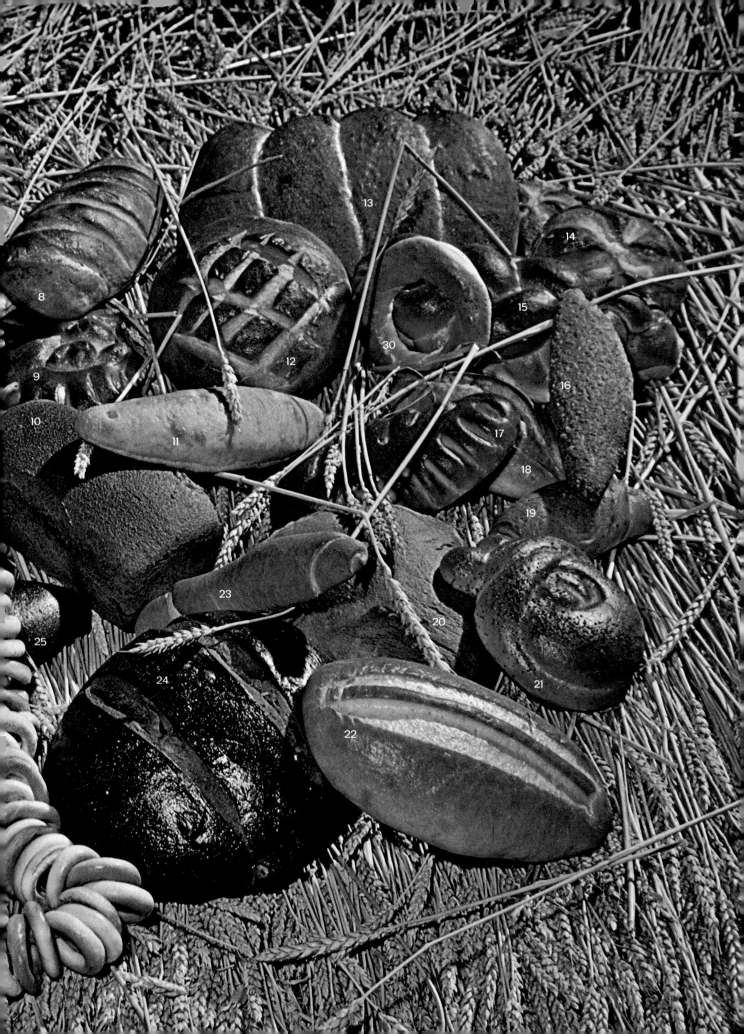

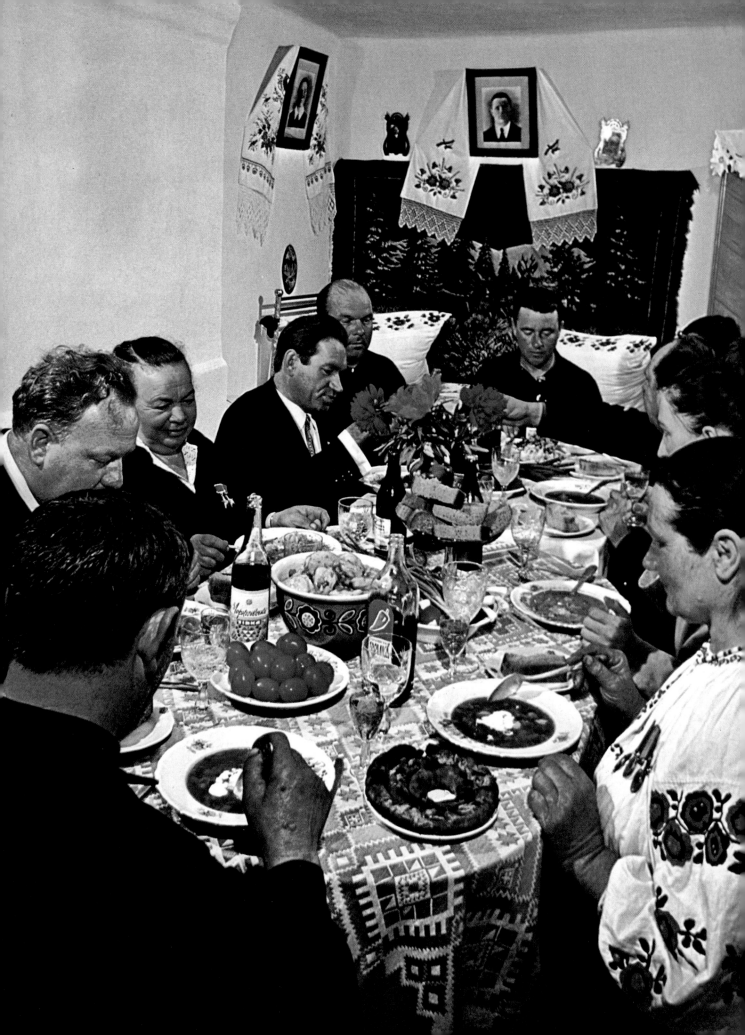

Unanswered questions and open disputes abound. Some cooks use nothing but wheat flour for their *varenyky* dough, while others add buckwheat flour, mashed potatoes or cottage cheese beaten or sieved to creamy smoothness. The liquid for the dough may be milk or water or a mixture of both (which raises another question—cool or lukewarm?), with or without either whole eggs or egg yolks. Does the addition of a pinch of sugar, baking powder, cream of tartar or a spoonful of melted fat improve the dough? To complicate the matter, country women who learned the art of the *varenyky* two or three generations ago make *yeast*-dough dumplings as light as thistledown.

Once made, the dough is rolled thin (but should it be rolled on a cloth or on a board?), then cut into squares or circles three or four inches wide. A spoonful of the filling is placed slightly off center on each piece, the dough is folded over to make a triangle or half moon, and the edges, which must be free of the slightest morsel of the filling are pinched firmly together—very firmly. *Varenyky* that burst are not *varenyky,* and the one who made them is not a cook—no question about *that* at least.

The well-sealed dumplings are slipped into a large pot of boiling, salted water. When they float to the top they are done, and may be removed with a slotted spoon and set on a plate, preferably without overlapping.

If the dough is right, the filling will taste right. It may be sauerkraut, mashed potatoes, cabbage, chopped mushrooms, ground meat, fish or—most common of all—dry cottage cheese mixed with egg. To complete the dish, the *varenyky* are garnished with buttered crumbs, browned chopped onions or bits of crumbled bacon, and eaten with liberal dollops of sour cream.

Visiting friends at a *dacha,* or summer cottage, outside Kiev we had dessert *varenyky* with a fruit filling. Our hostess picked plums from a dooryard tree. While they boiled in honey and water, she casually tossed together a *varenyky* dough of four cups of flour, two of water and three egg yolks. In less than 15 minutes, 10 people were enjoying meltingly tender dumplings, each containing a single plum like a precious jewel in rich purple syrup.

The mystique of *varenyky* dough, I said to myself, was surely all nonsense. Just to be sure I asked my friend, "You just use flour and water and egg yolks. Nothing more?"

"Absolutely nothing. But of course the flour *must* be ground from hard wheat, and of course freshly drawn spring water is the best liquid."

The eggs, I gathered, could be either brown- or white-shelled.

While *varenyky* are universal throughout the Ukraine, each area of the Republic also has its own specialties, developed from particular local products. Thus, many dairying regions produce distinctive cheeses. From some regions comes a rich, hard, almost orange cheese; dairymen in the western plains produce a mild, creamy variety; the highlanders of the Carpathians make both an aged cheese called *brynza* from sheep's milk, and a cheese of the Emmenthaler type, but firmer and slightly smoky.

Odessa is famous for fish—herring mashed to a smooth butter, whole grey mullet crisped in butter, carp simmered in *kvas* and lemon rind. It is also famous for roast veal served in a lily-gilding sauce made of its own juice enriched by a generous portion of caviar *(Recipe Index).*

Hazel grouse in sour cream is a specialty of Poltava, traditionally a town of such excellent food and talented cooks that many restaurants elsewhere

Her guests have assembled and Khristina's supper party begins. On the table are plates of *borshch* (each topped with a dollop of sour cream), sausage and *varenyky,* pickled tomatoes, scallions, radishes, bottles of mineral water—and, of course, good Ukrainian bread. Khristina's husband Nikolai Zagorodni (back to camera), a carpenter at the collective farm, has vodka and Ukrainian wine to offer when proposing toasts.

An Artistic Buffet for a Sculptor's Feast in Kiev

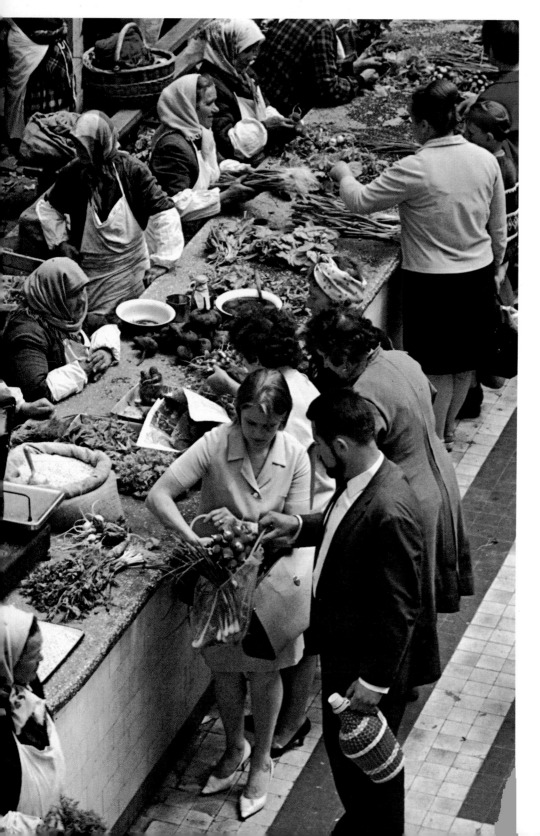

Unlike Khristina Djima *(page 120)*, who can get fresh vegetables right at her collective farm, Irena Cynkiewicz must depend on a local market, in this case Kiev's Central market. It is supplied both by state-operated truck farms and by private gardeners who bring their own produce to sell. At left Irena, the wife of sculptor Julius Cynkiewicz, is buying the food for an evening reception to celebrate the completion of a major work—a monument to the victims of the Babi Yar massacre in Kiev during World War II. Her husband holds the family shopping bag and a jug of wine while Irena stuffs in radishes.

In the cluttered studio that her husband shares with fellow-sculptor Mikhail Gritsyuk, Irena Cynkiewicz arranges her buffet as early arrivals chat outside. She has already sliced a baked ham and a lean pork sausage called *balik (left foreground)*. In the center is the table's main attraction, a roast of beef prepared with garlic. Other home-made sausages, as well as cheese, herring, salad, bread and butter and cottage cheese, have been set out. There is vodka and wine to drink and, for dessert, big bowls of fresh cherries and strawberries.

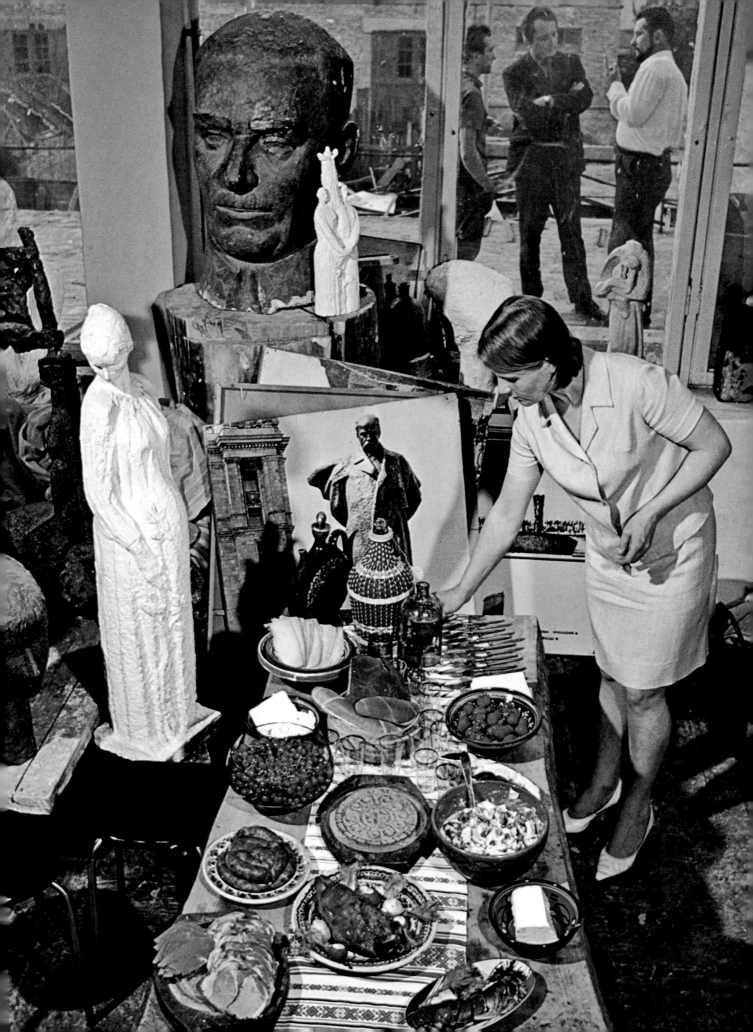

in the Soviet Union are called "The Poltava" as a kind of implicit compliment. Kharkov is known for veal *shashlyk,* the Carpathians for lamb soup—each region, each town, indeed many a small village boasts some distinctive dish. The best known of them all, undoubtedly, is Chicken Kiev—and what better place to eat it than in the city of its origin?

Kiev is an old city, and in the words of a well-known adage, "St. Petersburg (Leningrad) may be the head, Moscow the heart, but Kiev is the mother of Russian cities." It is also a beautiful city and an astonishingly clean one: every one of its streets is washed twice daily and once at night. Locust, poplar and oak trees line the wide streets and broad squares; parks are everywhere, some extending for miles along the bank of the Dnieper River, others consisting of pocket-sized gardens tucked into urban corners. Although some 7,000 buildings were destroyed by German troops in 1941, careful restoration has preserved the old city's character, and through some alchemy of light and façade the luminous glow of medieval Russia still lingers.

New suburban areas ring the city, now the third largest in the Soviet Union, and the markets, shops, museums and theaters are invariably crowded. Kiev has also opened many new restaurants, including several specializing in traditional dishes. Friends invited us to dinner at one called the Vitriak, "The Mill," on the outskirts of the city. Set on the bank of the Dnieper, the Vitriak is a large, romanticized version of the hundreds of wind- or water-turned mills that once dotted the landscape. Inside, the long tables were filled with merry parties served by waitresses in traditional Ukrainian dress, one of the most flattering costumes ever devised, with soft leather boots, full skirt, embroidered blouse, and a crown of flowers with fluttering ribbons.

Like Russians, Ukrainians begin dinner with *zakuska,* but they generally include some regional favorites along with the usual dishes. We sampled several Ukrainian sausages: fat, spicy *sardelky;* a long, thin, hard "hunter's sausage"; and a mild delicate "milk sausage" made from veal. There was a *pashtet,* or loaf, of veal, pork and lamb; pickles in honey, providing a piquant sour-sweet note; a salad of tart apples and fresh cabbage in a sour-cream dressing; and a dish of pickled peppers stuffed with chopped vegetables, parsley, carrots and celery. A special treat was a goose neck, boned and stuffed with chopped giblets, crumbs, neck meat and onions, boiled and served cold.

Steaming bowls of *borshch* followed *(Recipe Index).* "Ukrainian *borshch,*" our hosts pointed out. "Very different from Russian *borshch.*"

Ukrainians insist that they were the originators of *borshch,* and since there was a Kiev when Moscow was "a wheel track in the forest" they may be right. Actually, the question of who may justly claim the first—or, for that matter, the best—*borshch* may never be answered, for there are now more versions than can be counted or tasted. In general, Ukrainian *borshch* is distinguished from Russian by the presence of tomatoes, pork as well as beef, and a greater variety of vegetables, including garlic. But we must have enjoyed half a dozen different kinds of *borshch* while we were in the Ukraine—meatless ones made with mushrooms, a *borshchok* with almost no vegetables other than beets, Poltava *borshch* with fowl, *borshch* made with young beets and their green tops, and a clear *borshch* with the fat and vegetables removed.

In the Ukraine *borshch* is most frequently eaten without any accompaniment, but a plate of *pyrizhky*—brought to our table at the Vitriak for those who had ordered chicken bouillon—was generously shared. These small, glistening rolls, two (well, perhaps three) bites long, are made of yeast or, less frequently, pastry dough, stuffed with meat, mushrooms, chopped green onions, cabbage or cottage cheese.

Now we had our Chicken Kiev. In the United States, for some inexplicable reason, the dish has become the particular favorite of indifferent cooks, who have evolved so many time-saving, calorie-cutting "improvements" on the original that it is often indistinguishable from a sho' 'nuff Southern-fried chicken. Happily, none of these improvements has reached Kiev as yet. We were served the classic composition: chilled fingers of sweet butter wrapped in boned, flattened chicken breasts with the ends neatly tucked in, the whole dipped in seasoned flour, beaten egg and bread crumbs *(Recipe Index)*. It was fried and served in all its crisp, golden beauty, ready at the touch of a fork to release jets of butter on the unwary.

Our dessert was a torte of rye-bread crumbs and almonds, bathed in a wine syrup made from Crimean muscats. As I finished it and lingered at the table over tea, I came to the conclusion that the hallmark of Ukrainian cuisine is the golden crumb. In cake, *pashtet*, meat, fish, vegetables and desserts—everything is touched by the magic of grain. But when I expounded my theory to my friend she disagreed.

"Oh, no. We make many things that don't contain wheat. Pickles, for instance." She thought for a moment, then added: "But come to think of it, when I eat a pickle I usually have some bread and butter with it."

As we waited in the airport to leave Kiev we saw some final pieces of evidence for my theory. There was a souvenir counter full of postcards depicting a pretty kerchiefed harvester against a field of grain and bearing the slogan, "All Honor to the Breadmakers." Our last glimpse of the airport as the plane wheeled around included the emblem of the Ukrainian Republic, with its proud symbol of bearded stalks of wheat—and waving goodbye at the gate, a little boy munching on a roll.

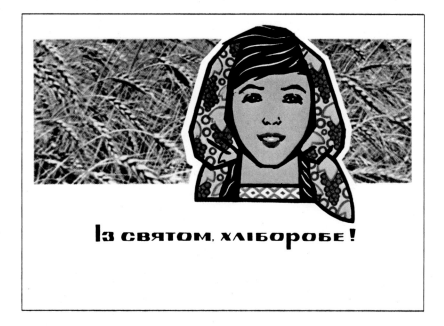

Із святом, хліборобе!

"All honor to the breadmakers" reads the legend on a postcard from a souvenir stand in Kiev. The words reflect the almost mystical regard accorded wheat—and its many delectable incarnations—by the well-fed people of the Ukraine.

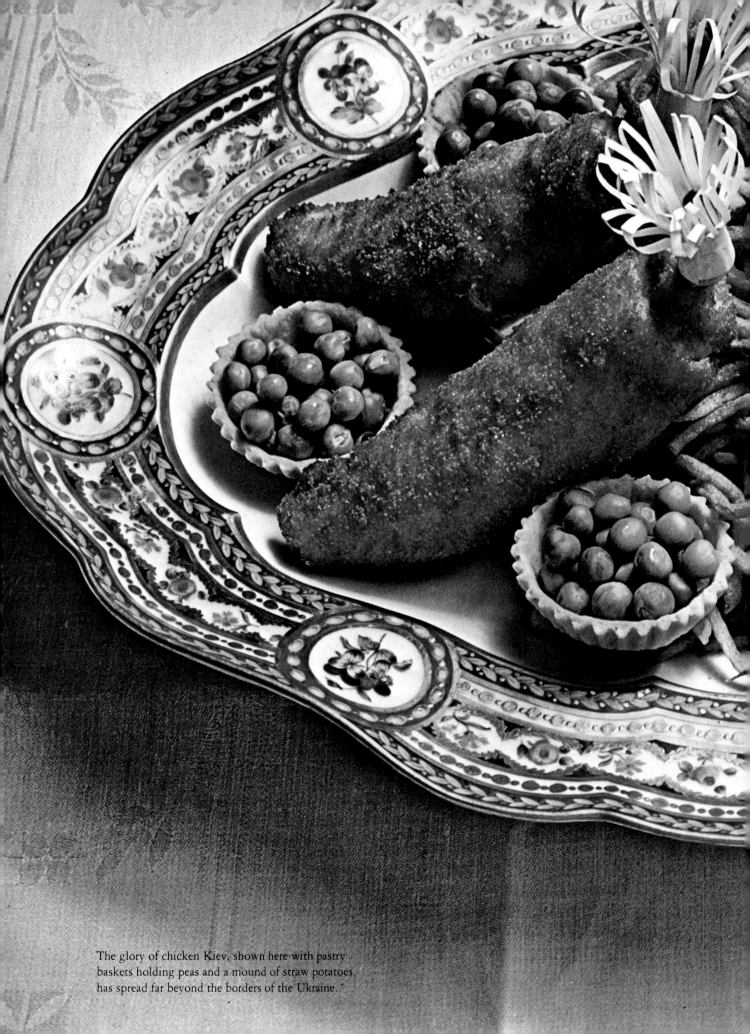

The glory of chicken Kiev, shown here with pastry
baskets holding peas and a mound of straw potatoes,
has spread far beyond the borders of the Ukraine.

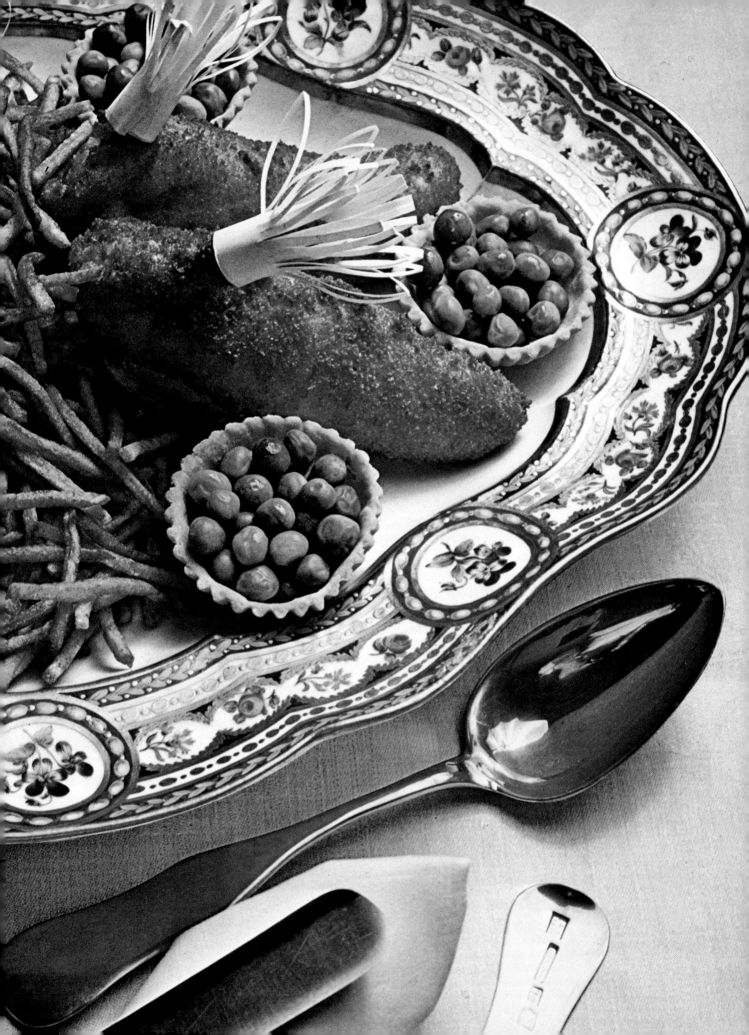

Kotlety po-Kyivskomu

DEEP-FRIED CHICKEN CUTLETS WRAPPED AROUND BUTTER (CHICKEN KIEV)

Chicken Kiev is one of the great classic Soviet dishes that has achieved international fame. The traditional Ukrainian recipe calls for boned pounded chicken breasts —fresh, never frozen—rolled around fingers of unseasoned butter. Less traditional are the herb seasonings suggested at left, which add a note of interest to an otherwise bland, though typical, dish.

To serve 4

4 whole fresh chicken breasts, ½ to
   ¾ pound each, with or without
   the wing bone attached
12 tablespoons chilled unsalted
   butter (1½ sticks)
2 eggs
Flour
2 cups fine, dry white bread crumbs
Vegetable oil for deep-frying
Salt
Freshly ground black pepper

OPTIONAL SEASONING
1 teaspoon fresh, strained lemon juice
1 teaspoon finely cut fresh chives
   or tarragon
1 tablespoon finely chopped
   parsley
2 teaspoons salt
Freshly ground black pepper

To skin the chicken breasts, start at the pointed end of the breast, insert your thumb under the skin, and strip it off. Bone and halve the breasts as described in the diagram at the top of page 138. To prepare the chicken breasts with the wing bone attached, cut off the wing tip and its adjacent bone and leave only the short leglike bone attached to each breast.

Place the 8 halved breasts smooth side down on a cutting board. With a small, sharp knife and your fingers, remove the small fillet from each breast. Lay the breasts and fillets, one pair at a time, on a sheet of wax paper. Cover the breast and fillet with a sheet of wax paper and, with the flat side of a cleaver or a metal meat pounder, pound them to a thickness of ⅛ inch. If holes appear in the flesh, overlap the edges of the tear slightly, cover the patch with wax paper, and pound gently until the meat joins together.

Cut the 1½ sticks of butter into 8 equal parts. Shape each piece of butter into a cylinder about ½ inch thick and 3 inches long. Wrap them in wax paper and chill until firm. (Or, cream the butter by mashing it against the side of a bowl with a wooden spoon and beating into it the optional seasoning—lemon juice, chives or tarragon, parsley, salt and pepper—and cut and shape the butter as described above. Chill until firm.)

To assemble the cutlets, gently peel off the wax paper and sprinkle the chicken lightly with salt and freshly ground black pepper. Wrap the chicken breasts and fillets around the butter fingers as shown on pages 138-139.

In a small bowl, beat the eggs just long enough to combine them. Spread flour and the bread crumbs on two separate strips of wax paper and, one at a time, dip the cutlets into the flour. Shake each one gently free of excess flour and, cradling it in your palms, pat the cutlet into a long cylinder tapering slightly at each end. Now dip the cutlet into the eggs, making sure its entire surface is coated, and roll in the bread crumbs, again making sure it is thoroughly coated. Arrange the cutlets side by side on a platter and refrigerate for 1 or 2 hours before frying.

About 30 minutes before you plan to serve the chicken, preheat the oven to 200°. Line a shallow baking dish with a double thickness of paper towels and place it in the oven. Pour enough oil to rise 3 or 4 inches up the side of a deep-fat fryer or a heavy saucepan into which a frying basket will fit. Set the pan over high heat until the oil registers 360° on a deep-fat thermometer. Fry the cutlets, 4 at a time, in the frying basket for about 5 minutes, or until golden brown, then transfer them with tongs or a slotted spoon to the lined baking dish. Fry the remaining cutlets similarly. The finished cutlets may remain in the low oven for no longer than 10 minutes before serving or they will lose their freshness and their butter may escape.

Traditionally, chicken Kiev is served accompanied by peas and by *kasha* (*Recipe Index*) or straw potatoes (*opposite*).

Medivnyk
SPICED HONEY CAKE

NOTE: *Medivnyk* should be made 1 or 2 days before you plan to serve it, to allow the flavor to develop properly.

In a 1- to 1½-quart saucepan bring the honey to a boil over moderate heat, stirring almost constantly with a wooden spoon. Stir in the cinnamon, cloves, nutmeg and baking soda and set aside to cool to room temperature.

In a large bowl, cream the 4 tablespoons of butter and the sugar together by mashing and beating them against the sides of the bowl with a large spoon until they are light and fluffy. Then beat in the egg yolks, one at a time, and stir in the cooled, spiced honey. Combine 1¾ cups of the flour with the salt and baking powder and beat them into the sugar-and-egg mixture, ¼ cup at a time. Combine the raisins, currants and walnuts in a separate mixing bowl and toss them with the remaining ¼ cup of flour until each piece is coated. Fold into the batter.

Preheat the oven to 300°. Beat the egg whites in a large bowl with a whisk or a rotary or electric beater, until they form stiff peaks on the beater when lifted out of the bowl. With a rubber spatula, gently fold the egg whites into the batter, using an over-and-under folding motion rather than a mixing motion. With a pastry brush and 2 tablespoons of the softened butter, coat the bottom and sides of a 9-by-5-by-3-inch loaf pan. Coat both sides of a sheet of brown paper with the remaining tablespoon of butter and line the sides of the pan with it. Pour the batter into the pan and bake in the center of the oven for 1½ hours, or until a toothpick or cake tester inserted into the center of the cake comes out clean. With a knife, loosen the sides of the cake from the pan and invert the cake onto a cake rack. Let the cake cool to room temperature, then cover loosely with wax paper and set aside for 1 or 2 days at room temperature before slicing.

To serve 6 to 8

¾ cup honey
½ teaspoon powdered cinnamon
¼ teaspoon powdered cloves
¼ teaspoon powdered nutmeg
1 teaspoon baking soda
4 tablespoons unsalted butter, softened
½ cup dark brown sugar
3 egg yolks
2 cups flour
¼ teaspoon salt
1 teaspoon baking powder
10 tablespoons raisins
6 tablespoons dried currants
½ cup finely chopped walnuts
3 egg whites
3 tablespoons butter, softened

Kartoplia Solimkoi
DEEP-FRIED STRAW POTATOES

Peel the potatoes and cut them into straw-shaped strips, about 2½ inches long and ⅛ inch thick. Drop them into a bowl of ice water and set them aside until ready to fry. Drain the potatoes in a colander, spread them out on a double thickness of paper towels and pat them thoroughly dry.

Pour enough oil into a deep fryer to come 3 or 4 inches up the sides of the pan. For the first frying of the potatoes (there will be two in all), heat the oil until it reaches a temperature of 370° on a deep-frying thermometer. Drop the potatoes into the frying basket and immerse the basket in the hot oil, shaking it gently from time to time to prevent the potatoes from sticking together. Fry them for about 15 seconds, or until the potatoes are tender and a pale golden brown. Drain on a double thickness of paper towels, then fry and drain the remaining potatoes similarly. The potatoes may now rest for as long as an hour before refrying and serving.

Immediately before serving, reheat the oil until it reaches a temperature of 385° on a deep-frying thermometer. Drop all the potatoes into the basket and, shaking the basket occasionally, fry for 15 seconds, or until the potatoes are crisp and brown. Drain on paper towels and transfer to a large platter or bowl. Sprinkle lightly with salt, and serve at once.

To serve 4 to 6

4 medium-sized baking potatoes (about 2 pounds)
Vegetable oil for deep-frying
Salt

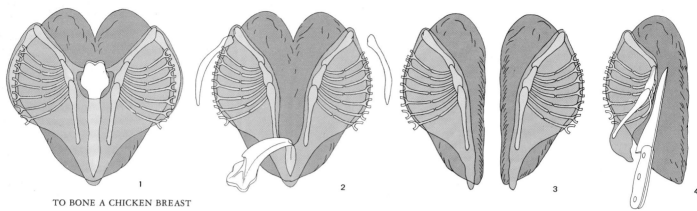

1   2   3   4

TO BONE A CHICKEN BREAST

Hold the breast skin-side down and bend it back in half until it is flat *(1)* and the spoon-shaped keel bone in the center pops up. Pull it out *(2)*, cut the breast apart *(3)*, and peel off the skin. Slip the point of a sharp knife under the base of the slender rib bone *(4)* attached to the rib cage. Press the flat of the knife up against the bone and gently pull the bone up toward you, meanwhile scraping away the flesh adhering to the adjacent ribs. Continue to scrape and cut until the entire rib cage and adjacent bones have been detached from the flesh. If you choose to prepare the more classic, elaborate version of chicken Kiev pictured opposite, purchase chicken breasts with the wing bone attached and bone them as above.

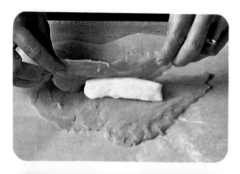

Cut off the narrow fillet attached to the breast and place fillet and breast between wax paper. With a cleaver or meat pounder, pound the meat thin. Center an oblong of butter on the breast and cover with the fillet.

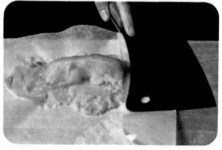

Fold the bottom sheet of wax paper over the edges of the breast and pound the meat flat again. The thinner the edges, the more firmly they can be sealed, thus preventing the butter filling from escaping.

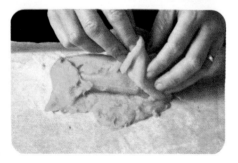

Bring one of the wide ends of the breast up over the fillet, and fold in the two ends. Then bring up the other wide end. The breast is now ready to be dipped in its coatings of flour, egg and bread crumbs.

The Classic Version of Chicken Kiev—with Wing Bone Attached

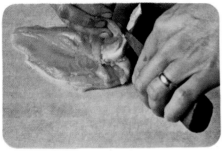

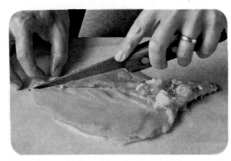

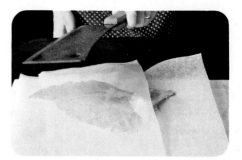

Breasts with wing bone attached are boned as opposite. Cut off wing tips, leaving short bone attached, then cut away its flesh.

With a small sharp knife, cut off the narrow fillet attached to each boned breast and place it alongside the breast itself on a sheet of wax paper.

Cover fillet and breast with wax paper and pound with the flat of a cleaver or meat pounder until they are no more than ⅛ inch thick.

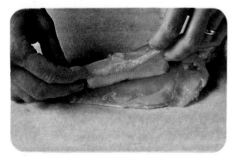

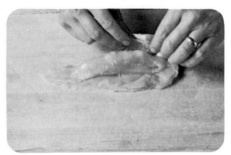

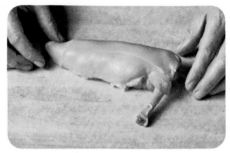

Lay an oblong of the butter in the center of the flattened breast, cover it with the fillet, and fold one wide side of the breast up over it.

Twist the wing-bone of the breast around to seal it and prevent butter from seeping through when the meat is fried. Fold in the other ends.

The folded chicken breast is now ready to be dipped in flour, egg and bread crumbs. It can be patted into its final shape after flouring.

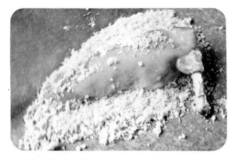

The rolled cutlet, dipped in flour and in eggs, is rolled in bread crumbs *(left)*. The cutlets must be refrigerated an hour or two before frying. As the prongs of a fork pierce the crisp golden coating of the deep-fried chicken cutlet *(below)*, the diner should be greeted by a spurt of melted butter.

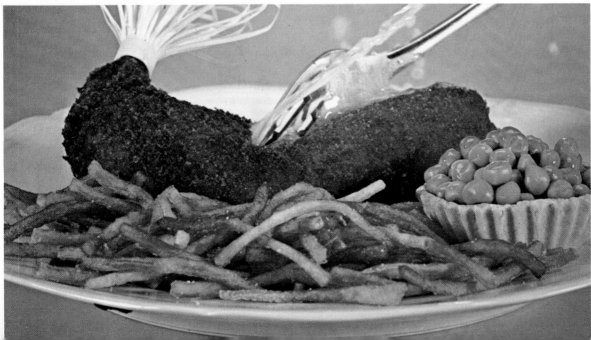

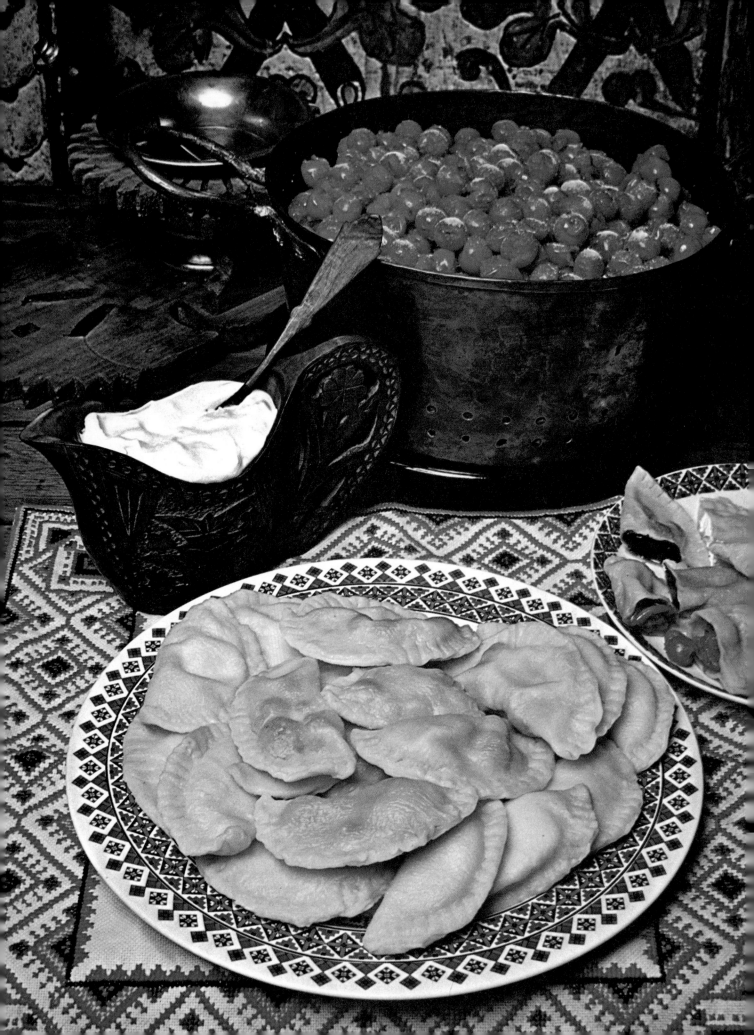

Borshch Ukraïnsky
UKRAINE-STYLE BEET SOUP

Drop the tomatoes into boiling water for 15 seconds. Run them under cold water and peel them. Cut out the stem, then slice them in half crosswise. Squeeze the halves gently to remove the juices and seeds then chop them coarsely and set aside. In a heavy 10- to 12-inch skillet or casserole, melt the butter over moderate heat. Add the onions and garlic and, stirring frequently, cook 6 to 8 minutes, or until they are soft and lightly colored. Stir in the beets, celery root, parsley root, parsnip, half the tomatoes, the sugar, vinegar, salt and 1½ cups of the stock. Bring to a boil over high heat, then partially cover the pot and lower the heat. Simmer for 40 minutes.

Meanwhile, pour the remaining stock into a 6- to 8-quart casserole and add the potatoes and cabbage. Bring to a boil, then simmer partially covered for 20 minutes, or until the potatoes are tender but not falling apart. When the vegetable mixture has cooked its allotted time, add it to the casserole with the remaining tomatoes and the meat. Simmer partially covered for 10 to 15 minutes, until the *borshch* is heated. Taste for seasoning. Pour into a tureen, sprinkle with parsley and serve accompanied by sour cream.

Varenyky
DESSERT DUMPLINGS FILLED WITH CHEESE

NOTE: Recipes for *varenyky* filled with fruit or sauerkraut may be found in the Recipe Booklet.

DOUGH: Pour the flour into a large mixing bowl and make a deep well in the center. Drop in the egg, milk and salt. With your fingertips or a large spoon, slowly mix the flour into the liquid ingredients, then mix vigorously until the dough is stiff enough to be gathered into a compact ball. If the dough crumbles add an additional 1 to 2 teaspoons of milk to make the particles adhere. Dust the ball with flour, wrap in wax paper, and chill 30 minutes.

CHEESE FILLING: Purée the cheese in a food mill, or rub it with the back of a large spoon through a fine sieve set over a bowl. Then beat in the sugar, egg yolk, melted butter and salt, and stir in 1 cup of the sour cream, ¼ cup at a time. Continue to stir until the ingredients are thoroughly mixed. Taste for seasoning; if you prefer the filling sweeter, stir in additional sugar.

On a lightly floured surface, roll the dough into a circle about ⅛ inch thick. Cut out as many circles as possible with a 3½- to 4-inch cookie cutter. Then gather the remaining scraps into a ball, roll out again, and cut out additional circles. With a pastry brush, coat each circle with a light film of the beaten egg white. Drop 1 tablespoon of the cheese on the lower half of each circle. Bring the exposed half of the circle up over the filling and press the edges all around the dough firmly with the back of a fork. Make certain that the edges are thoroughly sealed to prevent the filling from seeping through. Set aside, loosely covered with a towel, until ready to cook.

Bring 4 quarts of salted water to a boil in a 5- to 6-quart pot and drop in 6 dumplings. Lower the heat and simmer the dumplings uncovered for 8 to 10 minutes, or until they float to the surface of the water. Remove with a slotted spoon and transfer to a heated platter. Cover loosely with foil to keep them hot while you cook the remaining dumplings similarly. Moisten with melted butter and serve with the remaining sour cream.

To serve 6 to 8

4 medium tomatoes
4 tablespoons butter
1 cup finely chopped onions
2 cloves garlic, peeled and finely chopped
1 pound beets, trimmed of leaves and coarsely grated (2 cups)
½ celery root, peeled and coarsely grated (1 cup)
1 parsley root, peeled and coarsely grated (1 cup)
1 parsnip, peeled and coarsely grated (1 cup)
½ teaspoon sugar
¼ cup red wine vinegar
1 tablespoon salt
2 quarts beef stock, fresh *(see shchi, page 90)* or canned
1 pound boiling potatoes, peeled and cut into 1½-inch chunks
1 pound cabbage, cored and coarsely shredded
1 pound boiled brisket *(see shchi, page 90)*, or 1 pound boiled ham, cut into 1-inch chunks
3 tablespoons finely chopped parsley
½ pint sour cream

To make about 16 dumplings

DOUGH
2 cups all-purpose flour
1 egg
½ cup milk
1 teaspoon salt

CHEESE FILLING
1 pound large-curd cottage or pot cheese
2 tablespoons sugar
1 egg yolk
1 tablespoon melted butter, cooled
½ teaspoon salt
2 cups sour cream
4 tablespoons melted butter, hot

The dessert dumplings called *varenyky* may be filled with fruit or cheese.   141

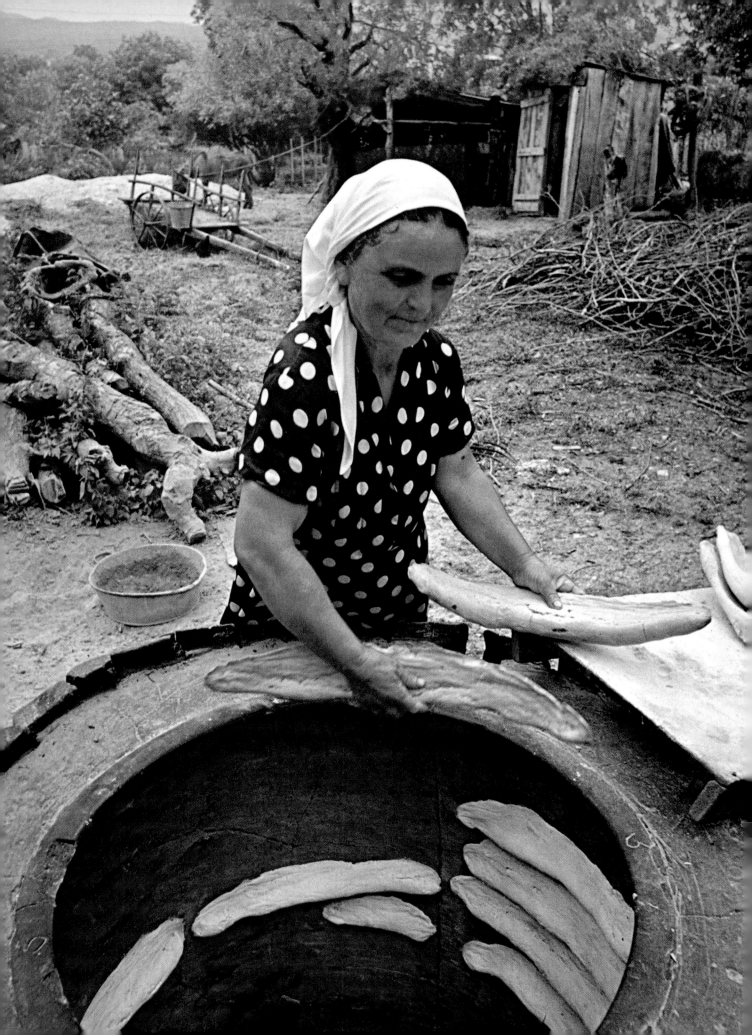

VI

The Caucasus: A Mountain World

On the Tsvelianaga Collective Farm in southeastern Georgia, Amira Kiladze removes baked loaves of bread from a *toné*. The ancient baking implements and methods that Mrs. Kiladze uses have survived all political upheavals. Her *toné* is a brick-lined pit, preheated by a fire of grapevine prunings and chunks of hardwood. The dough is slapped against the hot, inner wall of the *toné*, and clings there while baking.

This book has two authors, and now it is time for the second one to have his say.

When my wife and I planned the chapters of the book I said to her, "Suppose you write the sections on Russia, the Ukraine, the Baltic and Central Asia. I will do all of the Caucasus."

"All?"

"Well, Georgia and Armenia."

"But that's not an equal division of territory. The Russian Republic alone is 200 times larger."

"True. But we have 200 times as many dishes in the Caucasus. So. . . ."

"I know. 'So it comes out even.' "

I was born in Georgia. Ever since my first day in the United States I have been explaining that *my* Georgia is not the state below the Mason-Dixon line, but a country on the southern slope of the Caucasus Mountains, between the Black and Caspian Seas. Once an independent kingdom, Georgia became part of the Russian Empire in 1801 and is now a Soviet Republic.

Despite these geographical and political links with Russia, we Georgians are not Slavs. Anthropologists find it difficult to classify us and our customs. Our traditions are quite different from those of Russia, and so is our language, which no more resembles Russian than it does English. For something like 7,000 years we have lived in our mountains, and we have a legend that tells how we came here.

On the eighth day of Creation, so the story goes, God divided men into nations and told them to select a place for their country. After everyone was sat-

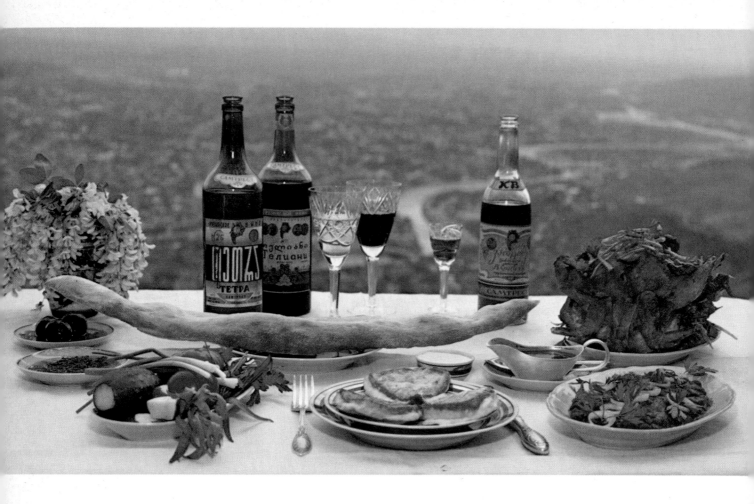

A supper of regional dishes awaits guests at the Mount David Restaurant, high above the Georgian capital of Tbilisi (Tiflis). The entrée, chicken *tabaka (Recipe Index)*, is at the upper right; its accompaniments include a kidney-bean dish called *lobio*, a plate of crisp deep-fried cheese *(suluguni)*, and a long loaf of *deda's puri*, or "mother's bread." The bottles in the background contain *(from left)* red wine, white wine and brandy, all locally produced and —though little known in the Western world—all excellent.

isfied and had settled down, God started home. On the way, He passed the Georgians, who were sitting around a table in an arbor by the roadside.

God scolded them. "While you sat here eating and drinking, singing and joking, the whole world was divided up. Now nothing is left for you."

The Tamada, as we call the head of the table, apologized. "It was very wrong, we know. But God, while we enjoyed ourselves we didn't forget You. We drank to You to thank You for making such a beautiful world."

"That's more than anybody else did," God said, "so I'm going to give you the last little corner of the earth—the place I was saving for myself because it is most like Paradise."

Two parts of the story at least are true. Georgians do spend hours around the table, not just for the food and drink, but also to enjoy the company of their friends. And Georgia is indeed beautiful, with eye-filling landscapes that range from towering peaks to tropical coastal valleys. If you could roll the country flat it might cover all of Europe, but since 90 per cent of it stands on end the total area is less than 27,000 square miles, which is less than half the size of the American state of Georgia.

Both the east-west line of the Caucasus, bordering upon Russia, and a north-south spur, the Surami, which divides Georgia itself, are high and steep. Below their peaks lie rocky ridges slashed by deep canyons and narrow gorges. Farther down are rugged slopes covered with dark pines and

144

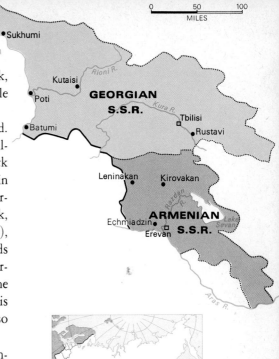

thickets of rhododendron. They in turn give way to lower forests of oak, beech, box chestnut and walnut, which thin to high pastures, where cattle and sheep grow fat on sweet summer grass.

The flora and fauna of the high country are unusually rich and varied. Ibex, mouflon and two kinds of mountain goat, the chamois and the smaller bouquetin, live on the crags; in the valleys there are bear, deer, roebuck and the rare gazelle. Wild boars root for mast, the fruit of the forest trees, in the beech woods. From the clearings, game birds call: snow and stone partridges, quail (delicious when cooked with green grapes), heath-cock, mountain turkey (which we roast and eat with a sauce of pounded nuts), black grouse and jewel-crested pheasants. Wild swan, geese and mallards come to the high pocket lakes. These lakes, too, are full of fish—carp, barbel and the *kramuli*, which has no English name since it is found only in the Caucasus. Ten inches long, white-fleshed and delicately flavored, *kramuli* is a special treat that we boil in spring water and eat unseasoned, without so much as a pinch of salt.

Our agricultural land, though limited, is wondrously fertile. In the temperate eastern half of the country, grapes and wheat have been cultivated for 6,000 years. Berries, nuts, figs and all the stone fruits flourish, and many grow wild. West of the Surami spur is a subtropical area with glossy citrus groves and tea plantations.

With such an abundance at hand, it might be thought that even in the old days all Georgians ate like kings. In fact we did not, because land was so scarce. My father, who was a farmer, had only three acres. The best farms belonged to princes who spent their time in St. Petersburg and taxes and rents were crushing.

In bad winters we lived mostly on beans and bread. But then, as we say, "Better beans and corn bread at home than cake and wine in the land of strangers." And fortunately, no Georgian ever tires of beans, for we have as many ways to prepare them as there are days in a week. My own favorite, I think, is a dish made with very young green beans, cooked whole. Well drained, they go into a buttered dish, and eggs whipped to a froth are poured over them and baked until set. The finished dish looks like a flower meadow—all green and white, flecked with gold—and tastes of spring.

As for corn, it is so important in our diet that some of us feel we must have eaten it from the beginning of time. Indeed, I had a friend who insisted that corn originated in our mountains, and nothing would change his mind. One day I showed him an encyclopedia article on maize, which said flatly that American Indians developed corn. "It only proves," he said, "that those Indians were lost Georgians who somehow got to America, with corn in their pockets."

Wherever corn came from we made it our own. We roast green corn on skewers, we simmer fresh shelled kernels and add walnut sauce, and we even pop corn, calling it *badi-budi* because that's what the grains say as they explode. Our corn bread, called *mchadi*, we make from finely ground yellow meal mixed with water and a little salt. The stiff dough is shaped into a flat, round cake and baked in a pottery dish set in the fireplace. Eaten hot, *mchadi* is soft and slightly moist; when cold, the texture sometimes approximates that of cement but this matters little. Fresh or stale, every crumb of *mchadi* has a grainy sweetness that lingers on the tongue and in the memory. Un-

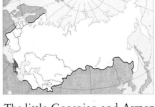

The little Georgian and Armenian Republics, shown on this map, are traversed by mountain ranges, most notably the great Caucasus Mountains, and much of their limited arable land is devoted to such cash crops as tea, citrus fruits, cotton, almonds and olives, which are not generally grown in the European parts of the U.S.S.R. Livestock raising is equally important. Though Georgia and Armenia together comprise less than half of one per cent of the total area of the U.S.S.R., the two Republics produce more than five per cent of the nation's wool, some four per cent of its goats and an important share of its cattle, sheep and milk.

Continued on page 148

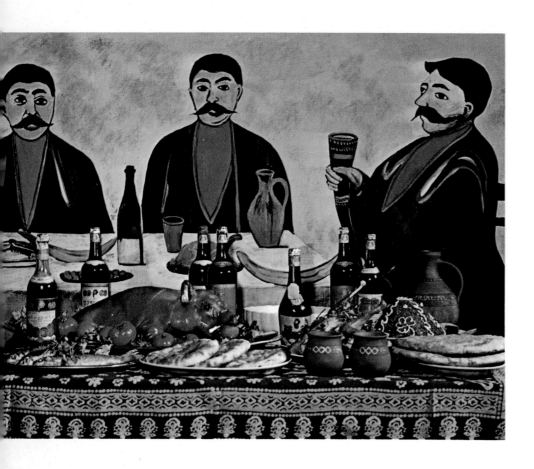

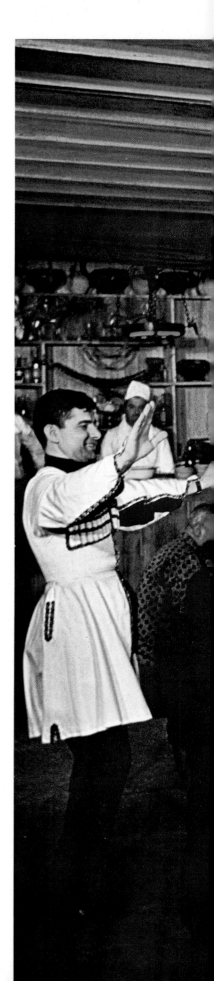

Banqueting in Georgia
Yesterday and Today

The classless workers of modern Georgia eat as intently and as well as the princes of old Georgia, to judge from the mural shown above—called "The Carousing Princes"—at the Darial Restaurant in Tbilisi. The table of modern foods set before the painting includes broiled fish, a roast suckling pig, chicken *satsivi (Recipe Index)* and a mound of *pkhala* (a kind of edible grass) in walnut sauce; the two breads served with the meal are *khachapuri* and *mchadi*. All of these foods have been popular in Georgia for centuries, and might well have been eaten by the princes depicted in the mural; even the shapes of wine jugs and bottles have changed little over the years. Other murals based on paintings by the same artist, a famous Georgian primitive, Pirosmanishvili, cover the walls of the restaurant. Some are visible in the busy scene at right, in which the restaurant's musicians have joined a party of diners. Primarily a masculine gathering place, the Darial serves about 500 customers a day.

146

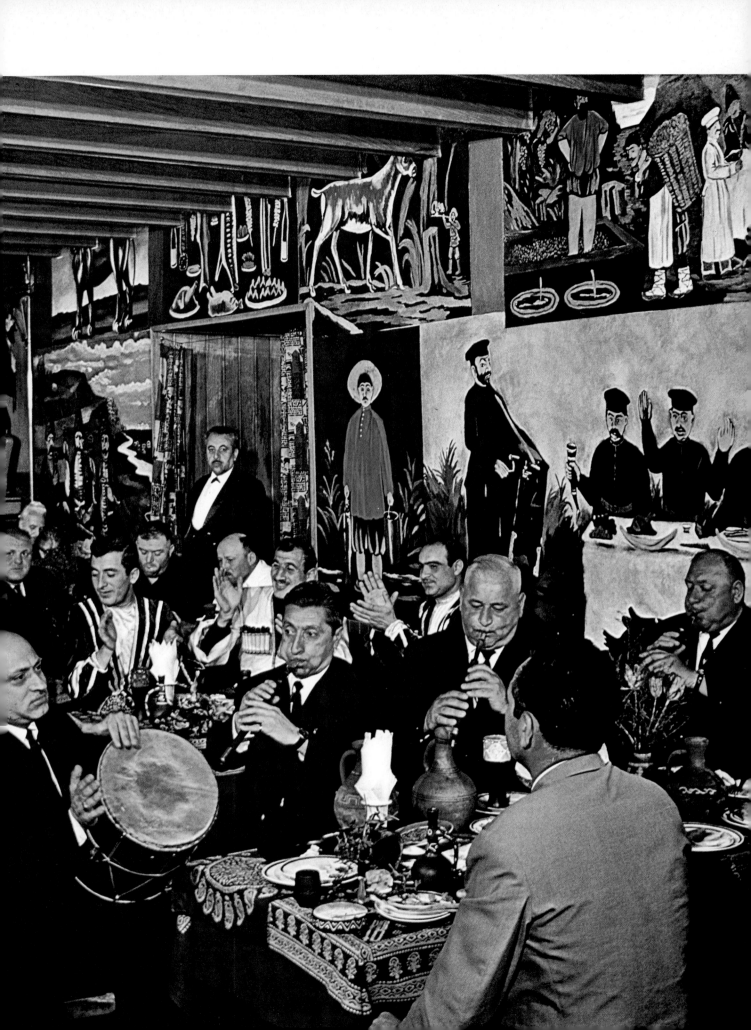

like *mchadi,* which bakes quickly, our wheat bread takes time and loving care. We bake it in a brick-lined outdoor oven we call the *toné,* which resembles the clay *tandoor* oven of India. When a man builds a new house the first thing he does is build a *toné*—one so good that not only his wife, but also —God willing, his son's wife and his son's son's wife can use it. The average *toné* is like a shallow well, about three feet across and four feet deep and three quarters of its four-foot depth is set below ground. A wooden platform surrounds the open top.

On baking day, the women of the houses build a fire of dried grape prunings topped by hardwood logs in the bottom of the *toné.* When the wood burns down, the coals are raked smooth. In the meantime whole-grain, stone-ground wheat has been mixed with water, salt and a starter from the previous baking, kneaded and left to rise. What gives our *deda's puri,* or "mother's bread," its distinctive flavor is the mountain-grown wheat and the starter, or leaven. In our village a bride's mother always gave her a jar of starter to take to her new home. The new housewife used half the gift in her first bread; the remainder was deposited in a stone crock and "fed" with new flour and water, to be dipped into every week for a lifetime. If, by some mischance, the starter was lost (my pet bear, I remember, once tipped over our crock) the housewife had to go to a neighbor for a fresh supply. We knew every bread in the village—sour, bland, sweetish, nutty, milky, slightly narcotic (that woman never cleaned all the poppy seeds from her grain), resinous (from a pine dipper)—and we borrowed our new starter to suit our taste.

When dough and oven are ready, a tray of slightly elliptical loaves is carried outdoors to the *toné* platform. There is no floor or rack in a *toné* to slide the loaves into. Instead a loaf is carefully hefted and slapped hard against the wall of the oven, to hang there and bake. (Before a woman learns the trick of making the loaves stick, more than one falls into the coals and burns to a cinder.) When the loaves are all sticking fast the top of the oven is covered (usually with a basket woven of filbert branches). Because the loaf hangs from the *toné* wall as it bakes, or perhaps because of the slap as it goes in, the lower part is always thicker than the upper, and one may choose to eat the soft *khiré* part or the crusty *kakknatsela.* To this day, though I am now half a century in time and half a world in space away from a *toné,* a symmetrical loaf always looks out of shape to me.

Our winter fare in Georgia might be beans and bread, but the spring brought young nettles, mallow, sorrel, sarsaparilla for soup or fresh greens. We hunted for wild onions that kept their sharp pungency even when fried brown and baked in corn bread. Wild asparagus grew in the hedgerows —bright green, pencil-thin stalks that we sautéed in bubbling clarified butter.

Best of all the wild greens was a succulent we called *donduri.* Imagine my pleasure when I discovered it in the United States as purslane—and then my shock at learning that an eminent horticulturist had described it as "a mischievous weed that Frenchmen and pigs eat when they can get nothing else." The trouble, I think, is that few Westerners know how to prepare purslane. It should be picked young, washed in seven waters, snapped into one-inch lengths and cooked in boiling, salted water until tender but not soft. After it drains, a dressing of oil, lemon juice, minced garlic and salt will enhance the peppery buds; on a hot day no dish could be more refreshing.

Of course we did not depend on wild foods. Every house in the village had a garden encircled by a basket-willow fence. One corner was dedicated to the herbs and greens we cannot live without—tarragon (which we ate by the handful), coriander, dill, purple and green basil, oregano, thyme, savory, mint and heavy-headed, deep-hued marigolds. (We strung marigold blossoms into garlands and hung them to dry; the dried petals, making an inexpensive substitute for saffron, are not only colorful but intensify other flavors without imposing their own.) Always there was a row of inconspicuous clover-like plants that have neither taste nor aroma until the blue flowers fade; but then a single dried cluster is enough to flavor a whole pot of *kharcho,* a beef, onion and tomato soup-stew. We called this spice, an uncommon variety of fenugreek, "the-fragrance-that-came-from-far-away."

Beyond each garden was an orchard, and the summer was heavy with fruit —sweet, flat, black-red cherries; satin-skinned pears; small, crisp, mountain apples; quinces, which we chop and bake with lamb; figs, black or green and ripe to bursting; bright-red, many-seeded pomegranates ("Tell me where," asks a Georgian riddle, "in a scarlet dome, 10,000 make their home"); and persimmons, each as round and bright as a little sun.

In the fall we collected nuts—filberts for candy, chestnuts to roast and eat in the winter while we told stories, Persian walnuts for our two great sauces, *satsivi* and *bazha,* and for the sweet called *chuchkella.*

Making *chuchkella* called for time and patience. Perfect, unbroken walnut halves were strung on a heavy thread that was knotted at one end and tied in a loop at the other. These strings were dipped into the juice of sweet grapes that had been boiled and slightly thickened with flour; they were next hung to dry, then re-dipped and re-dried until the *chuchkella* was about an inch thick. In the autumn every balcony and arbor was trimmed with rows of drying tapers, their fruity sweetness filling the air and attracting swarms of tipsy bees and expectant children. Finally, the *chuchkella* were sliced, each piece transformed into a perfect intaglio of convoluted ivory set in a circlet of glowing jasper.

Compared to *chuchkella,* the nut sauces were simple concoctions. Both *bazha* and *satsivi* began with walnuts pounded to a smooth paste in a mortar along with garlic cloves, salt and red and black pepper. For *satsivi* finely chopped onions fried in clarified butter went into the paste, together with enough strong bouillon to thin the sauce to the consistency of buttermilk if it was to be served with meat or fish, somewhat less for vegetables. Crushed dried fenugreek and chopped green coriander were added to taste.

For *bazha* the oil was squeezed from the pounded nuts, which were then rubbed through a fine sieve and rinsed in bouillon. Fried onions, perhaps half the amount used in *satsivi* were sometimes added. Just before serving, a few crushed marigold petals were added for color, and enough of the oil was restored to give the sauce the thickness of heavy cream. *Bazha* accompanied meat, fish and fowl; less frequently it was used with vegetables.

We made sauces of many other things—tomatoes, garlic, barberries, aloeberries, green grapes, pomegranates and even sour bread. My own favorite is *tkemali (Recipe Index),* made of rosy, tart wild plums stewed with whole coriander plants, then put through a colander and simmered with fresh coriander leaves, red pepper, garlic and salt until thick and smooth.

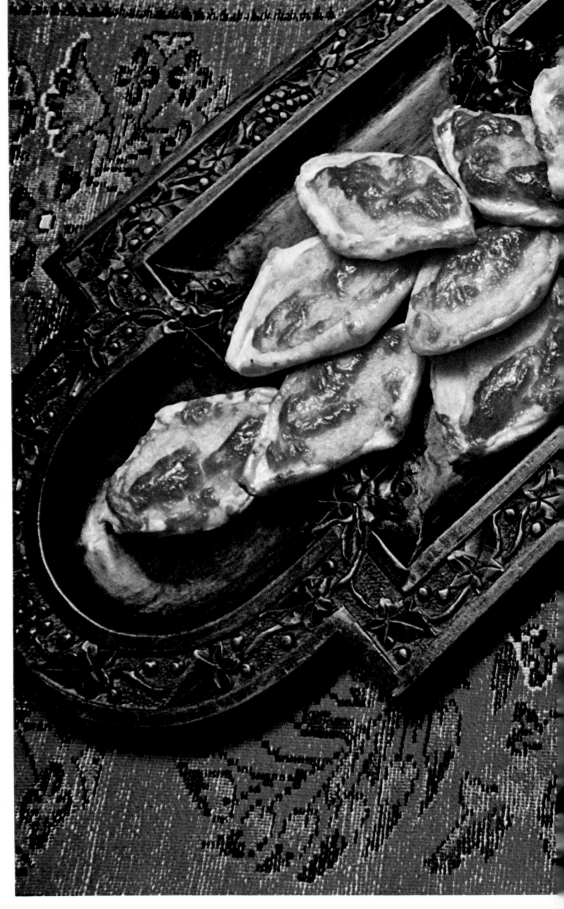

Khachapuri, or Georgian cheese bread *(Recipe Index)*, is one of the most delightful of all Caucasian specialties. It is made in many shapes and sizes, but the large round loaf and small diamond-shaped tartlets shown here are by far the most popular. Both adapt easily to Western eating: Slices of the bread make unusual brunch or teatime treats; the smaller versions go well as accompaniments for cocktails or soups, or as part of an informal buffet.

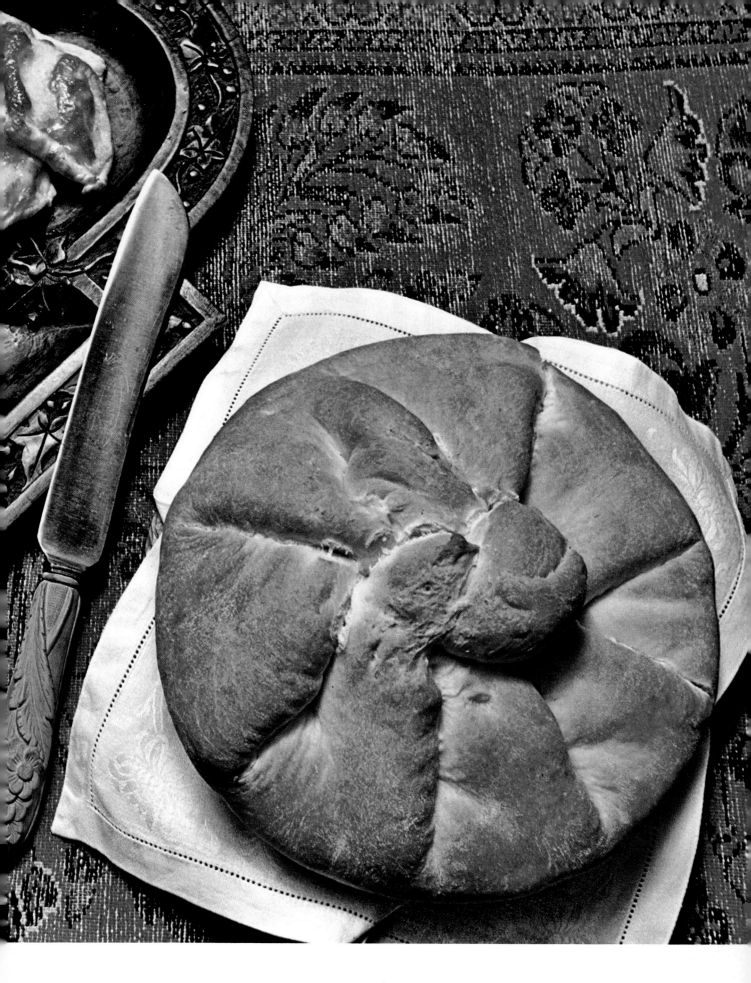

"I would not be surprised," a Russian chef once said to me, "to learn that Georgians eat sauce on sauce," He was almost right: we often fortify fruit sauces with a little *satsivi*.

Except when times were very bad almost every family had a cow and, for plowing, a water buffalo. We used their milk for a cultured clabber called *matsoni*. A quart of whole milk (that of the water buffalo, very rich and sweet, works better) is brought to a rolling boil and poured into a crock or wide-mouthed jar. Then, when the milk cools to lukewarm, a half cup of starter from a previous batch is stirred into it with a wooden spoon (the temperature of the milk is important, for the culture is a living thing and likes a pleasant climate). The vessel is covered and put into a warm place where it rests undisturbed for three hours or until it thickens. It may then be refrigerated. The process can be repeated indefinitely, using culture from old *matsoni* (well, not more than 10 days old) in new milk. We ate *matsoni* plain, and used it as a base for soup or, mixed with garlic and fresh herbs, as a sauce for vegetables. If we had any extra, we drained it into a linen bag to make curd cheese.

All these everyday dishes became special treats at holiday time. We kept many holidays in Georgia, but the most important of all was New Year's Day. Long before dawn the father of the family formed a one-man cere-monial procession around the outside of his house, carrying a newly burnished copper tray loaded with sweets. When he came in he went from per-son to person, inviting them to share the bounty of his burden: *gozinakh*, a candy of roasted almonds and filberts in an amber brittle; *chuchkella* slices; rai-sins in clustered bunches still sweet from the sun; stacks of paper-thin bread, and honey in pointed combs, meant to be touched to the lips of each child to insure a sweet new year.

Early in the morning the visiting began; heaped tables were everywhere we went for New Year's Day is the traditional day of friendship. By ancient law, a man must visit all his neighbors on that day; if he has an enemy, he must make peace with him before the sun falls so that the day will, in truth, usher in a New Year, and everyone can sit down at evening with a happy heart to sing and feast.

We had hot corn bread, of course, and heaping bowls of pickled vege-tables, including heads of cabbage with the leaves folded back to make them look like giant roses. Always there was chicken—roasted with *satsivi*, boiled whole and splashed with pomegranate sauce, or best of all, cooked as *chakhokhbili*. This dish consists of young pullets cut into serving pieces, rolled in finely chopped onions and fried in butter until the skin is golden. Then the pieces are put into a deep pot between thick layers of fresh to-matoes, peeled and quartered, with salt and pepper but not a drop of water. The pot simmers on a fire just hot enough to make the lid jump now and then and in an hour the lucky diner sits down to a blushing *rosé* chicken, sweet to the last morsel clinging to the coral bones.

When I returned to Georgia for a first visit after many years in the United States, I wondered if I would find the foods I remembered, prepared and served in the traditional ways. Was the table still the heart of the house? Did family and friends gather to eat and drink, to make toasts and sing, to enjoy each other? Or had the TV dinner, the packaged mix and the quick snack ar-rived there to destroy the culinary world of my youth?

152

I need not have worried. Half an hour after our plane landed we were at my sister's house, seated at a table covered with such a profusion of dishes that I wondered whether she feared I had not eaten at all since the last meal I took in Georgia. And if some of the songs were new to me (and some of the singers, too), the toasts and the spirit they expressed were as old as our country's history.

Later, I was to discover the Caucasus had indeed changed. Throughout the Republic there are new buildings, factories, libraries, theaters, hospitals and schools in every village—including mine, where once hardly anyone could read and write. Tbilisi, the capital, has modern hotels and a vigorous university. On each of many subsequent visits we saw improvements in housing, roads, and water and electrification systems. Irrigation and drainage have expanded the arable land, and farming is increasingly mechanized. But happily, the old ways of preparing food persist.

"Can it really be true," my sister-in-law asked me on my first visit, "that people in the United States eat frozen food?"

When I told her they did, she shook her head. "You should never have left home," she said.

My sisters and cousins believe that food must be bought and used fresh. They like to go to market every day, looking over the stalls to see which fish is the liveliest and which melon the most fragrant, and they carefully select every egg, fig and slice of sausage they intend to use.

"Cousin Tamara does more comparison shopping for a chicken," my wife once said, "than most people would for a car."

These early-morning trips to the markets are one of the joys we look forward to when we visit Georgia. I well remember the old bazaars, with rotting vegetables underfoot, and dirt and flies everywhere. The new markets are as clean and fresh as a garden after a rain, their tables piled high with perfect fruits, polished vegetables and all the greens we Georgians like so well. A beekeeper offers a honeycomb in a heart-shaped frame, and a cheese seller lures us with a nibble of briny *tushuri*. The last stop on one of these forays is always the counter laden with linen bags of dried herbs and spices, from which we assemble the *suneli*, or bouquet, for a particular dish.

Such a shopping trip always precedes one of our family dinners—which is an important event indeed and requires careful preparation. Guests are invited for 7 o'clock—which means that they come at 8 o'clock, which is when the hostess expects them. Twenty or 25 adults plus a half dozen children around a table is not unusual at such a dinner, with the young, unmarried guests congregated at one end and children tucked in here and there, often on a lap or the corner of a grownup's chair.

On the table for one typical dinner platters were piled high with greens —peppery cress, tarragon, scallions, parsley, coriander—and we stuffed handfuls of them with brined cheese into a pocket of the thin, white bread called *lavashi*. At the corners of the table were dishes of long white radishes, tomatoes quartered and dusted with dill, and tiny cucumbers still beaded with dew and almost seedless.

Now the hostess, my sister, brought in what she called "a bite of fish" —sturgeon smoked over hickory, sturgeon boiled and wreathed in tarragon, and mountain trout fried crisp in batter. The "poor man's caviar" *(Recipe* *Continued on page 157*

153

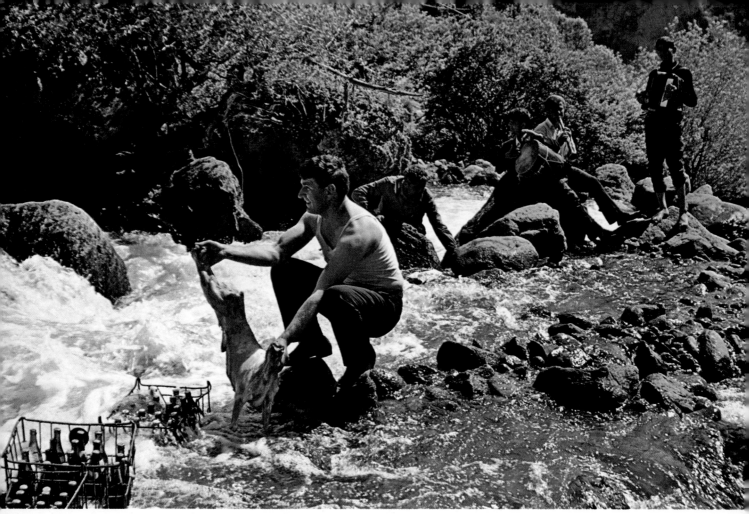

A picnicker rinses a slaughtered lamb while an impromptu band makes music with accordion, clarinet and a native drum, the *doola*.

A Mountain Picnic
on a Grand Scale

The banks of Armenia's swift mountain streams provide exhilarating settings for outings and outdoor dining. Large parties are popular: the picnic shown here featured a meal for 45 people, all grapegrowers and their families from Shenavan, a collective farm near Armenia's capital of Erevan. Provisions for the picnic included three live lambs, a plentiful supply of the Armenian bread called *lavash*, raw vegetables, cheeses and homemade vodka, beer and lemonade. Though the occasion had no religious significance, the picnickers followed a custom derived from an ancient Armenian Christian ritual of animal sacrifice when they slaughtered the lambs at the site of their feast.

Before the picnic meal begins, the women place folded sheets of *lavash* on a cloth-covered square of heavy canvas that will serve as a table. *Lavash*, like Georgian *deda's puri* (mother's bread), is baked against the walls of an oven. Unlike *deda's puri*, however, *lavash* is unleavened, and is rolled before baking into thin sheets.

154

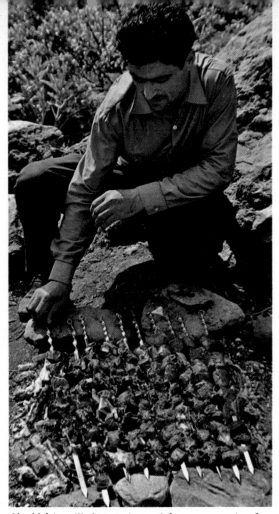

Shashlyk is grilled over charcoal from a grapevine fire.

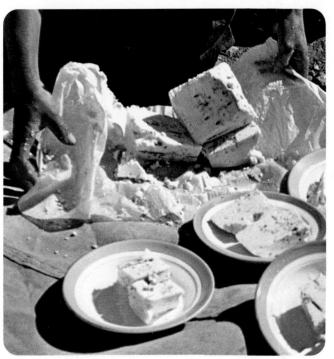

Plates of a blue cheese made from ewe's milk are set out for the picnickers. Armenians eat cheese, usually made from the milk of sheep or goats, as snacks. More formally, cheese is served at breakfast, at lunch, and at dinner, as a first course and—with fruit—a dessert.

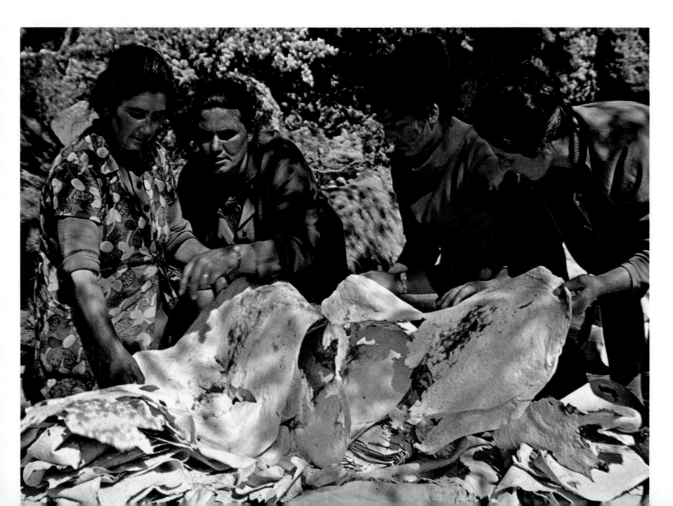

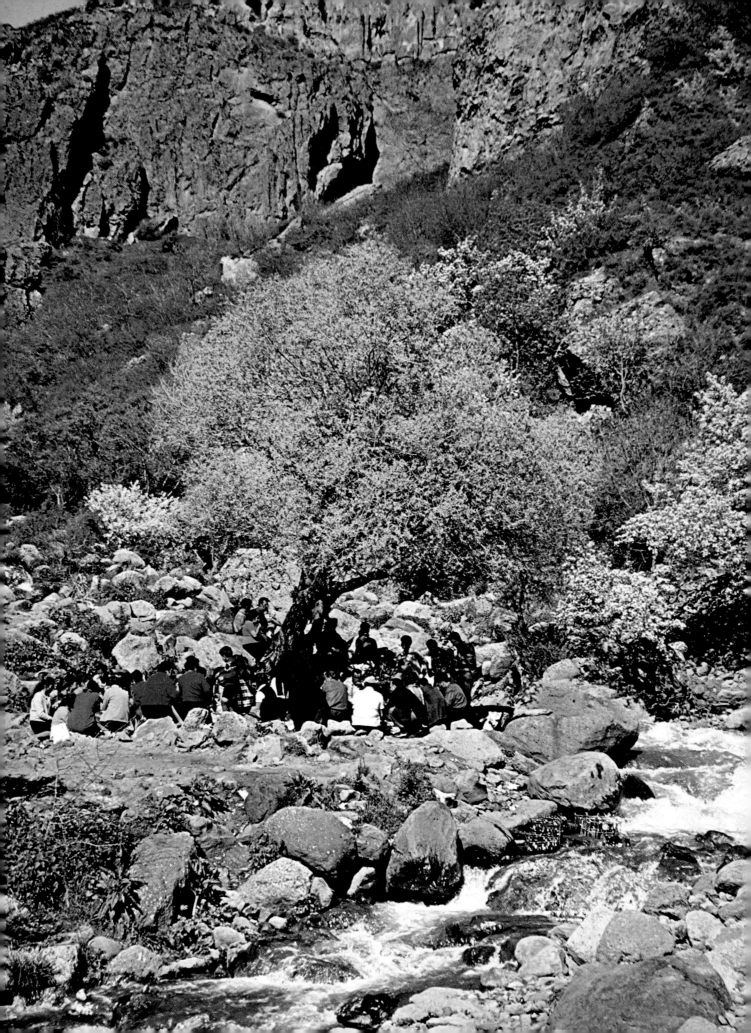

Index) that followed was not from the ocean but the garden. Whole baked eggplants were scooped from their purple skins, mashed with finely minced scallions, garlic, lemon juice, oil and coriander and then shaped into a fish with glittering pomegranate-seed eyes.

With all the guests seated but still unfed, it came time to select the Tamada, the head of the table. This high office calls for a man who remembers names and family relationships, for before the party is over he must offer a toast, well and roundly phrased, for every one of us and for our families in all their widespread branches. The Tamada must also know how to change the mood of the table, when to move from gaiety, gossip and jokes to serious concerns, how to divert the guests with music and dancing. He must be a diplomat, for he will have to decide arguments that may range from the best way to shoe a colt to the exact phrasing in the score of a ballet. If he can also recite portions of the Georgian epic, "The Man in the Panther's Skin," in the full rolling diction the poem demands, all the better. Finally this paragon must have a stomach for food and a head for wine, for upon him lies the trust of making the guests eat and drink by his happy example.

Chosen at last by popular acclaim, our Tamada for the feast, Uncle Davit, rose to his feet. "Friends," he jovially announced, "I drink this little glass for . . ." and the meal began.

For those who wanted to start with a glass or two of spirits there was a decanter of *chachis araki*, a very dry, sharp-edged grape spirit distilled from the lees of pressed grapes. It went untouched, for most Georgians are wine drinkers. Archeological evidence indicates that they have been so since the Neolithic Age. The delicate balance of soil and sunshine, slope and moisture that are needed to produce fine wine grapes occurs in many parts of the Caucasus, and "the honey-sweet wines of Colchis" enjoyed a great reputation in the ancient world. In modern times, unfortunately, Caucasian wines have been little known outside Russia because of limited production and distribution. But modern Georgian wines are full-bodied, brisk and possessed of a distinctive personality derived from trace elements in the Georgian subsoil—or perhaps in the Georgian heart. They well repay a trial.

Of course I am prejudiced, but I believe that no wine compares with that from the vineyard of my cousin in Mukran. Twelve generations have loved those sunny fields, have weeded and pruned them, have set new stock with careful hands, and have taught children and children's children to cherish the vines, gather the harvest, press the grapes. The wine is not stored in cellars or caves, but tenderly buried in earthen crocks beneath the arbor, there to ripen right under our feet. These years of love and labor have given every glass an unsurpassed bouquet. This is what we drank as the Tamada raised his glass and toasted "the home we are in and the host and hostess who have made it so happy a place for us."

The hostess gracefully acknowledged the raised glasses and vanished to return with hot *khachapuri* bread *(Recipe Index)*, a rich raised dough rolled flat, its center filled with a mixture of cheese and eggs, its sides brought up and over to the center and sealed.

It is our custom at a party to have one dish of beans on the table—partly to remind us of how we lived in hard times and partly because we like beans. This time it was *lobio (Recipe Index)*, a dish of red kidney beans with

Against a background of flowering jasmine, an age-old tree shades the picnickers as they form a circle around their spreads of food, ready to begin a serious attack on the *shashlyk*, cheeses and drinks. Their appetites have been whetted by the vigorous steps of an Armenian circle dance, the *butchari*, in which all joined while the *shashlyk* was grilling.

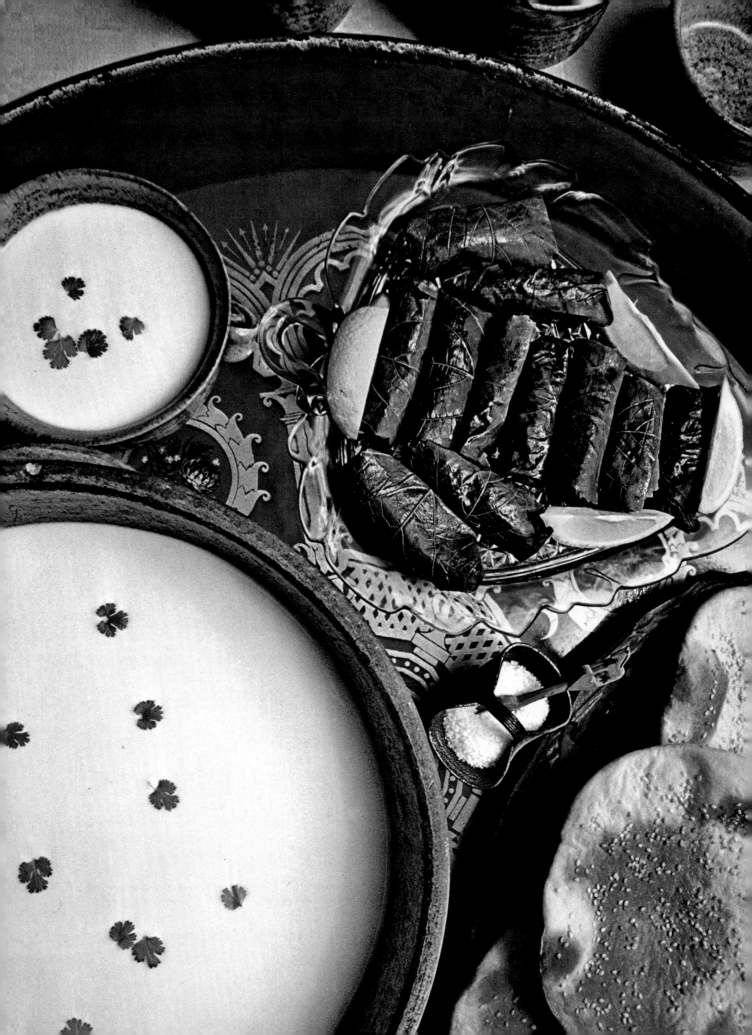

thin slivers of scallions, chopped coriander, a dash of tarragon vinegar and a very light film of olive oil. ("Oil is a priest to marry," says a Georgian proverb, "not a king to rule.") Then we were served the soup called *chikhirtma* *(Recipe Index)*—rich chicken stock with egg yolks, saffron and lemon juice, stirred in carefully just before serving so as not to curdle.

A roast turkey with *satsivi* came next, and with it a mound of *ghome*, which is cornmeal porridge cooked for hours over a slow fire. *Adzhersandal*, eggplant baked with fried onions and tomatoes, was passed among us. There was talk, more toasts, a song, and another song, this one gay enough to stimulate some dancers—a man and woman who circled the room in a symbolic pattern of flight and pursuit.

A new cloth was laid; new plates appeared. Preceded by a mouth-watering aroma, a young suckling pig roasted to a crackling brown came to the table. For the hardy there was a garlic sauce that had all the deceptive mildness of the center of a hurricane. The youngest child at the feast was ceremoniously presented with the pig's ear to remind him to listen to his elders. As dish followed dish, the pace and mood vary but never go too fast. Each food had its glass of wine; each glass of wine its word. One learns to eat sparingly and wait. We drink a glass for peace and understanding, another for absent friends. We dip a crust of bread in the wine and drink for those who have died.

Presently our host left the table and we were soon invited into the garden, where he was grilling meat for us. We protested. "Just a stickful," his wife said, and we went to watch.

Of *mtswadi*, or grilled meat, there are two kinds. One, called *basturma*, is marinated meat for a hunter who must save his bag until the next lucky day —a functional dish for a special situation. For pleasure there is a *mtswadi* of fresh, tender, well-fleshed meat—lamb, fat-tailed sheep or mountain kid—untouched by spices, vinegar or lemon juice. The broiling sticks are whips of new hardwood trimmed of bark. ("No man is fit to marry," says the proverb, "until he can cut a *mtswadi* stick with no more than three knife strokes.") We watched the meat spitting at the fire. In minutes it was done and we returned to the table.

Georgians eat few sweets for dessert. Our dessert was fruit on a copper tray. For the ladies there were tiny glass saucers, each holding perfect pieces of apricots, cherries or melon rind in syrup. Now the last toast was drunk: "For our safe departure and our safe return." After that we drank "Qelas Mindas," "All Saints," the last wine of the day.

From that feast at my sister's we went to Erevan, the capital of Armenia, in search of another, very different meal. I hoped to keep an engagement I made 50 years earlier with my friend Haik Sarafian, who served with me in the Russian army during World War I.

Haik and I were companions of the army mess, such as it was. In those days, soldiers had tea and bread in the morning. In the late afternoon, soup and meat for four men were ladled into a pot. We sat on the ground, Haik and I and the two Russians who made up our quartet, pulled our spoons from our belts and ate in turn from the same pot. Over the years I have often heard our *soldatsky borshch* described as good, honest fare, and for all I know it might have been—if the officers had used the commissary funds to

The dishes shown on the tray, all made from traditional Armenian recipes, reflect Armenia's culinary ties with the lands of the Middle East. The courses of a very similar meal could be found in almost any Middle Eastern home or restaurant —under different names. The yoghurt soup with barley and herbs is called *spas* in Armenian; the grape leaves stuffed with lamb and rice are *yarpakh dolmasy;* the unleavened bread with sesame seeds is *churek.*

159

get proper ingredients instead of to pay their gambling debts or buy horses. The only thing that could be said for our rations is that, after eating them for four years, I never complained of anything I ate the rest of my life.

Day after day in Erevan, as the army *borshch* grew thinner and thinner, Haik and I described good dinners to one another. "How about a trout from our Lake Sevan, Georgi? Fresh, six pounds—no, smaller is better—nicely cleaned and dropped into a pot of spring water to simmer. I pinch the steam and when it feels sticky, out comes our fish, and we eat it with some vegetables—green tomatoes, yellow peppers, cucumbers and cauliflower straight from the pickle tub. . . ."

"The pickles sound fine, but I think we should fry the fish."

"In that case it should not be a trout, but a whitefish, with a grating of orange rind and red pepper, rolled in flour and dropped into deep fat. Unless fish *plaki* suits you better—fresh fish covered with chopped celery, carrots, parsley, tomatoes and oil and baked. My mother adds potatoes, too."

The two Russians would stop eating long enough to call us crazy, and maybe we were—but we passed the time most pleasantly and the dinners we described grew better and better. We lovingly discussed the soup called *matsunabur* (made with Armenian *matsun*, or yoghurt, which is a cousin to Georgian *matsoni*), with an egg stirred in gently, then noodles and browned onions added just before serving and chopped mint sprinkled over the bowl. Next we decided to have *yarpakh dolmasy (Recipe Index)*, which is grape leaves stuffed with chopped lamb, onions and rice, simmered and served with cinnamon-flavored yoghurt. Or should we have stuffed squash or eggplant or tomatoes instead? Or should we have all of these dishes and the fish too?

When the Russians laughed and called us fools, Haik said, "Never mind. When the war is over my mother and sisters will make Georgi and me a week-long feast fit for a king's marriage."

On our brief leaves from the army Haik and I would venture into the country and find a farmer who could sell us some vegetables and meat for a few kopecks and lend us a pot for nothing. On the spot, we made the Armenian dish called *tureli givech*, frying the meat first and then tossing in an eggplant, onions, squash, carrots, green beans, okra, fresh tomatoes and whatever else came to hand, all cut fine. While it bubbled over our fire we gave the farmer a hand at his chores, and in that way we made some friends. Soon the farmers were sharing with us half the nothing they had: an egg; a piece of beef sausage sharp with hot pepper, allspice, cinnamon and cumin; or thin slices of *basturma*—salted beef, wind-dried, brined with fenugreek and dried again.

To give something in return Haik and I saved our weekly ration of a half pound of sugar and handed it over to our new friends. They were delighted, for red roses were in bloom, and with our sugar they could make jam. We helped carry baskets of dusky petals that were tossed into a pot and covered with sugar and boiling water. After steeping, a soggy gray pulp remained, but when the liquid was drained and touched with lemon juice, back came the color and fragrance of the roses.

I wonder still at some of the dishes we ate—dishes made of almost nothing and cooked over a few smoldering faggots, but generously shared. We ate soul-warming pilafs of wheat, and of rice given savor by herbs and the smallest bit of meat or chicken. If there was meat it was chopped and fashioned into stuffed meatballs—*kiufta*—fried or boiled. Each dish seemed a triumph. It might be thought one cannot judge the cuisine of a country impoverished and at war, but the contrary is true. It is when food is precious that cooks display all their skill and ingenuity. At one time, for example, we had nothing but a single pumpkin. It provided no less than three delicious meals—one stewed with garlic, tomatoes and mint leaves; a second baked with butter; and a third of the boiled and roasted seeds, which we cracked and ate like pistachios.

In the last year of the war I was sent to the Persian front. As Haik and I parted I heard his last words, shouted after the truck that was carrying me away: "Remember, after the war . . . a feast . . . *liulia kebab! . . .*"

Now here I was back again, so many years later. The Erevan I remembered, a few mud houses sprawled beside a dirty river, was gone; in its place I found a beautiful city with shady streets, fine buildings, splashing fountains, banks of flowers, a university and a library of invaluable manuscripts. But —this was my problem—the city had grown to 650,000 people, and among them the name "Haik Sarafian" seemed to be as common as the name "John Smith" in New York.

How to find my friend? In 50 years a man's face, size and business may alter, but one thing never changes. So I made the rounds of the best restaurants, asking waiters and chefs for word of Haik. On the evening of the fourth day I found him exactly as I had left him—eating.

As he promised, his sisters—now he had a wife, daughters and granddaughters as well to help—gave us parties, each one better than the next.

I remember string cheese beaded with brine; flaky *burek,* or cheese-filled turnovers; *peda,* a dimpled, crusted yeast bread; home-cured peppered green olives; cucumbers in *matsun,* fragrant with mint; cold boiled leeks, glistening with oil; bowls of lamb-and-spinach broth afloat with wheat-ball dumplings; rosy lentil soup, thick enough to support a bouquet of chopped tarragon on its surface; and more kinds of *kiufta* and pilaf than I knew existed.

Haik's grandson grilled shish kabobs which, unlike my Georgian *mtswadi,* are marinated in chopped onions, oil, lemon juice and tomato paste, then threaded on the skewers with the unexpected addition of onions, finger eggplant, green peppers or tomatoes. And we had, as Haik had promised, *liulia kebab,* which is ground lamb broiled on sticks and tasting as hot from its spices as from the coals.

Many of the Armenian dishes resembled those of Georgia, but there were noticeable differences, too. Where Georgians use corn, walnuts and dried beans, Armenians prefer cracked wheat *(bulghur),* pine nuts and chick-peas, and they have many more pastries and desserts—coffee cakes, twists, rolls, cakes stuffed with flour, butter, nuts and sugar crumbs, others layered with sesame paste, and a cookie called *gurabia,* so short it had to be eaten in one bite lest it fall to crumbs.

Haik's sisters made their Armenian *baklava* in the traditional way, rolling the dough with a broomstick into circles a yard or more wide and practically as thin as a shadow. A few huge rounds of dough were stacked on a flat copper pan, then covered with chopped nuts and painted with clarified butter. More pastry was added, and more nuts. The top sheet was scored, a final coating of butter was painted on, and the pastry went into the oven. Just before

Continued on page 165

161

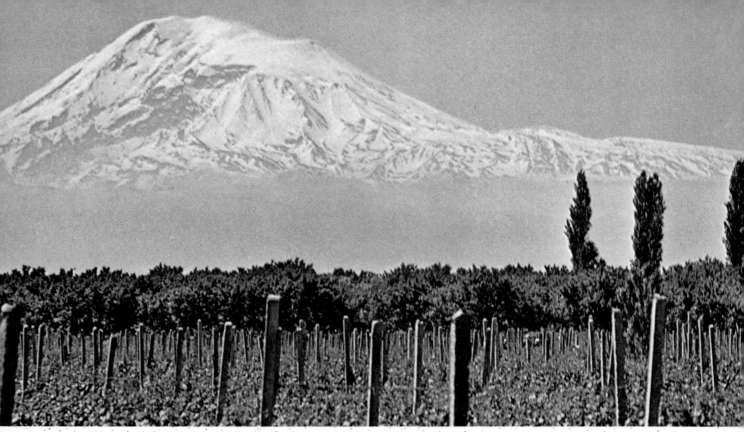

Wine grapes flourish in a sun-drenched vineyard at the foot of snow-capped Mount Ararat, which lies partly in Armenia.

From the High Caucasus, Wines for Connoisseurs

The mountain slopes, soil and sunshine of the Caucasus combine to produce some of the world's finest wine grapes. Most of the wines made from them are consumed within the region, for though some Western connoisseurs have ranked Georgian wines and Armenian brandies equal to those of Germany and France, the country has not yet mastered the problems of transportation and distribution involved in a large-scale export trade. In the art of making wine, however, the peoples of the Caucasus are heir to an ancient tradition. According to the Old Testament, one of the first things Noah did after his ark landed on Mount Ararat was to plant a vineyard, and some of the earliest recorded accounts of grape growing come from Armenia. Much Caucasian wine is still made at home but commercial wineries are now an important source. The bottles of brandy at right, for example, were produced in Erevan; the barrels in the background contain brandy that is still in the aging process.

162

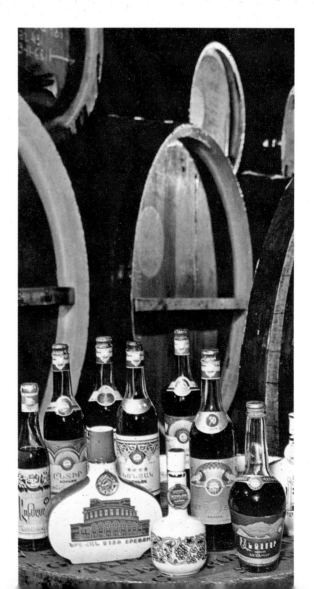

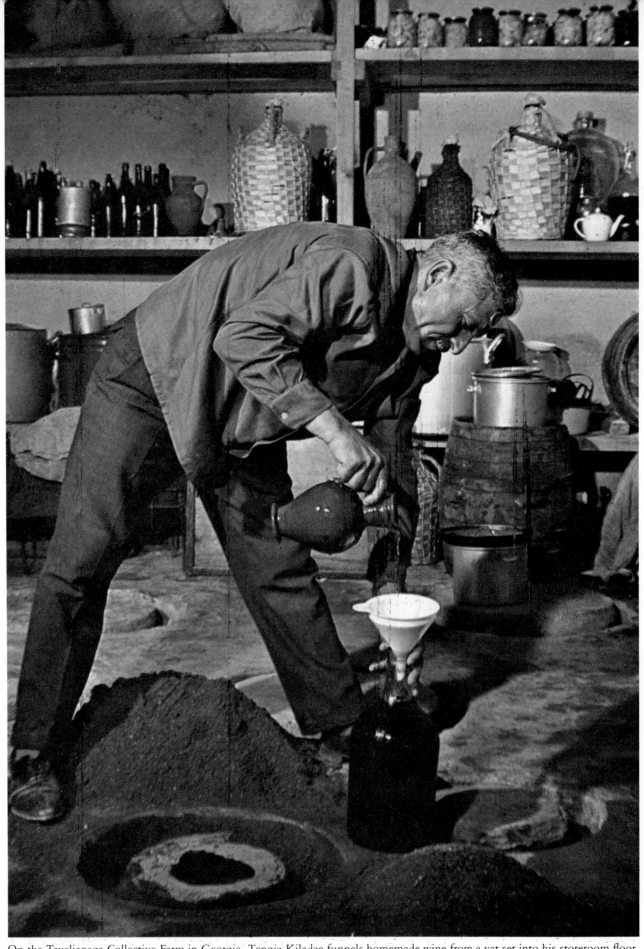

On the Tsvelianaga Collective Farm in Georgia, Tengiz Kiladze funnels homemade wine from a vat set into his storeroom floor.

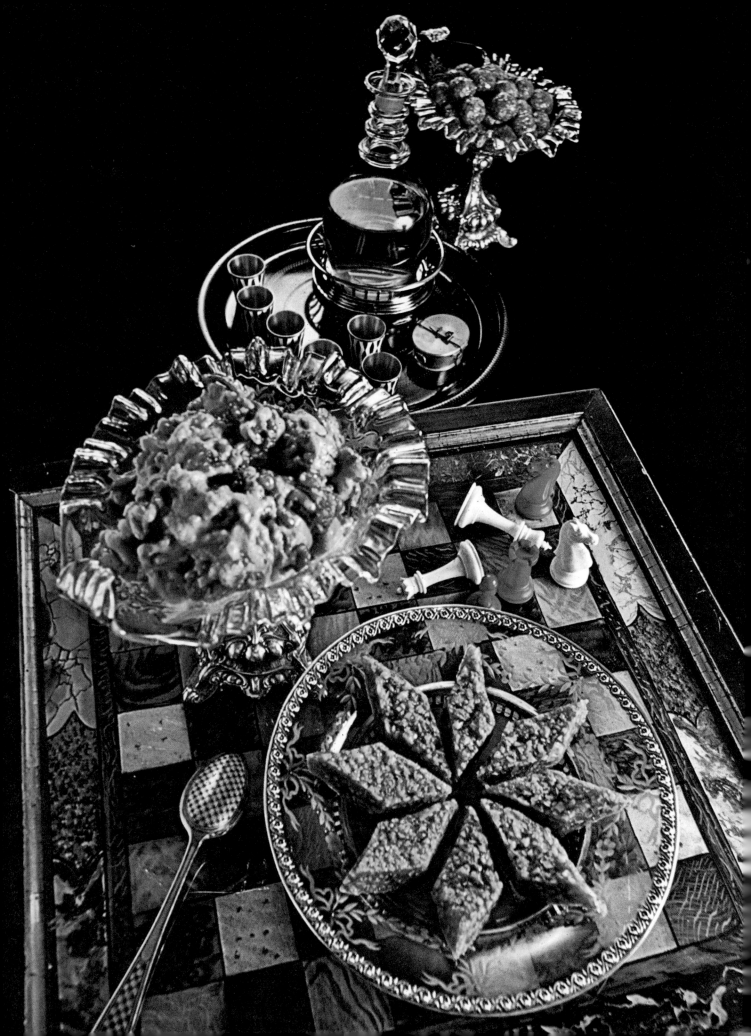

serving it was drenched, or perhaps a better word is drowned, with honey.

My favorite of all the sweets was *ekmek,* a pudding made of bread but by no means a "bread pudding." A thick, trimmed piece of yeasty white bread was toasted golden, dipped quickly in milk and drained. Then it was dropped into a boiling syrup of sugar, honey and butter for three minutes, drained again and served with *kaimak,* a special cream skimmed from very rich milk, simmered for three hours and left to stand overnight. If we ate too much or ended our meal by sampling too many kinds of Armenian brandies ("But it won a gold medal . . ." Haik always said), then we greeted the next morning with a guaranteed restorative—big dishes of tripe stewed with garlic, pepper and salt and finally simmered in a broth that was fortified with beaten egg and lemon juice.

Haik showed me the sights—or, at least, all the sights connected with food. We went to Lake Sevan, 6,000 feet up the slope of the Caucasus, and ate fresh trout, both steamed and broiled, with a sauce of pomegranates and an accompaniment of wine from the local Garandmak grapes. Elsewhere, we visited canning factories, wineries, distilleries and fields where girls picked roses for jelly by the basketful, as they have always done—except that the jelly is now made in steel vats inside tiled factories. To this restaurant and that one we went; each one had its specialty, and who knew better than Haik what the specialty was. In this way we sampled *kharput kiufta,* a complex affair of ground lamb, minced lamb, pine nuts and cracked wheat, boiled and served in chicken broth; *kashlama,* which is lamb shoulder boiled with vegetables; grilled lamb liver; dried apricot soup—and another gold-medal winner of a brandy.

On our last day together, a Sunday, Haik decided that we would go to Echmiadzin, the ancient capital of Armenia and the residence of the head of the Armenian Church, for a picnic in the park. The walkways were crowded with families going to the church services and visitors from all over the world eager to see the frescoes, easel paintings and carvings in the Fourth Century basilica. Children passed by, some leading beribboned animals—sheep, goats, chickens—to the church for ritual blessing and marking, others returning through the throng still steering their charges, now bedaubed with vivid streaks of carmine.

We skirted other picnic parties that already had their kettles boiling on portable stoves, and found a secluded spot under the trees where we unpacked our baskets. We ate our flat bread spread with ground meat, herbs and minced vegetables, and drank our amber wine. And as we ate and drank, we spoke once again of the old days and all that had happened to us since. For that little while we were young again.

"You must come to visit us in the United States," I said.

Haik shook his head. "It's a long way. I am an old man."

But I knew how to win Haik over. I simply described a very good American dinner, from clam chowder to apple pie. "And with this pie, you know, you will have a piece of sharp cheese or some vanilla ice cream, whichever you like."

"Cheese *or* ice cream? Well . . . I would have to try both of them, I suppose, before I could decide."

He'll come.

Armenians and Georgians often indulge a national sweet tooth with brandy sipped while nibbling sweets. *Gozinakh,* made in the shape of diamonds or small balls, is a confection consisting of only three ingredients—chopped nuts, honey and sugar. Armenian *khalva,* center, is composed of toasted walnut halves with a custard coating. Recipes are in the Recipe Booklet.

Khachapuri

GEORGIAN CHEESE BREAD

To make 48 cheese tarts or 1 large
loaf

DOUGH

2 packages active dry yeast
½ teaspoon plus 1 tablespoon sugar
1 cup lukewarm milk (110° to 115°)
3½ to 4 cups all-purpose flour
2 teaspoons salt
8 tablespoons butter, softened (¼-
pound stick)

FILLING

2 pounds sweet Muenster cheese,
finely grated by hand or in a blender
2 tablespoons butter, softened
1 egg
1 egg, lightly beaten (for tarts)
2 tablespoons finely chopped
coriander *(cilantro)* (optional, for
the tarts)

Georgian cheese bread is made either as individual open tarts or large round or ob-long loaves. (The small tarts are so popular in the Caucasus that they are sold by street vendors.) Both the loaves and the tarts are well-suited to brunch or breakfast. Sprinkle the 2 packages of yeast and the ½ teaspoon of the sugar over ½ cup of the lukewarm milk in a small, shallow bowl. Set aside for 2 or 3 minutes, then stir until the yeast is thoroughly dissolved. Place in a warm, draft-free spot (such as an unlighted oven) for 5 to 8 minutes, or until the mixture has doubled in volume.

Pour 3 cups of the flour into a large mixing bowl and make a deep well in the center. Add the remaining ½ cup of milk, the yeast mixture, the remaining 1 tablespoon of sugar, 2 teaspoons of salt and 8 tablespoons of butter. With a large spoon, slowly beat the flour into these ingredients and continue to beat vigorously until smooth. Gather the dough into a ball and place it on a lightly floured surface.

Knead the dough by folding it end to end, then pressing it down, pushing it forward with the heel of your hand and folding it back. Knead in this fashion for at least 10 minutes, sprinkling the dough every few minutes with small handfuls of as much of the remaining flour as you need to prevent it from sticking to the board.

When the dough is smooth and elastic, place it in a large, lightly buttered bowl. Dust the dough lightly with flour and cover the bowl loosely with a kitchen towel. Let the dough rise in the warm, draft-free place for about 45 minutes to an hour, or until it has doubled in bulk and springs back slowly when gently poked with a finger. Then punch the dough down with a blow of your fist and set aside again to rise for another 30 to 40 minutes or until it again doubles in bulk.

Meanwhile, prepare the cheese filling. In a large mixing bowl, combine the grated cheese, softened butter and the whole egg. Beat vigorously with a large spoon until smooth, then purée in a food mill or rub with the back of a spoon through a fine sieve set over a large bowl.

Preheat the oven to 375°. To make the round loaf, punch the dough down with a sharp blow of your fist, then roll it on a lightly floured surface into a circle about 22 inches in diameter.

Following the illustrations on the opposite page, use the dough to line a buttered layer-cake tin 9 inches round by 1½ inches deep. Then fill it with the cheese mixture, and fold in the ends of dough. Set the loaf aside to rest for 10 or 15 minutes, then bake the bread in the center of the oven for 1 hour, or until golden brown. Turn the bread out onto a wire cake rack and cool a little before serving.

To make individual tarts, roll the dough into a 24-inch-wide circle and with a 4½-inch cookie cutter, cut out 48 rounds. Following the illustrations opposite, fill and shape the rounds. Set them side by side on buttered cookie sheets and brush the dough with lightly beaten egg. Let the tarts rest for 10 minutes, then bake them in the center of the oven for 20 to 25 minutes, or until golden brown. With a wide spatula, transfer the tarts to a serving platter, sprinkle with chopped coriander, if you like, and serve warm.

"Khachapuri": A high-rising Georgian Cheese Bread for Hearty Diners

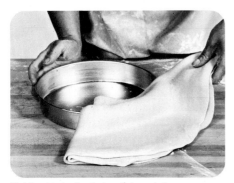

Fold a 22-inch circle of dough into quarters and place the point of the wedge at the center of a 9-inch tin.

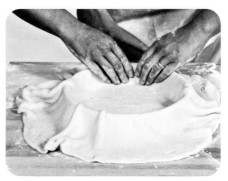

Unfold the dough, draping the outer rim of the circle over the edge of the pan. Smooth out the center.

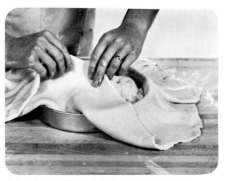

After mounding the cheese filling high in the center begin to fold in excess dough hanging over the tin.

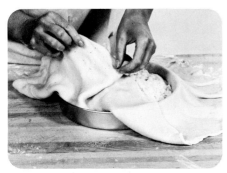

Draw the sides of the dough up over the filling into the center, pleating the dough into loose folds.

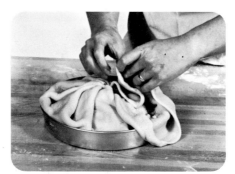

Rotate the tin as you continue to pleat the dough. Try to make the pleats even all around the tin.

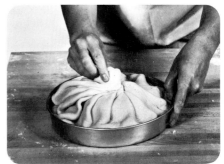

Gather together the ends of the dough that meet in the center and twist them into a small knob.

A Delicate "Khachapuri" Tartlet for Cocktails or Soup

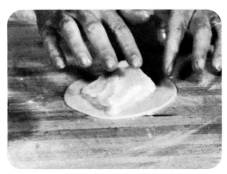

Place 2 tablespoons of the cheese filling on a 4½-inch circle of dough and form the cheese into a diamond.

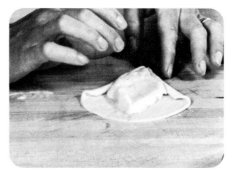

With your fingers, roll the edges of the dough up over the edge of the filling, following the diamond shape.

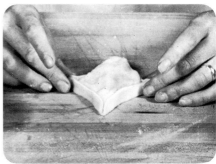

Perfect the final shape of the tartlet by pinching each of the four corners of the diamond to a sharp point.

To serve 4

1 large onion, peeled and finely grated
1 tablespoon strained fresh lemon
    juice
1 tablespoon olive oil
1 teaspoon salt
¼ teaspoon freshly ground black
    pepper
2 pounds boneless leg or shoulder
    of lamb, trimmed of excess fat
    and cut into 1- to 1½-inch cubes
2 medium onions, cut into ¼-inch-
    thick chunks

GARNISH
2 medium firm, ripe tomatoes, cut
    into eighths
10 scallions, trimmed
1 lemon, quartered

To serve 4 to 6

1 pound fresh string beans, trimmed
4 tablespoons butter
2 cups thinly sliced onions
1 small green pepper, seeded, deribbed
    and cut into ½-inch pieces
3 medium tomatoes, peeled, seeded
    and coarsely chopped (see borshch
    ukraïnsky, page 141)
1 tablespoon finely chopped sweet,
    fresh basil leaves, or substitute
    1½ teaspoons dried crumbled basil
1 egg
1 cup sour cream
1 teaspoon salt
Freshly ground black pepper

To make 1½ cups

2 cups water
½ pound sour prunes (about 24)
1 clove garlic, peeled
3 tablespoons finely chopped
    coriander (cilantro)
¼ teaspoon salt
⅛ teaspoon cayenne pepper
2 tablespoons strained fresh lemon
    juice

Shashlyk
GEORGIAN SKEWERED LAMB

In a large mixing bowl, beat together the grated onion, lemon juice, olive oil, salt and pepper. Add the meat and let it marinate for at least 3 hours at room temperature, tossing it about in the marinade every hour or so to keep the pieces well moistened.

Light a layer of coals in a charcoal broiler and burn until a white ash appears on the surface, or preheat your kitchen broiler to its highest point.

String the cubes of lamb tightly on 4 long skewers, alternating the lamb with the chunks of onion; press them firmly together. Broil 4 inches from the source of heat, turning the skewers occasionally, until the lamb is done to your taste and the onions are brown. For pink lamb, allow about 10 minutes; for well-done lamb, more typical of Georgian cooking, allow about 15 minutes. Slide the lamb and onions off the skewers onto heated individual plates, and serve with the raw tomatoes, scallions and lemon quarters.

Karabakh Loby
STRING BEANS IN SOUR CREAM AND TOMATO SAUCE

In a 4- to 5-quart pan, bring 3 quarts of lightly salted water to a boil over high heat. Drop in the string beans a handful at a time and bring back to a boil. Lower the heat and cook uncovered for 8 to 10 minutes, or until the beans are tender but still slightly resistant to the bite. Drain the beans, wash them under cold running water and set aside.

Melt the butter in a heavy 10- to 12-inch skillet or 2-quart casserole set over high heat. Add the onions and green pepper, lower the heat and, stirring occasionally, cook 5 to 8 minutes, or until the vegetables are tender but not brown. Stir in the tomatoes and basil, raise the heat to high, and boil rapidly for 1 or 2 minutes, until most of the juices in the pan have evaporated. Stir in the green beans and simmer 1 or 2 minutes until heated through.

In a mixing bowl, beat together the egg, sour cream, salt and a few grindings of black pepper. Taste for seasoning and stir into the vegetables. Transfer to a serving bowl and serve at once.

Tkemali
SOUR PRUNE SAUCE

Bring the 2 cups of water to a boil in a 1-quart saucepan and drop in the prunes. Remove from the heat and set aside for 10 minutes, then bring the water back to a boil over high heat. Cook briskly uncovered for 10 to 15 minutes, or until the prunes are tender. Pour the contents of the pan into a sieve set over a small bowl and set the liquid aside.

With a small, sharp knife cut out and discard the prune pits and combine the prunes, garlic and coriander in an electric blender. Pour in ¼ cup of the reserved prune liquid and blend at high speed, gradually adding the remaining prune liquid. The blended sauce should have the consistency of sour cream.

With a rubber spatula, transfer the sauce to a 1½- to 2-quart saucepan and stir in the salt and pepper. Bring to a boil over high heat, then, off the heat, stir in the lemon juice. Cool to room temperature and serve with shashlyk (above) or tabaka (Recipe Index).

A tripod of shashlyk, grilled skewered lamb, is served with fresh vegetables.

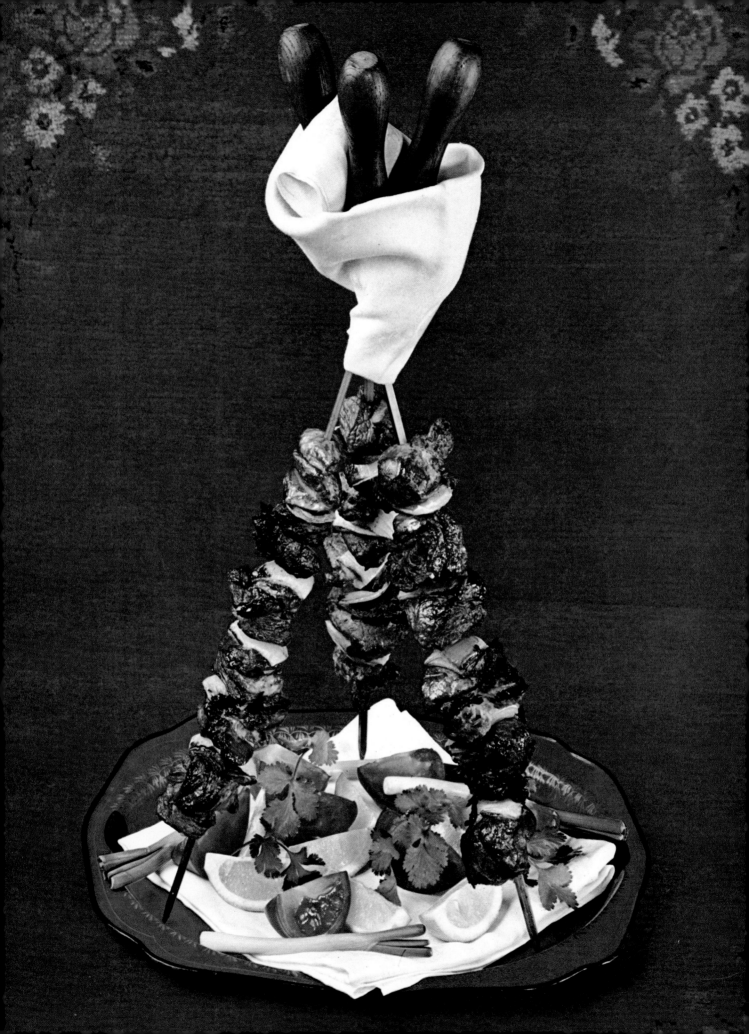

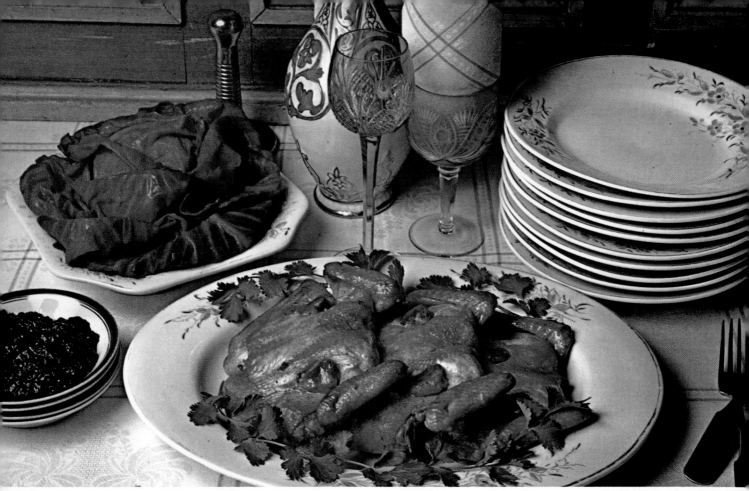

Chicken *tabaka*, flattened and fried to a juicy crispness, is served with a tart prune sauce and an artfully arranged pickled cabbage "rose."

PREPARING PRESSED CHICKEN:
Beginning at the neck end *(1)*, insert a boning knife alongside the backbone and cut along its length. Turn the chicken over and cut along the other side of the backbone, freeing it *(2)*. Break it away from the spoon-shaped bone connecting the breasts, and pull out both bones and the white cartilage *(3)* below them. Loosen the skin around the leg and thigh *(4)* and push it back, exposing the thigh joint. Cut halfway into the joint *(5)* to straighten it, pull the skin into place and repeat on the other leg. Insert the tip of a knife *(6)* into each breast below the ribs, to make a slit. Cover the chicken with wax paper *(7)* and flatten it by pounding with a cleaver or with a meat pounder. Twist the legs into the inside and bring them out through the holes in the breasts *(8)*.

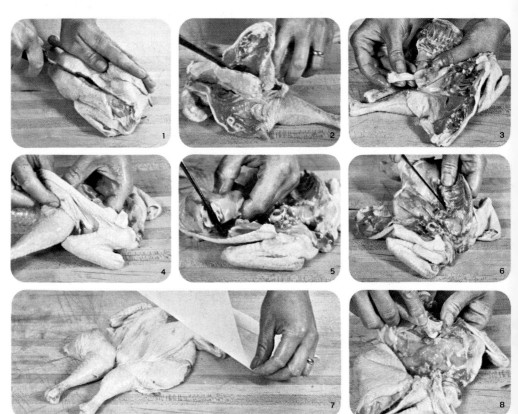

Tabaka

PRESSED FRIED CHICKEN

Georgians prepare small chickens in this unusual fashion—the backbone removed, the chicken flattened and then fried under a weight—so that the birds brown and cook quickly, and retain their shape.

Pat the chickens thoughly dry with paper towels. Following the illustrations below, remove the backbone, flatten the chickens, and draw their legs up through slits in the breasts.

Clarify the 6 tablespoons of butter in the following fashion: Melt it slowly in a heavy 10- to 12-inch skillet set over low heat, without letting it brown. Skim off the foam with a large spoon as it rises to the surface. Remove the pan carefully from the heat, let it rest 2 or 3 minutes, then spoon off the clear butter and discard the milky solids (whey) at the bottom of the pan.

Preheat the oven to 250°. Sprinkle both sides of the chickens liberally with salt and spread the flesh sides evenly with half the sour cream. Pour 2 tablespoons of the clarified butter into a heavy 10- to 12-inch skillet set over high heat and when the butter begins to brown, place 2 of the chickens skin-side down in the pan. Set a heavy weight—such as another skillet laden with cans of food—on top of the chickens, reduce the heat to moderate, and fry for 8 to 10 minutes. Then turn the chickens over with tongs, brush them with half of the remaining sour cream, and fry—again under the weight —for 10 minutes, or until they are a deep golden brown. Watch for any sign of burning, and regulate the heat accordingly.

When the chickens are done, place them skin-side up on an ovenproof platter. Keep them warm in the oven while you add the remaining butter to the skillet and proceed to fry the other chickens as before. Serve 1 whole chicken per person, accompanied by a bowl of *tkemali* sauce.

To serve 4

4 squab chickens (1 to 1¼ pounds each)
Salt
4 tablespoons sour cream
6 tablespoons butter, clarified *(below)*
1 cup *tkemali* sauce *(page 168)*

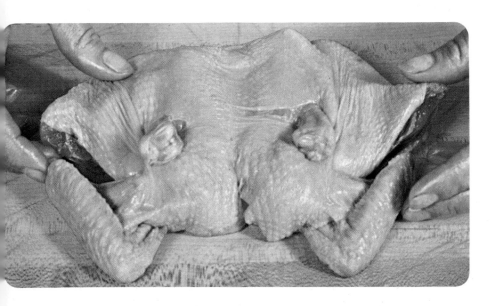

The flattened whole chicken, with the breast bone removed and the legs drawn through the openings in the breasts, is ready for frying. During the frying process *(see recipe, above)* the chicken will be further flattened by weighting it with a heavy object. Traditionally, the ideal weight was a flat iron, but a heavy skillet makes an acceptable substitute.

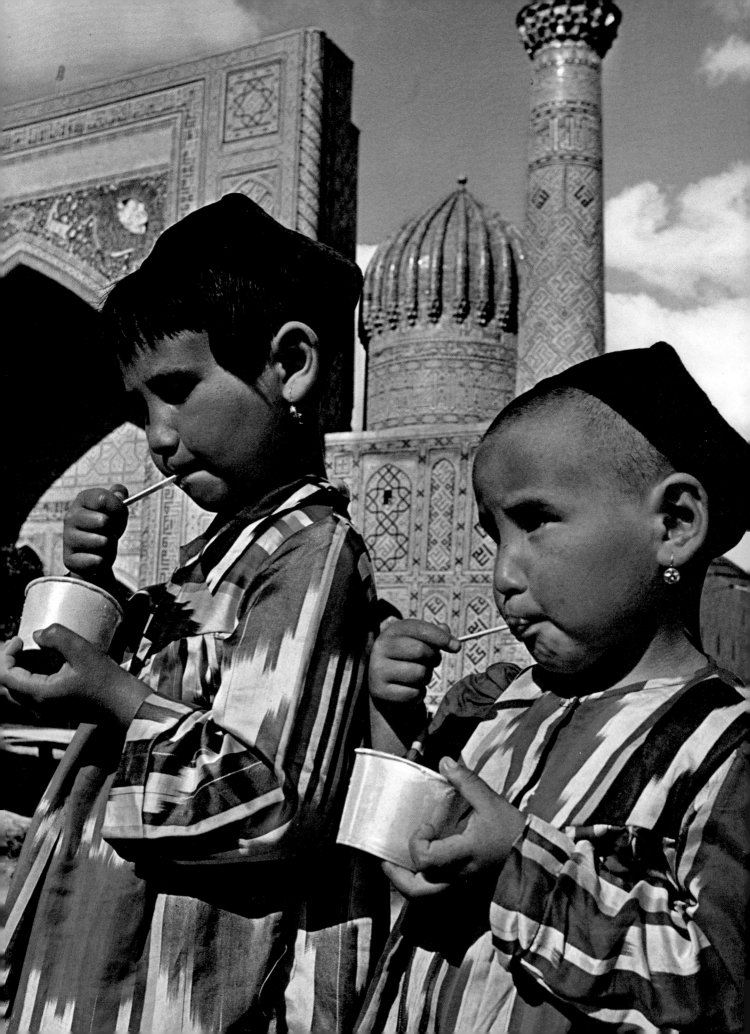

VII

From the Steppes of Central Asia

Samarkand! Tashkent! Bukhara! Just reciting the names of the cities lying ahead in Soviet Central Asia filled our minds with romance. Here was the old Silk Road, the ancient caravan route that brought the fabled riches of the Orient to Europe. Alexander marched through in the 4th Century B.C., Genghis Khan in the 13th Century. Tamerlane made his headquarters here, and Marco Polo stopped by on his way to China. One of the oldest, for centuries one of the richest, civilized regions in the world, it has been half forgotten in recent years. But now it is one of the most vigorous and fascinating sections of the U.S.S.R.

Changes that took generations in the West erupted here in decades. Factories, schools, sports pavilions rose—and yet ancient blue-domed mosques were lovingly restored. Women were emancipated—and returned to traditional dress. The automobile came—and the horse stayed. Food is different, too, and yet in many places delightfully old-fashioned.

While irrigation projects and collective farms, expanding cities and mining operations have absorbed parts of the old grazing lands, modern wells and water-storage facilities have opened new pasturage. The herds, greatly increased by winter-feeding programs and scientific care, still move to pasture, but the cattle are more numerous, the camels fewer, and the herdsmen usually members of a collective farm with a permanent base. Service in distant pastures may be rotated among them.

Inevitably the cities have grown more cosmopolitan and large restaurants are more proud of their Russian dishes than their Asian ones. One evening in an Alma Ata hotel we ordered *besh barmak*, a thick Central Asian soup

173

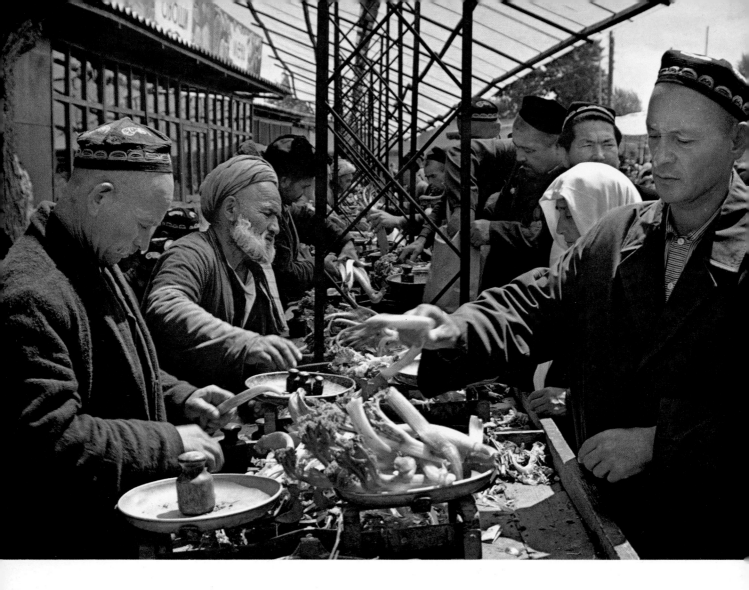

Fruit vendors at a market in Tashkent *(page 176)* sell rhubarb by the stalk. Rhubarb grows well in the nearby mountains (the plant is a native of Asia); besides going into jellies and compotes, it is eaten raw by devotees with a sour tooth.

that invariably includes a hefty amount of meat. At an adjoining table a party of Kazakhs were celebrating some momentous event and before long we were invited to join them to toast the guest of honor, a lively, laughing woman. By the time we discovered that she was a plant geneticist who had just won a government award, we were members of the party. Our *besh barmak* was whisked away and we were offered a Russian dinner—*zakuska, borshch* and *kotlety pozharskie*.

I asked the lady sitting next to me why the food of Kazakhstan was not served, and she seemed surprised.

"But this is a party!" she said.

The statement baffled me for a moment, but then I remembered the day we arrived in Moscow. Friends immediately took us to lunch at one of the most popular places in the city—the Uzbekistan restaurant, which specialized in authentic Central Asian dishes. Everywhere in the world, obviously, the novel and exotic have a certain charm.

But in similar Central Asian restaurants and in private homes the old dishes are still served and the rhythm of the old meals remains largely unchanged. The day usually begins with *kumys*, a clabber that resembles a sour yoghurt, or with a sharp creamy cheese, inevitably accompanied by a dish of the flat bread called *non*, warm from the oven. A summertime lunch is light—cheese,

174

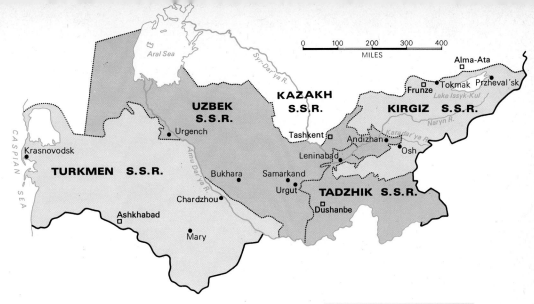

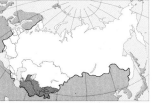

The four Central Asian Republics
—Turkmen, Uzbek, Tadzhik and
Kirgiz—occupy the fabled land of
ancient caravans and exploration
between the Caspian Sea and the
Chinese border, lying south of the
huge Kazakh Republic. In area,
all five of these states rank
among the largest of the 15
Republics in the Soviet Union, but
their semiarid land and harsh climate
have kept their populations low.

greens, *non* again, fruit and tea. In winter it might be a hearty soup, thick, pungent and well spiced, bread—and of course tea.

Tea is in fact a round-the-clock affair. Every block or two has its *chaikhana*, or tea house, a roofed pavilion where dignified, bearded men sit on low platforms, with their bowls of tea in hand, engaged in endless conversations. The women have their tea at home in enclosed gardens or within cool, thick-walled houses.

Whenever we visited a household the steaming pot and bowls appeared, along with a *dastarkhan*, or "offering tray," containing all manner of little things—*non; patyr*, which are round cakes of sour-milk dough; *samsa*, pastries filled with chopped greens, onion, eggs and scallions or with pumpkin or ground walnuts. The best preserves were there too: translucent melon rind, grapes and pears in syrup, rose-petal jam as fragrant as the flower itself, dried fruits, strawberries, white mulberries and slices of quince. There were the candies that Central Asians dearly love: *yanchmish*, balls of roasted ground walnuts; *khalva;* and *bukman* made of thick, concentrated, sweetened cream and browned flour. A bowl of fresh fruit, as vital to the region as air itself, was always on the table—pomegranates, small purple grapes, apricots, satin-skinned pears and plums with their violet bloom unmarred. Lavish as they were, such snacks never seemed to interfere with the evening meal, usually eaten at home and consisting of meat or a *palov*, followed by fruit or a sweet, depending on the region.

The great regional diversities may make a bewildered traveler wonder where he will find the best food in Central Asia. There are as many answers to that question as there are cities, or villages, or perhaps even families. For my part, I would go to Bukhara in summer to eat the long, smooth-skinned melons of that place. The markets are full of their perfume, and men discuss texture, taste and aroma with the expertise of wine growers, identifying not only the variety of a melon but the area in which it grew, the sun, the slope and the quality and quantity of the irrigation. On our visits to Bukhara we reveled in fresh melons with such names as *chogare*, or *bukharka* and *sara-guliabi*. Some growers sun-dry their melons and twist the dried melon slices into long ropes. We sampled these, too, and found them, like all the fruits of Bukhara, lusciously sweet.

Continued on page 180

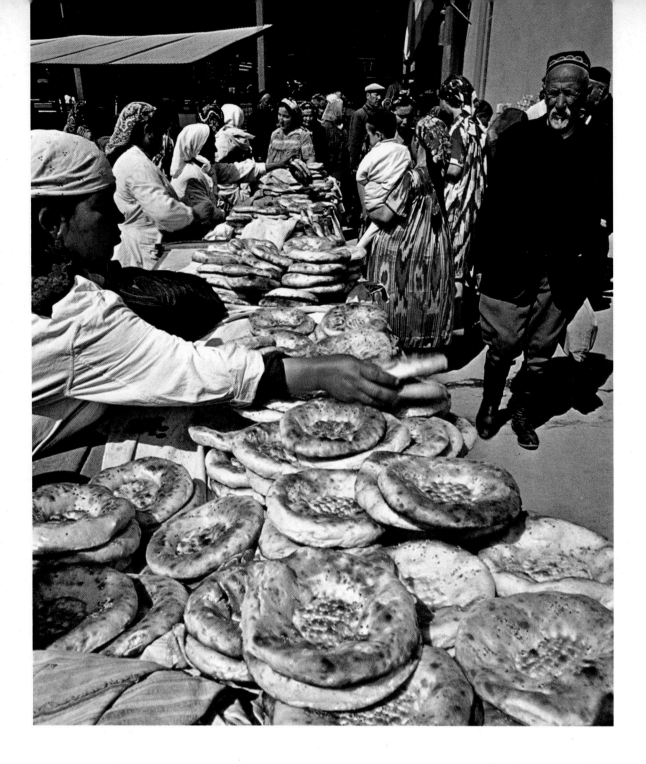

Private Enterprise in an Uzbek Market

The outdoor markets of Tashkent, the largest city in Soviet Central Asia, still retain the loud and aromatic ambience of ancient Oriental bazaars. The vendors are private entrepreneurs, who set the prices of their wares to meet the competition and flourish or fail accordingly. (Like all Soviet cities Tashkent also has state-owned retail stores, where prices are government controlled.) In the picture above, sellers compete for the attention of customers who appear to be making their choices among identical-looking discs of Uzbek bread.

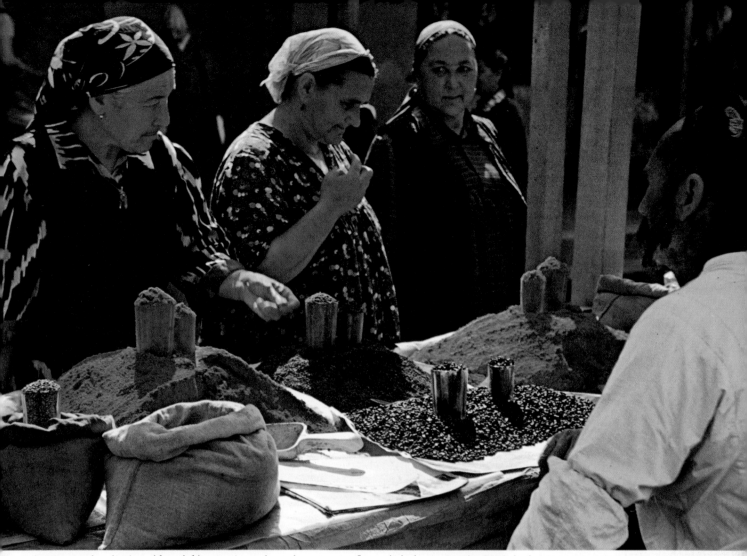

A spice vendor displays *(from left)* caraway seeds, red pepper to flavor kabobs, aniseed, dried barberries and minced dried apricots.

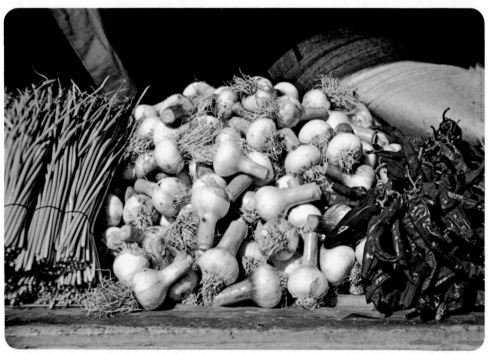

Green garlic leaves, fresh garlic and dried red peppers are offered for sale in a vegetable stall.

Overleaf: An enormous variety of fruits flourishes in Uzbekistan, including almost all that grow in temperate and semitropical areas of the Western world. Some were brought to the region in the course of exchanges with neighboring regions: peaches probably came from China, grapes from around the Caspian Sea; figs from Arabia and the Mediterranean coast. The melons, apples, cherries, plums and pears are indigenous to Central Asia. Of them all, the melons—little known in the West—are probably the most remarkable for quality and variety. More than 1,000 varieties are produced in the Republic.

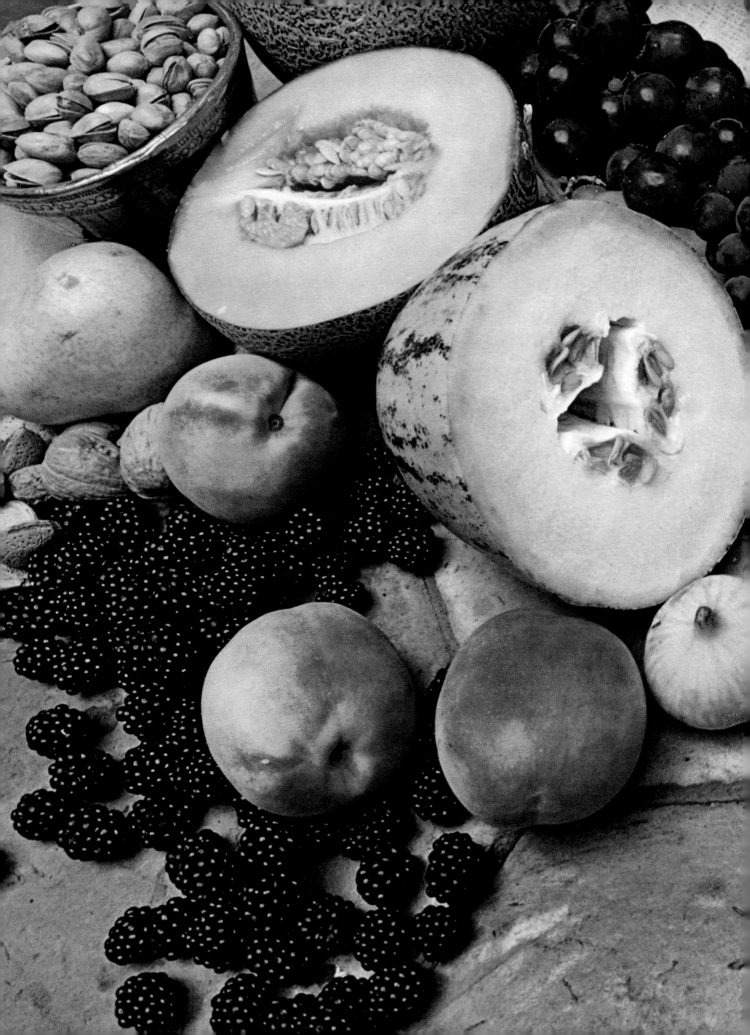

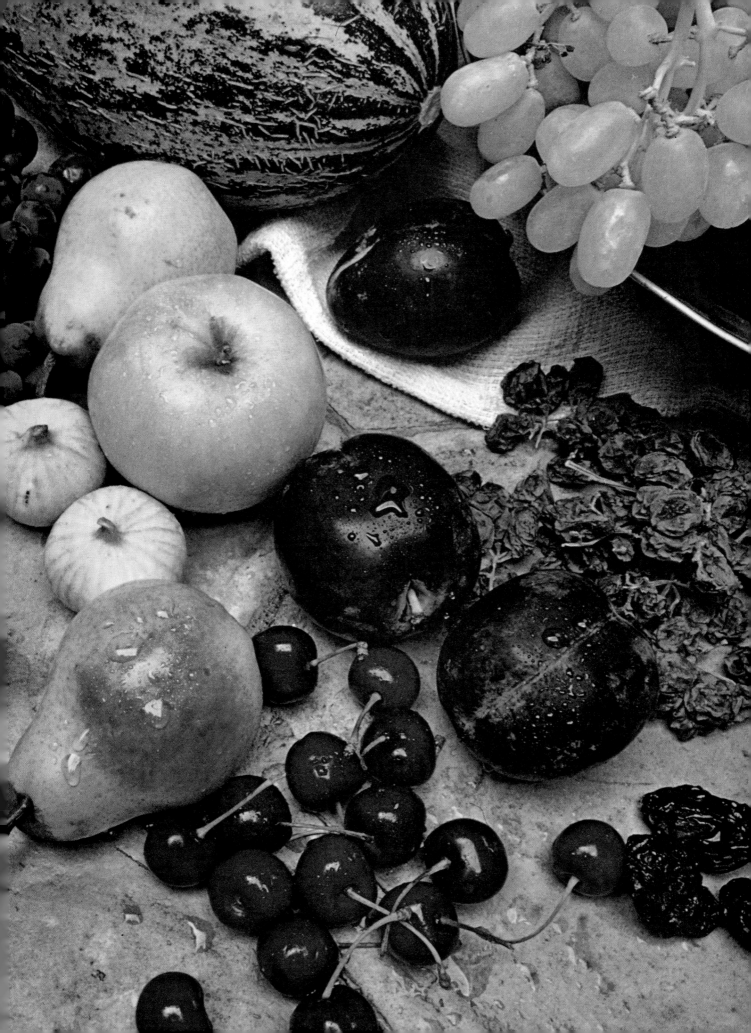

Fall is the time for Alma Ata. It is a lovely season there; the mountains are crowned with the season's first snows, but down in the valley the days are golden. Our visit took us through the apple orchards, past trees heavily hung with many varieties: yellow-green *kandils*, red *aports*, pale *limonovkas*. At Lake Issyk-Kul (which is actually just over the border, in the Kirgiz Re-public) we ate grilled fish and the truly authentic version of the *besh barmak* we had tried at the hotel. In the Turkic languages the word means "a dish of food eaten with all five fingers"; and it is just that. *Besh barmak* is made of thinly sliced meat (the Kazakhs use lamb, beef or horsemeat; the Kirgiz, lamb or mutton) and square-cut (Kirgiz) or diamond-cut (Kazakh) noodles, served with a bowl of the meat broth.

Another popular dish in Kazakhstan is a steamed dumpling called *manty* (*Recipe Index*). One day, taking a short cut through the Alma Ata market, we glanced through an open door at the back of a building and saw what looked for all the world like a ballet practice session. A figure bent down and rose up, another moved forward and back, a third turned in a half circle. We stopped and looked in. Moving with rhythmic grace was a corps of seven or eight *manty* makers. We watched the perfectly synchronized performances of the onion peeler, the meat chopper, the dough roller, the meat mixer, the dumpling assembler and the dough pincher. Then we went through to the front counter of the establishment and ate one of the finished *manty* just fished out of the steamer—a pouch of tender dough filled with peppery ground lamb swimming in its own juice. A single one made a good and ample lunch.

May is the time for Uzbekistan. Tashkent is still cool and in Samarkand the locust trees that line the streets are hung with blossoms. Musicians play in the parks and children dance. Torrents of water rush through open viaducts, fountains leap and every courtyard has a *khauz,* a small pool that reflects the glory of the spring.

In Tashkent we had a superb evening meal at the "Chaikhana of the Elders," a new restaurant done in the old style. The moon shone into a garden pool and on a row of glowing braziers laden with roasting *kebabs.* Inside were low platforms with bright rugs for the older generation, tables and chairs for the young and for European guests. An Uzbek orchestra played the haunting Oriental melodies of the region. A higher platform at one corner of the room was designed as a podium for a reader who, following a very old custom, sometimes recited or read excerpts from literature, folklore, newspapers or political texts—a reminder of the days not so long ago when literacy was rare in Uzbekistan.

We sat down to plates of melon—white, pink, orange and green—pots of tea and monumental bowls of *palov*. In Central Asia a *palov* is not a casually assembled collection of odds and ends supplemented by rice, but a structure based on exact principles and assembled in a rigid time sequence. First into the pot go pieces of the grainy fat from a fat-tailed sheep. The time it takes for the fat to render is just long enough for raw mutton to be cut into pieces and tossed in. Again, in the time the meat browns, the cook peels and slices the onions for the dish. While the onions simmer, wild yellow carrots are washed and chopped. (I should note that a vociferous carrot-before-onion faction does exist.) Then the rice is run through the fingers grain by grain to

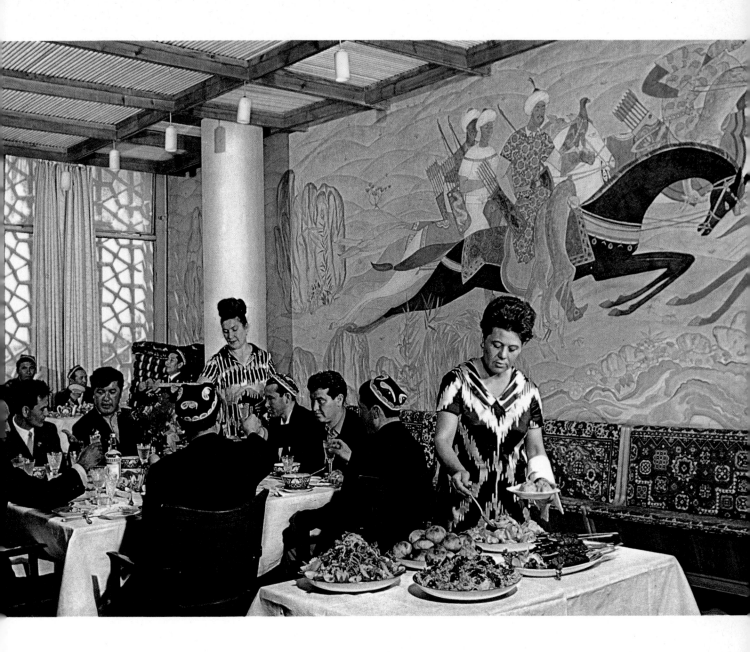

remove any bit of chaff or seed, and rubbed to remove its starchy coating. (A good cook does this job so rapidly that it looks as if he were stringing seed pearls.) The cleaned rice is washed with cold water, drained, slowly poured into the fat and turned a few times; finally, water is added to the level of two fingers above the rice. Now the pot is covered and left undisturbed until the food is done.

In the old days the great pot was set on the floor or a low table; each guest dipped his right hand into the *palov,* scooped up a handful of food, and dexterously molded it into a compact ball, a manageable mouthful, before bearing it to his lips. Nowadays plates and forks generally preclude this tactile pleasure, but in some rural regions of Uzbekistan where old manners linger on, one is occasionally made to realize how clumsy and ridiculous a fork really is for certain foods.

Improvisations on the basic *palov* theme are many. We had *palovs* that con-

A waitress in a Tashkent restaurant assembles a portion of *manty (Recipe Index),* the steamed lamb-filled dumplings that form an Uzbek national dish. Also on the serving table, going clockwise from the *manty,* are *shashlyk, palov, kaurma lagman* (a fried-noodle-and-meat dish) and *samsas* (served here in the form of meat pies). The diners have already begun their meal with wine, appetizers and soup. The mural depicts a scene from an heroic Uzbek poem of the 15th Century.

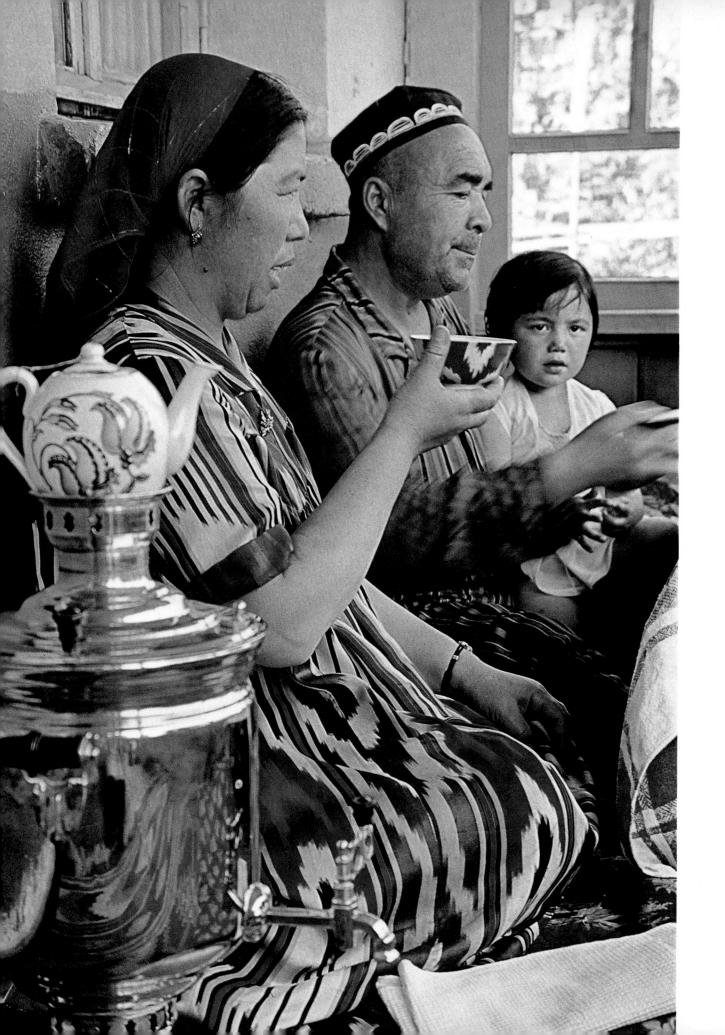

tained quinces, succulent pumpkin, eggs, meatballs, chicken, garlic and dried peas. In Bukhara, Uigur chefs made us a golden *palov* based on pheasant. At the Chaikhana in Tashkent the chef was also an Uigur, and in his mutton *palov* he gave us a multicolored medley of rice, butter, raisins, dried apricots, onion rings and red peppers. For dessert we had fruit and *rokhati dzhon,* a syrup of dried apricots poured over a mound of shaved ice.

That such bountiful tables can be set for a guest is itself a wonder, for Central Asia is a spectacularly bleak land. The region resembles no other territory in the Soviet Union, and its uniqueness derives from harsh, even savage extremes of climate and terrain. Sweeping eastward from the Caspian Sea all the way to the Chinese border is a shallow desert basin almost half as large as the continental United States. A band of grassy uplands forms its northern rim; on the east and south it is bordered by the Tien Shan and Pamir mountain ranges. Known once as Tatary, the region is now officially designated as Central Asia (comprising the Turkmen, Uzbek, Tadzhik and Kirgiz Republics) and Kazakhstan.

It is a dry land, and a hard one. Several large rivers flow across the central plain, but the country receives no more than 12 inches of rainfall a year in the northern grasslands and less than four in the deserts proper (the Mojave Desert, for comparison, gets up to five). Elsewhere in the world, water can be a nuisance to be alleviated by drains and levees; here it is more precious than food, gold or land. Winds blow unimpeded for hundreds of miles, gathering sand or snow along the way. Earthquakes, frequent and violent, level cities, move mountains and change the courses of the rivers. The extremes of climate are so great that Central Asians ask wryly, "Why should we travel when our land is Siberia in winter, Egypt in summer?"

The 30 million people of the region include many ethnic strains, with corresponding differences of occupation and cuisine. Thousands of years ago inhabitants of Turkic and Iranian stock intermixed with Mongolian and Chinese invaders to form major tribal groupings that survive today. Later arrivals included Jews, Gypsies, Dungans (Chinese Muslims), Indians and Arabs. In the 18th Century Catherine the Great sent many Tatars who had lived for generations in the Crimea to Kazakhstan to serve as teachers, traders and advance agents for Russia's future expansion. At about the same time, in a reverse movement, groups of Uigurs migrated west from China. Finally Russia's conquest of Central Asia, completed in 1885, brought Russian and Ukrainian settlers seeking new land.

Until the 20th Century these peoples of Central Asia were divided into two major groups. The peoples of what are now the Kirgiz, Turkmen and Kazakh Republics were nomadic herdsmen, called "black water" people because they depended on wells and underground sources of water. The majority of the Uzbeks and Tadzhiks—along with the Uigurs, Dungans, Tatars and Jews —were "white water" people, who lived in permanent settlements along rivers fed by mountain snows and glaciers.

The nomads followed a way of life almost inconceivable to members of a modern industrialized society. Their sole occupation was raising animals: horses, goats, camels, sheep and, in some areas, yaks and cattle. They spent the winter months in a sheltered spot on the bank of a river or at the base of the mountains. In the early spring an entire *aul,* or village—its people, tents,

Three generations of an Uzbek family drink tea in their kitchen at the Kizil Collective Farm near Tashkent. The people of Uzbekistan, young and old, rich and poor, drink great quantities of green tea every day. At every meal and between meals they assemble around the samovar, as ubiquitous in Uzbekistan as in Russia proper. By custom and for convenience, the samovar is placed beside the mistress of the house.

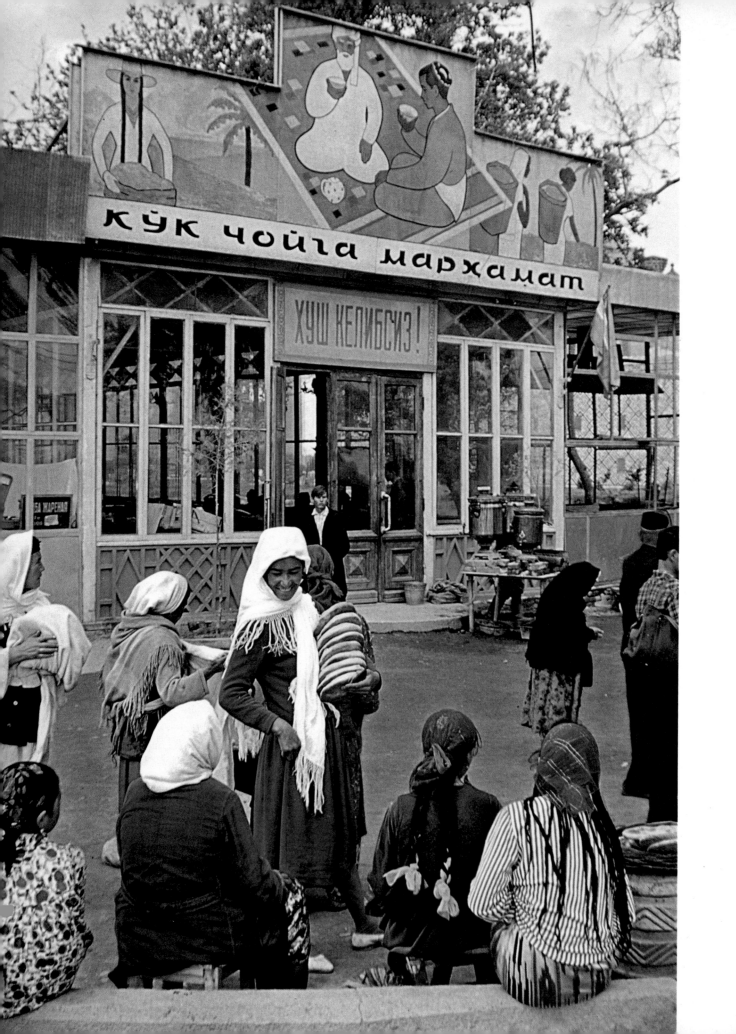

animals, equipment—began an annual trek toward fresh pasture, moving year after year over the same paths to the same resting places. Whether they made a 1,000-mile trek northward (and some did) or merely climbed from the plains to the mountain meadows, they followed such exact travel schedules that the arrival of an *aul* at a given location could be estimated to the day, almost to the hour.

Their dwellings, masterpieces of functional architecture, were domed tents called *yurts*, made of felt stretched over a collapsible, easily portable framework. The *yurt* provided shade, warmth and protection from wind and dust storms. Its furnishings were simple—rugs and pillows for sitting, sleeping and eating, with perhaps a chest or two and carpetbags for storage. Cooking equipment, the property of the women, consisted of homemade wooden bowls, ladles, flasks and leather sacks hung on the wall, along with a fine copper pitcher or two wrought by a professional smith.

In the center of the *yurt*, beneath an adjustable vent in the tent top, was the hearth, and over the fire a great pot stood on legs or hung from a tripod. This vessel served not only for cooking; when it was emptied of food and turned on one side, its upper edge supported a pothook arrangement that held a teakettle over the flames.

The nomads' cuisine was unique for its lack of variety. They seldom, if ever, sat down to a meal in the Western sense of the term, and they ate no bread, rice or grains of any kind, no fruit, and no vegetables other than an occasional wild carrot or the bulbs of the scarlet tulip. From March until October they lived almost exclusively on milk and milk derivatives—clabber, soured milk, and soft and hard cheeses. How the people thrived on this diet is a mystery; by modern dietary standards, milk alone cannot provide a human's minimum daily requirement of iron. Perhaps water drawn from deep desert wells contained this important mineral, for no traveler ever reported meeting a listless nomad.

Certainly, they made the best use of what they had. One of their hard cheeses, *kurt*, anticipated dried milk by a millennium or two. A ball of sun-dried *kurt* had the consistency and appearance of a marble sphere, and this self-packaged instant food could be stored almost indefinitely and reconstituted at any time by soaking crumbled bits in water. *Airan*, a favorite delicacy, consisted of still-warm milk from camels, sheep and goats simmered over a fire until it clabbered and grew sharp and somewhat acrid. It was said to taste cool even on the hottest days.

Those who had enough horses drank *kumys*, fermented mare's milk that has been described as a kind of desert champagne. A great mystique surrounded the drink. Along with the birth of the first foal in the spring, the brewing of the first *kumys* was a time of celebration in the *aul*. *Kumys* was served at weddings, funerals and receptions for honored guests. Among some tribes it was believed milk from white mares made the best *kumys;* in others, a roan or a gray was preferred.

In all cases, the beverage was prepared by adding a starter of old *kumys* (either liquid or in the form of a sun-dried brick mixed with a little fat) to fresh mare's milk. Lacking a starter, the bacterial process could be initiated with fresh horse skin, a bit of tendon from a slaughtered animal or even—lethal though it may seem—a copper coin encrusted with verdigris. The treated

A vendor on a Samarkand street sells loaves of *non*, the basic Uzbek bread, which she has baked at home. In the background, a garish Central Asian *chaikhana*, or teahouse—a roofed pavilion where patrons may sit for hours over tea and tidbits—invites the passerby. The sign above the door reads "Welcome!" and the one beneath the billboardlike painting reads "Welcome to Green Tea."

milk was left in a bag made of smoked horsehide for 24 hours, by which time it was usually bubbling nicely. Then fresh mare's milk was added, and the brew was churned steadily for a full hour. A second fermentation of a few hours and 15 more minutes of beating followed. During a third and final fermentation period, an expert tasted the *kumys* periodically to determine when the exact peak of alcoholic acidity was achieved. Even after that a mild beating might continue. A bag of the finished brew often hung outside the *yurt* for hospitable refreshment, and proper etiquette required that anyone who passed within arm's length should agitate the bag just to keep the *kumys* shaken up.

A fare so limited and bland did not produce gourmets, but it did produce connoisseurs. Near Alma Ata, in Kazakhstan, my husband and I caught a glimpse of the nomad past from a Kazakh woman who claimed she was 90 and could remember the days "before the Russians." Describing the food of her youth, she said, "One mouthful of *kumys* and I could name the mare from which it came."

"And sheep's milk?" I asked her. "Could you name the ewe from which it came?"

She laughed. "No, no. How could I? The sheep had no names. But I *could* tell how the ewe was fed and what flowers had bloomed where she pastured and the age of her lamb. . . ."

"Was this talent usual?"

"I think so. By tasting sheep's milk my grandmother could tell whether the ewe had borne a male or female, but my grandmother's tongue was bet-

Outside a Bukhara park, a *shashlyk* vendor hands three "sticks" of grilled meat to a passing customer. The outdoor grill is as common in the streets of Central Asia as the hot-dog stand in the United States. The vendors come to their posts with portable grills, skewered lamb, seasoned and usually marinated, and wood for fuel. A "stick," or minimum portion, may sell for as little as 25 kopecks (about 28 cents). Though ancient Bukhara now boasts modern facilities and buildings, its old food habits persist. A member of the youngest generation *(opposite)* demonstrates that the Bukharan taste for *shashlyk* is as strong as ever.

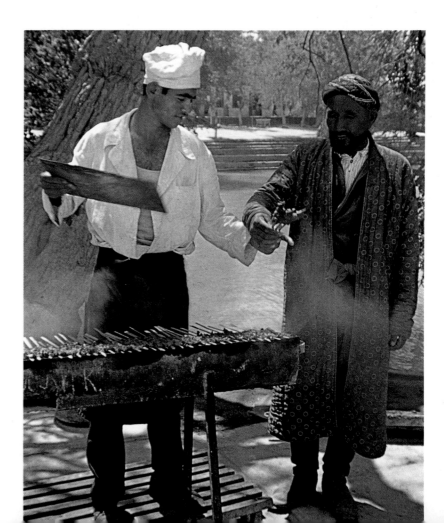

ter than most people's eyes and ears and nose together. One time, when she was still living in her father's *yurt,* a servant driving part of their flock to pasture sent back word that a certain sheep had borne a single lamb. But when the milk was brought in, my grandmother tasted *twin* lambs—and so it proved to be. The servant had intended to keep that extra lamb for himself. He was, you see, a Persian, and fond of meat.''

The nomads were equally discriminating about green tea, which they drank in copious quantity. More than 15 distinct kinds were brought by caravan from China to be sold in Central Asian bazaars, and choosing among them was no light matter. Before a buyer made his decision he first nibbled a single leaf that had been steeped in water. If he liked the taste and texture, he then ordered a pinch of the tea leaves brewed and savored a mouthful of the beverage. There were brews to suit the season, the mood, the company and, above all, the occasion—from everyday brick teas (coarse tea leaves and stems pressed into bricks) taken in the morning with milk and salt to a *lonka,* an Oriental blend of such intense bouquet and flavor that a single potent leaf sufficed for a bowl.

In the fall, when animals were well fleshed from a summer of ample pasturage, the nomads supplemented their milk diet with meat. A particular delicacy that, like *kumys,* only a man who had a surplus of horses could afford, was smoked horsemeat sausage. Camel and goat were boiled or roasted. The most common meat animal of the region, however, was probably the fat-tailed sheep. These lean, long-legged creatures have coarse hair rather than fleece and store fat in their hind quarters rather than throughout the body. (When pasture is poor the animal draws on its reserve of fat much as a camel draws on its hump, and its size diminishes.)

In the Syrian variety of fat-tailed sheep the fat is indeed concentrated in the tail, which attains tremendous size and weight, and becomes so unwieldy that shepherds sometimes attach a wheeled support to the tail, like a trailer, so the sheep can move about to graze. The Central Asian type, on the other hand, has its fat divided between the tail and a hump between the rump and the tail. Unlike ordinary mutton and lamb fat, which tends to be tallowy, the fat of this sheep does not completely liquefy when it is rendered, but retains a residue of minute, wonderfully flavored grains of crackling. The rendered fat can be used for cooking, and as a spread it equals (some would say surpasses) butter.

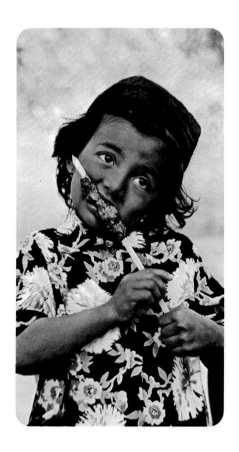

The ''white-water'' people of Central Asia and Kazakhstan enjoyed a more varied fare than the nomads. When the arid lands here are irrigated, they prove to be immensely fertile; around the lakes and along the river deltas, the early farmers built systems of canals and raised barley, millet and wheat. With these grains they made a simple bread in the form of flat disks with little or no leaven, baked in clay ovens. The bread served them as an edible plate, a scooping spoon and a napkin.

Rice was grown in Central Asia as early as 4000 B.C., but rice requires a low terrain and surplus water for flooding the fields in which it grows; therefore, the supply was limited, and for most people it was a luxury reserved for holidays. Vegetables—pumpkins, greens, peppers, onions, cucumbers, turnips and carrots—were all raised. Long yellow grapes, deep crimson peaches, white mulberries, jujubes, apricots and the cherry now known as the Tar-

tarian grew in walled gardens. Most famous of all were the melons, a relatively sophisticated fruit that only a skilled grower could bring to perfection and a connoisseur fully appreciate.

Central Asians, both the nomads and the oasis dwellers, might have enjoyed a more varied cuisine than they did. Their rivers and irrigation canals were so full of giant carp and pike that one enthusiastic traveler claimed he "could ride a horse over them," but only a few people ate fish. Other travelers saw wild geese, rabbit, hare, partridge and gold-winged pheasant in profusion, and often shot and cooked them—but the natives seemed for the most part uninterested. No one really knows why.

They were not ascetic. On the contrary, they liked to eat, and on occasion to overeat. A wedding celebration among them often included an eating contest, with professionals in the art of gorging on hand to demonstrate their prowess. Poets described local beauties in good-enough-to-eat metaphors: "rosy-apple chins," "almond eyes," "lips like cream," and—inexplicably, to me—"pistachio noses." We can only conclude that they liked what they ate and preferred to concentrate on it.

I began to get an inkling of the reasons why the Asians proved so conservative in their tastes only on the day before we left Samarkand, on our last visit to the region. We were invited to a farewell picnic. We took the old Silk Road that runs eastward toward China, a road worn eight feet deep below the adjacent fields by the shoes and hoofs and wheels of many millennia's caravans. Then we left the road, and climbed high in the mountains to a glade near a fast-running stream. There we spread rugs, built a fire for our *shish kebabs* and set melons and *shinni* (a fruit-syrup drink) to cool in the icy water. While we waited for the fire to burn down we ate cold lamb, cold chicken, *kazy* (sausage made of horsemeat), *damlama khasip* (a new Samarkand specialty, a smoked sausage made of lamb), tomatoes, radishes and *non*, the flat, round bread of Uzbekistan.

Uzbek *kebabs* are customarily made of lamb cut into small pieces, mixed with finely diced onions, fresh coriander or dill, ground black pepper and salt. The meat is often marinated in wine vinegar in an earthenware dish for several hours; then it is roasted over charcoal embers, five or six pieces impaled on a stick. Served with the sticks of *kebab* are quartered tomatoes or pomegranates, the juices being squeezed over the meat. No one, it appears, ever eats fewer than four sticks.

Uzbeks make *kebabs* not only of lamb, in chunks or ground, but also of quail, partridge and ptarmigan. The *kebabs* we had that day in the mountains, though they looked like lamb, turned out to be a surprise. Hot and smoking, they were pushed off the sticks into opened *non*, and a bright plume of coriander was tucked inside. With my first bite, I realized that I had never before tasted such delicious meat.

"What kind is it?"

"Fat-tailed sheep!"

I can only describe what was melting in my mouth as super-lamb or mutton-plus, as much superior to a well-finished Southdown as that aristocrat of sheep is to a middle-aged backyard billy goat. With that kind of raw material, it was not surprising that our *kebabs* turned out to be as fine as that finest of grilled-meat dishes can ever be.

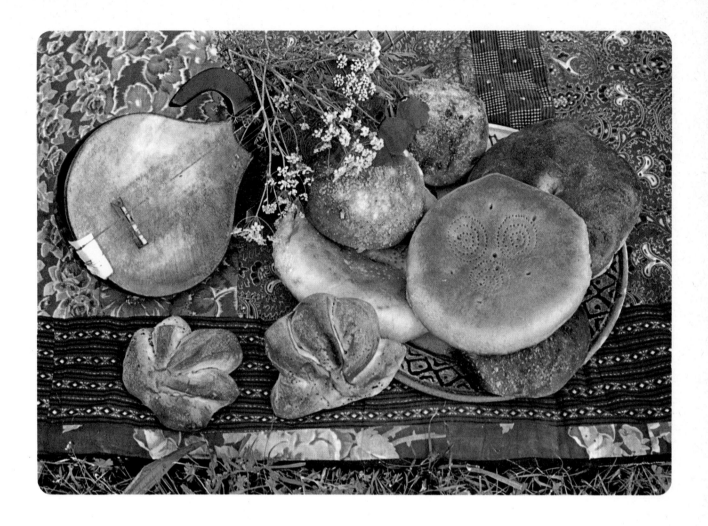

Bread, Lamb and Music for a Student Picnic

In Uzbekistan, as in the Caucasus *(see pages 154-156),* breathtaking scenery and fine weather entice groups of city-dwellers into the countryside for impromptu outdoor meals. The indispensable item on the menu is bread—half a dozen different kinds (shown above with another picnic essential, the native musical instrument called the *rubab)* were brought along for one carefree picnic in the mountains by a group of students *(overleaf).* These distinctive breads will accompany *shashlyk,* barbecued over a wood fire, and raw fruit and vegetables. When the students are ready for their meal, they eat this traditional food in a traditional way, sitting on brilliantly patterned rugs spread over the ground, with a spot in the middle of the picnic site covered with a tablecloth for the food. And after they have eaten, they follow another ancient Uzbek custom—singing folk songs and reciting lyrical poems to the music of the *rubab.*

Overleaf: Two young men of the picnic party light fires to cook *shashlyk* and *palov.* Spread on the cloth are rhubarb, radishes, green onions, garlic and bottles of wine and lemonade. An uninvited addition to the party *(center),* owner of the mud house in the background, is offering hospitality rather than receiving it; in the local custom, he presents bowls of sour milk to the sojourners on his land.

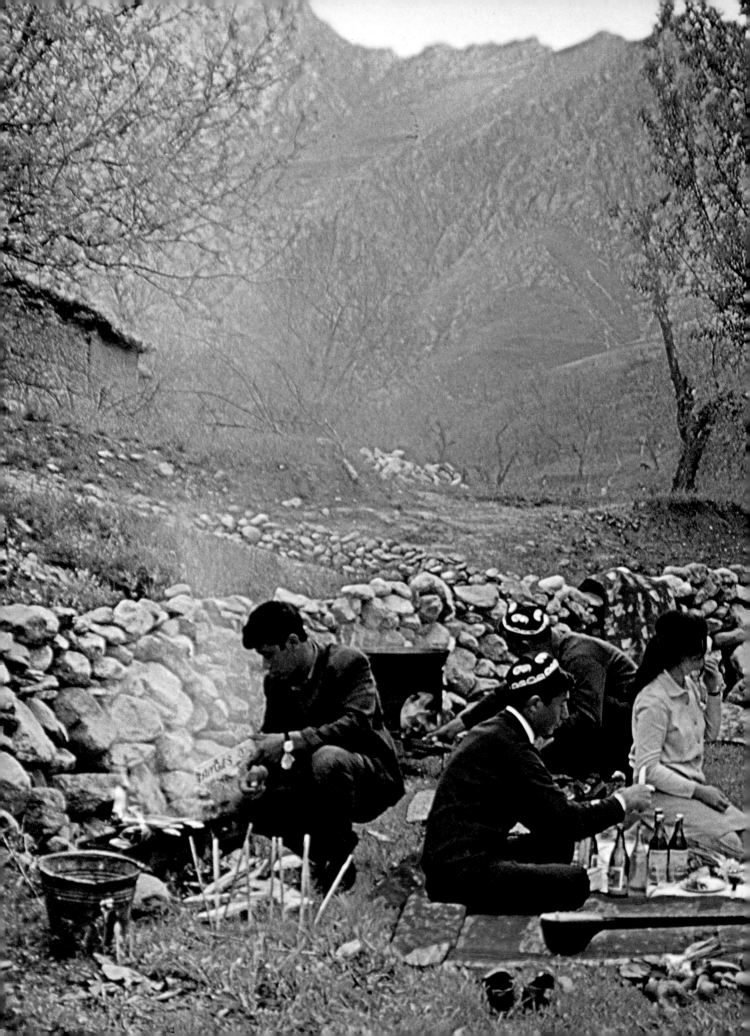

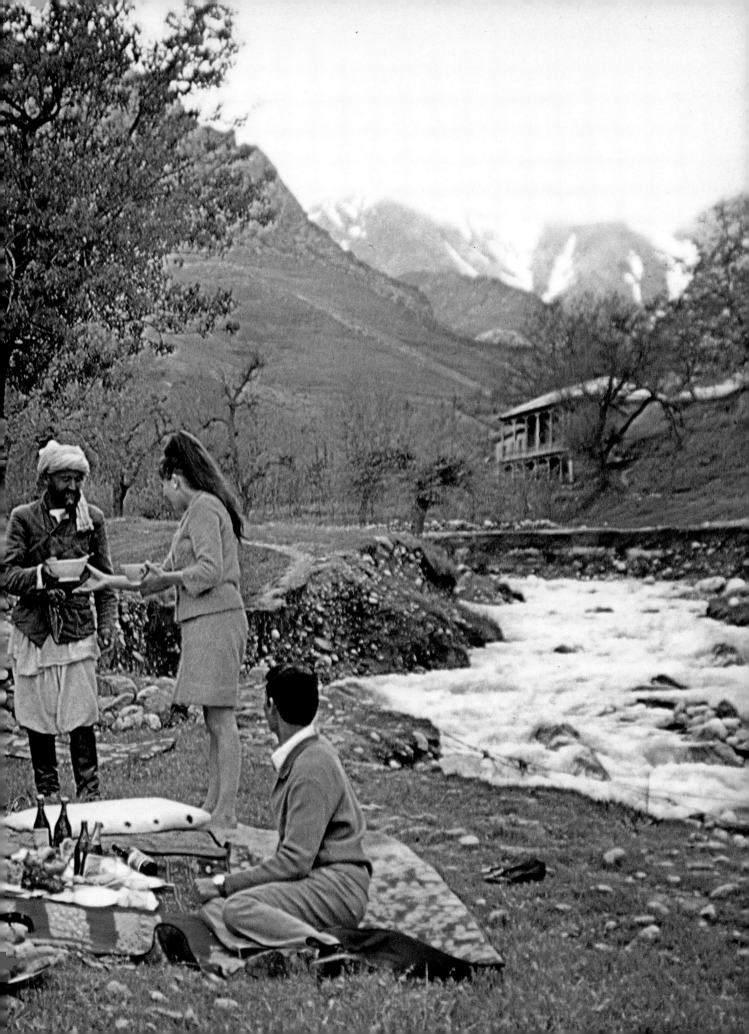

To make 16 breads

6 tablespoons butter
1½ cups finely chopped onions
¾ cup lukewarm water (110° to
   115°)
1 teaspoon salt
2½ to 3 cups all-purpose flour

Non

FLAT ONION BREADS

Melt 1 tablespoon of the butter in a heavy 10- to 12-inch skillet set over high heat. Add the onions, reduce the heat to low and, stirring occasionally, cook 3 to 5 minutes, or until the onions are soft but not brown. Transfer them to a bowl and cool to room temperature.

Melt the remaining butter in the skillet and pour it into a large mixing bowl. Add the lukewarm water and, with a large spoon, stir in the chopped onions, salt and 2½ cups of the flour, ½ cup at a time. If necessary, beat in as much of the remaining ½ cup of flour as you need to make a dough that does not stick to your fingers. Gather the dough into a large, compact ball and divide it into 16 pieces. With the palms of your hands, shape each piece of dough into a 1½- to 2-inch ball. Then, with a lightly floured rolling pin,

A hearty Uzbek dinner features a traditional lamb pilaf, strewn with raw onions and served with scallions and flat onion bread.

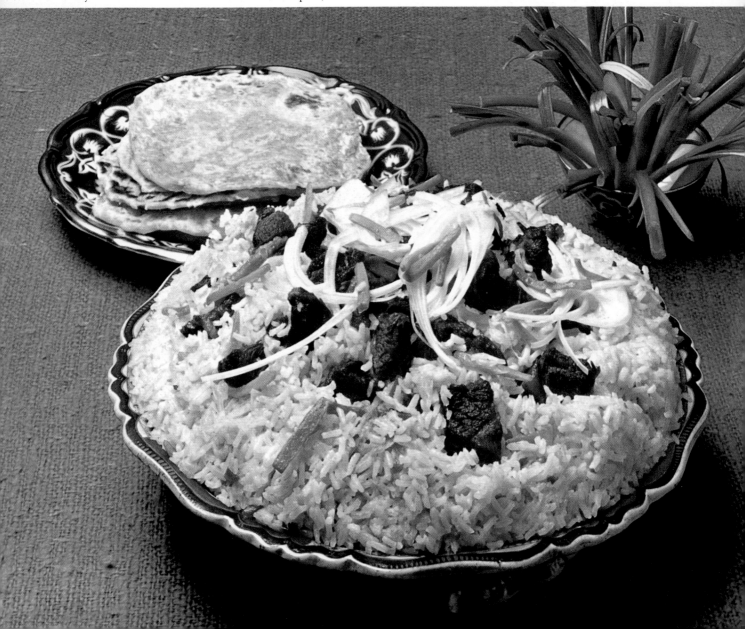

roll out the balls one at a time into circles that are about 8 inches in diameter. Set the rounds of dough aside.

Set a heavy 10- to 12-inch ungreased pan over high heat. When it is hot enough for a drop of water flicked across its surface to instantly evaporate, place 1 round of dough in the center. Brown for 3 or 4 minutes on each side, turning it over with your fingers or a wide spatula; do not be concerned if the bread does not brown evenly.

Transfer the bread to a rack to dry and proceed to fry and dry the remaining dough similarly. Serve the bread in a basket or other porous container. If for any reason the bread becomes limp after a day or so, place the rounds in a single layer on a cookie sheet and bake them for 5 to 10 minutes in a preheated 250° oven until they freshen.

Sabzi Piez

BRAISED ONIONS AND CARROTS

Melt the 3 tablespoons of butter in a heavy 10- to 12-inch stainless-steel or enameled skillet set over high heat. Drop in the onion rings and stirring frequently, cook over moderate heat for 8 to 10 minutes, or until they are golden brown. Add the tomatoes, raise the heat and boil briskly, uncovered, until most of the liquid in the pan has evaporated. Then stir in the carrots, salt and cayenne pepper.

Pour in just enough water (about ½ to ¾ cup) to barely cover the carrots, bring to a boil and cover the skillet tightly. Reduce the heat to low and simmer for about 10 minutes, or until the carrots are just tender. Transfer the carrots and the sauce to a heated serving bowl, sprinkle with chopped scallions and coriander or parsley, and serve at once.

To serve 4 to 6

3 tablespoons butter
1 medium onion, thinly sliced and separated into rings (1 cup)
1 large tomato, peeled, seeded and finely chopped *(see borshch ukrainsky, page 141)*
8 small carrots, scraped and sliced lengthwise into ⅛-inch-thick strips (2 cups)
½ teaspoon salt
⅛ teaspoon cayenne pepper
¼ cup finely chopped scallions, including 2 inches of the green stems
2 tablespoons finely chopped fresh coriander *(cilantro)* or parsley

Uzbek Palov

RICE PILAF WITH LAMB AND VEGETABLES

Heat the oil in a heavy 10- to 12-inch skillet over high heat until a light haze forms above it. Drop in the lamb cubes and fry them for 5 to 8 minutes, turning them constantly with a large spoon until they are lightly and evenly browned on all sides. With a slotted spoon transfer the cubes of lamb to a heavy 4-quart casserole.

To the fat remaining in the pan, add the carrots and 3 cups of the onions. Stirring frequently, cook the vegetables over moderate heat until they are soft but not brown, then stir in the rice. Reduce the heat to low and, stirring constantly, cook about 2 minutes, or until the rice becomes somewhat opaque and is thoroughly coated with the oil.

With a rubber spatula, transfer the contents of the pan to the casserole of meat and sprinkle with the salt and pepper. Toss lightly to combine the ingredients, then pour in 6 cups of water and bring to a boil over high heat. Reduce the heat to low, cover the casserole and simmer 20 minutes, or until the rice is tender and has absorbed most of its cooking liquid. Taste for seasoning.

Transfer the pilaf to a serving bowl or platter and scatter the remaining ½ cup of raw onions over the top. Serve at once, accompanied if you like by flat onion bread *(opposite)*.

To serve 6

¼ cup vegetable oil
1 pound boneless shoulder of lamb, cut into 1-inch cubes
3 large carrots, scraped and cut into strips ¼ inch wide and 2 inches long
2 large onions, peeled and cut into strips about ¼ inch wide and 2 inches long (about 3½ cups)
3 cups unconverted, long-grain white rice
2 teaspoons salt
½ teaspoon freshly ground black pepper
6 cups cold water

To serve 4

DOUGH

1 package active dry yeast
¼ teaspoon sugar
3 cups all-purpose flour
1 cup lukewarm milk (110° to 115°)

FILLING

1½ pounds beef, finely ground
¾ cup finely chopped onions
1 teaspoon salt
¼ teaspoon freshly ground black
  pepper
3 to 4 tablespoons butter
2 to 3 tablespoons vegetable oil

To serve 6

FILLING

1½ pounds lean lamb, finely ground
1½ cups finely chopped onions
2 teaspoons salt
½ teaspoon freshly ground black
  pepper
7 tablespoons butter

DOUGH

3 cups flour
1½ cups water

¼ cup finely cut fresh dill leaves or
  fresh mint
¾ cup unflavored yoghurt

Beliashi
KAZAKH FRIED PASTIES FILLED WITH MEAT

Sprinkle the yeast and sugar over ¼ cup of the lukewarm milk in a small bowl. Let the mixture stand for 2 or 3 minutes, then stir to dissolve the yeast completely. Set the bowl in a warm, draft-free place (such as an unlighted oven) for 5 to 8 minutes, or until the mixture doubles in volume.

Pour the flour into a deep mixing bowl, and make a well in the center. Pour in the yeast mixture and the remaining milk and gradually stir the flour into the liquid. Then beat vigorously until a firm dough is formed. Gather the dough into a ball and place it on a lightly floured surface. Knead it by pressing down and pushing it forward several times with the heel of your hand, then fold it back on itself. Repeat for about 10 minutes, or until it is smooth and elastic. Shape the dough into a ball and place it in a large lightly buttered bowl. Dust the top with flour, cover loosely with a kitchen towel and set aside in the warm, draft-free place for about 45 minutes, or until the dough doubles in bulk.

Combine the meat, onions, salt and pepper in a large bowl and knead with your hands or beat with a large spoon until smooth. On a lightly floured surface roll the dough into a circle about ⅛ inch thick, then cut out 16 circles with a 4½-inch cookie cutter. Place 5 teaspoons of filling on each circle and moisten the edges of the dough with cold water. Fold up all the edges of the dough, enclosing the filling and making a flat, round cake.

Preheat the oven to 250°. In a 10- to 12-inch heavy skillet set over high heat, melt 3 tablespoons of butter in 2 tablespoons of oil. When the fat begins to turn light brown, add half of the flat cakes and cover the pan. Reduce the heat to moderate and cook for about 10 minutes on each side, or until the cakes are crisp and brown. Then transfer them to an ovenproof platter and keep warm in the low oven while you cook the remaining cakes. Add additional butter and oil to the pan if necessary. Serve at once.

Manty
UZBEK LAMB DUMPLINGS

For the filling, mix the ground lamb, chopped onions, salt and pepper in a mixing bowl and beat with a wooden spoon until well combined.

Pour the flour into a large mixing bowl, make a deep well in the center and pour in the water. Mix vigorously until smooth, then gather the dough into a ball and transfer it to a lightly floured surface. Roll out into a rectangle about 1/16 inch thick. With a 4½-inch cookie cutter, cut out 18 to 20 circles of dough and spoon about 5 teaspoons of filling in the center of each. Top each circle with 1 teaspoon of the butter and draw up the sides of the circle so that they meet in the middle, enclosing the filling. Dip your fingers in water, pinch the top closed and twist it to form a small pouch.

Steam the *manty* in the following fashion: Pour enough water into a large kettle to come about 1 inch up the side. Bring to a boil over moderate heat and set a colander into the kettle. Place the *manty* in the colander, cover the kettle securely and lower the heat. Steam for 15 minutes, then transfer the *manty* to individual bowls or to a large serving bowl. Sprinkle with the dill or mint and serve with yoghurt, either as an accompaniment to soup or alone as a light luncheon dish.

194

Samsa

SWEET WALNUT FRITTERS

In a large mixing bowl, toss together the walnuts, 1½ tablespoons of butter and the sugar. Set aside at room temperature.

Place the flour in a deep mixing bowl and make a well in the center. Pour in the water, salt and 2 tablespoons of the butter and slowly stir the flour into the other ingredients until well absorbed. Then beat vigorously with a large spoon until a firm dough is formed. Gather the dough into a ball. On a lightly floured surface, roll it into a rectangle approximately 16 inches wide by 18 inches long. Brush the dough with the additional 2 tablespoons of butter and fold it into quarters. Roll it out again as thinly as possible and with a pastry wheel or small, sharp knife, trim the dough into a rectangle 16 inches wide by 18 inches long. Cut the rectangle into 2-inch squares.

Heap 1 teaspoon of the filling in the center of a square of dough and draw up the four corners to meet in the middle, thus enclosing the filling. Dip your fingers in water and pinch the corners firmly together to seal them. Fill and seal the remaining squares similarly.

Fill a deep-fat fryer or deep, heavy pot with enough oil to come 4 inches up the sides of the pan and heat until the oil registers 375° on a deep-fat thermometer. Drop in 10 or 12 fritters, turning them about occasionally with a slotted spoon, fry them for about 3 minutes, or until they are golden brown and crisp. Then drain them on paper towels while you fry the remaining fritters similarly. Arrange the fritters on a serving platter, sprinkle them with confectioners' sugar and serve.

To serve 8 to 10

FILLING

6 ounces walnuts, pulverized in a blender or ground in a nut grinder
1½ tablespoons unsalted butter, softened
1½ tablespoons sugar

DOUGH

1½ cups all-purpose flour
⅔ cup lukewarm water (110° to 115°)
½ teaspoon salt
4 tablespoons unsalted butter, softened

Vegetable oil for deep-fat frying
Confectioners' sugar

Chebureki

DEEP-FRIED LAMB DUMPLINGS

These fried lamb dumplings are a Tatar dish developed in the Crimea and brought to Central Asia, where many Tatars now live.

Melt the 3 tablespoons of butter in 1 tablespoon of vegetable oil in a heavy 10- to 12-inch skillet set over high heat. When the fat just begins to brown lightly, add the ground lamb. Mashing the meat constantly with a fork to break up any lumps, cook for 3 to 5 minutes, or until the lamb is light brown. Transfer to a large mixing bowl and with a large spoon or your hands, toss with the chopped parsley, coriander, salt and rice. Cool to room temperature.

On a lightly floured surface, roll the dough until it is about ⅛ inch thick. Lift the dough over the backs of your hands and spread your hands apart gently until the dough stretches almost paper thin. Lay it flat on the table and with a 2½- to 3-inch cookie cutter, cut out 76 rounds of the dough. Top half of the rounds with a heaping teaspoon of filling and flatten the filling slightly. Cover with the remaining rounds and seal the edges by pressing them firmly all around their circumference with the prongs of a fork. With a pastry brush, coat the edges of the dumplings with the beaten egg to seal them even more securely.

Heat the oil in a deep-fat fryer until it reaches a temperature of 375° on a deep-frying thermometer. Fry the dumplings, 6 to 8 at a time, for 2 or 3 minutes, turning them over in the fat until they are evenly browned. Drain on paper towels and serve hot, with soup or as a first course.

To make 38 dumplings

3 tablespoons butter
1 tablespoon vegetable oil
¾ pound lean lamb, finely ground twice
¼ cup finely chopped parsley
2 tablespoons finely chopped fresh coriander *(cilantro)*
2 teaspoons salt
3 tablespoons cold boiled white rice
1 recipe *pelmeni* dough *(see Recipe Index)*
1 egg, lightly beaten
Vegetable oil for deep-frying

Glossary

ABRAU-DURSO (ah-BROW door-SOH) CHAMPAGNE: Russian champagne created at the end of the 19th Century by the French agronomist and wine maker Georges Barberon from a selection of domestic and imported vines. This champagne is still produced in the Soviet Union in the cellars of Abrau-Durso, now a state farm.

ADZHERSANDAL (ah-zhehr-sahn-DAHL): Georgian eggplant baked with fried onions and tomatoes.

AGNAUTKA (ahg-nah-OOT-kah): A flat, whole-grained Ukrainian bread loaf.

AIRAN (eye-RAHN): Central Asian clabbered milk.

ALEKSANDER TORTE (AH-leek-sahnd'r TAWRT): Alexander torte; Latvian pastry strips filled with raspberry preserves.

APORTS (ah-PAWRTS): Central Asian variety of apple.

ĂVIŽINĖ KOŠĖ (ah-vee-ZHUH-ney KO-shey): Fermented oatmeal porridge of Lithuania; a traditional Christmas Eve dish.

BABA (BAH-bah): Tall, cylindrical Russian cake.

BADI-BUDI (BAAH-dee BOO-dee): Georgian popcorn.

BAGRATION (bah-GRAH-tyawn): An elegant Russian cream soup made with veal and sometimes asparagus tips.

BAKLAVA (bah-klah-VAH): A honey-drenched Armenian dessert of flaky, paper-thin layers of dough with crushed nuts.

BALABUSHKY (bah-lah-BOOSH-kuh): Small, sour-dough Ukrainian rolls.

BASTURMA (bah-stoor-MAH): Armenian dried, salted beef. Also Georgian grilled marinated meat.

BAZHA (BAH-ZHAH): Georgian walnut sauce used with meat, fish or fowl.

BEF STROGANOV (behf STRAW-gah-noff): Beef Stroganov; Russian sautéed beef, onions and mushrooms in sour-cream sauce.

BELUGA (bee-LOO-gah): Large-grained eggs (caviar) yielded by the sturgeon of the same name.

BESH BARMAK (BEHSH bar-MAHK): A thick, Central Asian meat soup.

BITKI (beet-KEE): Tiny, highly seasoned Russian meatballs or fish cakes.

BLINY (blee-NUH): Russian buckwheat yeast pancakes.

BORSHCH (BAWRSH): A Russian or Ukrainian beet soup to which can be added other vegetables and meat.

BOTVINIA (baht-VEE-nyah): Russian green vegetable soup with fish.

BRYNZA (BRIN-zah): An aged cheese made from sheep's milk in the Carpathian mountains of the Ukraine.

BUKHARKA (boo-HAHR-kah): Central Asian variety of melon.

BUKMAN (book-MAHN): Creamy Central Asian candy.

CHACHIS ARAKI (CHAH-chis ah-RAH-kee): A dry Georgian spirit distilled from the stems, pips, and skins of pressed grapes.

CHAIKHANA (chye-hah-NAH): An Uzbek tea house.

CHAKHOKHBILI (chah-hah-BEE-lee): Georgian chicken and tomato casserole.

CHARLOTTKA (shahr-LAWT-kah): Charlotte Russe; French-created molded dessert of ladyfingers with cream filling.

CHIKHIRTMA (chee-HEERT-mah): A tart Georgian chicken soup.

CHOGARE (chuch-GAH-ree): Central Asian variety of melon.

CHRISTOS VOSKRES (hrees-TOSS vahs-KREHS): "Christ is risen." A traditional Russian Easter exclamation that requires the response, "Voistinu Voskres" (vah-EES-tee-nah vahs-KREHS), "Truly, he is risen."

CHUCHKELLA (chooch-kel-LAH): Georgian grape-and-walnut candies.

DAMLAMA KHASIP (dahm-LAH-mah huh-SEEP): A Central Asian smoked lamb sausage.

DEDA'S PURI (dyeh-DAHZ poo-REE): "Mother's bread," the Georgian wheat bread baked in a *toné*, or outdoor oven.

DONDURI (dahn-doo-REE): Purslane, a pot herb favored by Georgians.

EKMEK (EHK-MEHK): Armenian pudding made of toasted bread boiled in sugar, honey and butter.

FABERGÉ EGGS: A series of jeweled eggs created for Easter gifts by Karl Fabergé between 1884 and 1894. The more elaborate eggs, with fantastic surprises inside, were commissioned annually by the Czar and are known as the Imperial Easter eggs. Simpler eggs were made for members of the nobility.

FORSHMAK (for-SHMAHK): A Russian dish of minced meat, herring and mashed potatoes.

GASTRONOM (gahs-traw-NOM): Soviet luxury food shop.

GHOME (HOM-EH): Georgian corn-meal porridge.

GOGOL-MOGOL (GAW-g'l MAW-g'l): Russian fluffy egg dessert.

GOZINAKH (guh-zee-NAHK): Georgian nut-and-honey candy.

GURABIA (goo-RAH-byah): Light, sugar-powdered Armenian cookies.

GUREV KASHA (GOO-ruhf KAH-shah): Russian sweet farina pudding with candied fruits and nuts.

HALUSHKI (HAH-loosh-kee): Ukrainian fluffy egg dumplings.

HOLUBTSI (HAH-loop-tsuh): Ukrainian packets of rolled cabbage leaves, filled with rice alone or with rice combined with meat and mushrooms.

KAIMAK (KYE-mahk): A rich Armenian concentrated cream.

KALACH (kah-LAHCH): An especially rich Ukrainian wheat bread.

KASHA (KAH-shah): Russian dry porridge made with grain, usually buckwheat.

KASHLAMA (kah-shlah-MAH): Armenian lamb shoulder boiled with vegetables.

KAZY (kah-ZEE): A Central Asian horsemeat sausage.

KHACHAPURI (hah-chah-POO-ree): A Georgian bread made as a large, round loaf or individual tartlets and filled with cheese.

KHARCHO (hahr-CHAW): Georgian beef, onion and tomato soup-stew.

KHARPUT KIUFTA (HAHR-poot KEEF-tah): Armenian cracked wheat and lamb, stuffed with minced lamb, pine nuts, chopped onions and parsley.

KHOLODETS (hah-lah-DYEHTS): Russian jellied beef, veal and chicken mixture.

KISEL (kee-SEHL): Russian puréed fruit dessert.

KIUFTA (KYOOF-tah): Armenian meat balls.

KOROVAI (kah-rah-VYE): Very large, richly ornamented Ukrainian cake.

KOTLETY (kat-LYET-tuh): Russian fried meat patties.

KOTLETY POZHARSKIE (kat-LYET-tuh puh-ZHAHR-skee-yeh): Russian ground meat patties named after their inventor, a tavern keeper called Pozharsky.

KRENDEL (KREHN-del): Pretzel-shaped Russian sweet bread.

KRUPNIKAS (KROOP-nee-kas): Honey-based liqueur, the national drink of Lithuania.

KUGELIS (KOO-gheh-lees): Lithuanian grated potato pudding.

KULENARIA (koo-lee-NAH-ryah): Store in the Soviet Union specializing in ready-to-eat or semi-prepared food.

KULICH (koo-LEECH): Russian cylindrical Easter cake with nuts and raisins.

KUMYS (KOO-muhs): Fermented mare's milk of Central Asia.

KURNIK (KOOR-nik): Creamy Russian dish of chicken and rice covered with a pastry crust.

KURT (KOORT): A hard, sun-dried Central Asian cheese made from sheep's milk.

KURZEMES (koor-ZEH-mes): Pork cutlet named after Kurzeme, now known as Kurmēn or Courland, a Latvian region.

KUTIA (koo-TYAH): Traditional Ukrainian Christmas dish of wheat grains combined with honey, poppy seeds and stewed dried fruit.

KVAS (KVAHS): Fermented and slightly alcoholic Russian beverage made from grain. Also used as a cold-soup stock.

KVHOROST (HVAW-rist): Crisp, buttery, twig-shaped Russian cookies.

LAVASHI (lah-VAH-shee): Thin, white Georgian wheat bread.

LEKAKH (LEH-kakh): Lithuanian honey cake.

LIGZDINAS (lehg-ZDEE-nas): Latvian meat patty.

LIIVA KOOK (LIV-ah KAWK): Estonian sand cake.

LIULIA KEBAB (LYOO-lee keh-BAHB): Armenian ground lamb patties broiled on skewers.

LOBIO (LAW-byoh): Georgian dish of red kidney beans with herb dressing.

LOKSHYNA (lawk-SHUH-nah): Ukrainian egg noodles.

MALOSSOL (mah-lah-SAWL): Russian for "little salt." Denotes the very mildly salted grades of caviar.

MANTY (MAHN-tee): Steamed Central Asian dumplings filled with ground lamb.

MASLENITSA (MAH-sleh-nee-tsuh): "Butter Festival"; the week that precedes the strict Russian Orthodox Easter Lent. During this week, dairy products are still allowed and Russians prepare for the long fast ahead by gorging themselves on *bliny,* the traditional buckwheat yeast pancakes.

MATSONI (mat-SON-ih): Georgian yoghurt.

MATSUN (maht-SOON): Armenian yoghurt.

MATSUNABUR (maht-soon-ah-BOOR): Armenian yoghurt soup.

MAZURKI (mah-ZOOR-kee):
Finger cookies or Easter cake of Polish origin.

MCHADI (MCHAH-dee): Flat, round Georgian corn bread.

MEDIVNYK (meh-DUHV-nuhk): Spiced Ukrainian honey cake.

MEDOVYE PRIANIKI (meh-DOH-vee-eh PREN-ee-kee): Crumbly Russian cakes made out of rye meal and honey.

MINOGA (mee-NAW-guh): Russian for lamprey.

MTSWADI (MTSWAH-dee): Georgian grilled meat.

NAKYPLIAK (nah-KUH-plyak): Steamed Ukrainian cabbage soufflé.

NALISTNIKI (nah-LIS-nee-kee): Crisp Russian pancakes stuffed with cheese.

NON (NAWN): Flat bread of Central Asia.

OKROSHKA (ah-KRAWSH-kah): Chilled Russia vegetable soup made with *kvas.*

OSETROVA (ah-see-TRAW-vah): The roe (caviar) yielded by a medium-sized species of the sturgeon family.

PALOV (pah-LAWF): Central Asian version of pilaf.

PANNKOOGID (PAHN-kawk-id): plural of Pannkook (PAHN-kawk); Estonian dessert pancakes.

PASHTET (pahsh-TYET): Russian molded paté.

PASKHA (PAHS-khah): Russian pyramid-shaped mold of pot cheese, candied fruit and nuts, a traditional Easter dish. Also Russian word for Easter.

PATYR (pah-TUHR): Small, round, sour-milk cakes of Central Asia.

PAUSNAIA (PAH-yoos-nah-yah): Russian pressed caviar.

PEDA (PEH-dah): Dimpled, crusted Armenian yeast bread.

PELMENI (peel-MYEH-nuh): Siberian meat-filled dumplings.

PERTSOVKA (peer-TSAWF-kah): Vodka fortified with black pepper.

PIROZHKI (pee-rahsh-KEE): Small Russian pasties filled with meat, mushrooms, fish, cheese or cabbage.

POLIANITSA (pah-lyah-NEET-sah): Round Ukrainian white bread, topped with a crusty cap.

PYRIZHKY (puh-ruhsh-KEE): Ukrainian equivalent of *pirozhki. (See above)*

PYSHKI (PIHSH-kee): Light, dry filled Russian fritters.

RASSOLNIK (rah-SAWL-neek): Russian sorrel soup often served with kidneys.

RASTEGAI (rahs-tee-GYE): Russian oval pastry filled with meat or fish.

ROKHATI DZHON (rah-HAH-tee-ZHAWN): Central Asian dessert of shaved ice topped with apricot syrup.

RUBINOVAIA (roo-bee-NAW-vah-yah): Vodka flavored with mountain ash berries.

SALAT OLIVIER (sah-LAHT ah-lee-VYAY): Russian chicken and vegetable salad created by the French chef Olivier. Often called *salade russe* outside Russia.

SAMSA (SAHM-sah): Central Asian pastries filled with chopped greens, onion, eggs and scallions or with pumpkin or ground walnuts.

SARA-GULIABI (SAHR goo-LYAH-bee): Central Asian variety of melon.

SATSIVI (saht-SEE-vee): Georgian walnut sauce used with meat, poultry, vegetables or fish.

SEVRUGA (see-VROO-gah): The roe (caviar) yielded by the smallest sturgeon.

SHASHLYK (shuh-SHLEEK): Georgian grilled lamb.

SHCHI (shee): Russian cabbage soup.

SKABA PUTRA (SKAH-bah POO-trah): Latvian sour milk-and-barley soup.

SMARODINOVKA (smah-rah-DEE-nawf-kuh): Vodka infused with black currant leaves.

SOLIANKA (sah-LYAN-kah): Russian fish or meat soup with salted cucumber.

STOLOVAIA (stah-LAW-vah-yah): Soviet luncheonette, offering short-order or ready-made dishes. Also
the Russian word for dining room.

SUDAK (soo-DAHK): Russian word for pike perch.

SUNELI (soo-NEH-lee): Bouquet of dried herbs Georgians use to flavor particular dishes.

ŠVIEŽIA DĒSRA (SVIEH-zha DEH-shah): Common variety of Lithuanian sausage.

TABAKA (tah-bah-KAH): Georgian pressed, fried chicken.

TKEMALI (KMAH-lee): Georgian tart sauce made from wild plums or sour prunes.

TONĒ (TAW-NEH): A brick-lined pit used by Georgians as an outdoor oven.

TSENTRALNAIA (tseen-TRAHL-nah-yah): Restaurant in Moscow founded in 1865 as the Filippov café.

TURELI GIVECH (too-REH-lee gih-VECH): Armenian meat fried with vegetables.

TUSHURI (too-SHOO-ree): Georgian hard cheese.

UKHA (oo-HAH): Clear Russian fish soup.

UKRAINKA (oo-krah-EEN-kah): Heavy, dark, rough-textured Ukrainian bread loaf.

VARENYKY (vah-REHN-uh-kuh): Ukrainian dumplings filled with fruit, cheese, or sauerkraut.

VATRUSHKI (veh-TROOSH-kee): Russian pastry shells filled with cheese.

VECHERNY TCHAI (vee-CHEHR-nee TCHYE): Evening tea; a light meal of cold cuts and tea served a few hours after dinner in traditional Russian homes.

YANCHMISH (yahnch-MEESH): Central Asian walnut candy.

YARPAKH DOLMASY (yar-pah DOLE-mah-see): Stuffed Armenian grape leaves.

ZAKUSKA (zah-KOOS-kah): Russian hors d'oeuvres.

ZUBROVKA (zoo-BRAWF-kah): Vodka flavored with buffalo grass.

Recipe Index: English

NOTE: An R preceding a page refers to the Recipe Booklet. Size, weight and material are specified for pans in the recipes because they affect cooking results. A pan should be just large enough to hold its contents comfortably. Heavy pans heat slowly and cook food at a constant rate. Aluminum and cast iron conduct heat well but may discolor foods containing egg yolks, wine, vinegar or lemon. Enamelware is a fairly poor conductor of heat. Many recipes therefore recommend stainless steel or enameled cast iron, which do not have these faults.

Recipe Index: Foreign

General Index

Numerals in italics indicate a photograph or drawing of the subject mentioned.

Credits and Acknowledgments

The sources for the illustrations that appear in this book are shown below. Credits for the pictures from left to right are separated by commas, from top to bottom by dashes.

Photographs by Eliot Elisofon pages—25, 38, 56, 57, 59, 67, 80, 81, 84, 85, 89, 92, 100, 105, 107, 108, 112, 120, 125, 126, 127, 128, 130, 131, 139 (bottom), 142, 144, 146, 147, 154, 155, 156, 162, 163, 169, 172, 174, 176, 177, 181, 182, 184, 186, 187, 189, 190, 191, 192. Photographs by Richard Jeffery pages—9, 28, 29, 31, 37, 62, 68, 69, 86, 87, 97, 98, 116, 119, 134, 135, 138, 139 (except bottom), 140, 150, 151, 158, 164, 170 (top), 178, 179. All other photographs cover—Fred Eng. 4—Charles Isaac—Henry Groskinsky, Monica Suder—Charles Phillips, Sebastian Milito. 12, 13 —Map by Charles Mikolaycak. 14, 15—Eric Schaal for TIME. 16, 17—Herbert Orth courtesy The New York Public Library. 19, 20, 21—Henry Beville courtesy of Mrs. Merriweather Post, Hillwood, Washington, D.C. 22, 23—Henry Beville courtesy of Mrs. Merriweather Post, Gift of Colonel C. Michael Paul to The Smithsonian Institution for Hillwood, Washington, D.C. 33 —Drawing by Matt Greene. 41 through 45—Lev Nosov of Novosti Press Agency, Moscow. 46 through 55—Brian Seed. 60, 61—Drawings by Robert Geissman. 64—Erich Lessing from Magnum courtesy State Historical Museum, Moscow. 72 through 75—Nosov of Novosti Press Agency. 76—Drawings by Matt Greene. 78, 79—Nosov of Novosti Press Agency. 94—Fred Eng. 103—Map by Lothar Roth. 115—Fred Eng. 122—Howard Sochurek. 123—Map by Lothar Roth. 138—Drawings by Matt Greene. 145—Map by Lothar Roth. 167—Fred Eng. 170 —Fred Eng (bottom). 171—Fred Eng. 175—Map by Lothar Roth.

Two people deserve special thanks for their contributions to this book. Miss Inessa Pushkin of the Novosti Press Agency accompanied the field photographer as interpreter throughout his travels in the Soviet Union and provided valuable information for picture captions. Prince Nicholas V. Galitzine provided much information and thoughtful advice based on his long experience in preparing and enjoying Russian food.

For their help in the production of this book the editors wish to thank the following: in the U.S.S.R., R. K. Dzarakhokhov, director, Sadko Restaurant, Leningrad; Pavel Gevorkyan, Chief of the North American Section, and Vladislav Shidlovsky, Novosti Press Agency; O. Gigineishvili; Gregory Pavlovitch Irmilian, chef, Moskva Restaurant, Moscow; Ivan Nemtsov, Gastronom No. 1, Moscow; Akaki Nijeradze; Mme. Anastasia Makarova, manager, Factory Bolshevik, Moscow; Mme. Taisija Vasilijevna Ivanova, deputy director, Management of Public Food Supply, Leningrad; and the Novosti Press Agency; in Montreal, Arnold Kagan; Gregory Schwartzberg; in Cambria, California, Michael Borodin; in Reading, Pennsylvania, Mr. and Mrs. Charles Muhlenberg; in Washington, D.C., Mrs. Merriweather Post, Hillwood, and Marvin C. Ross, Curator, Hillwood; Mrs. Nathalie P. Scheffer; in New York, Mrs. Liuba Solov Assade; Edward Berberian, Jr., Balkan Armenian Restaurant; Igor Damashkin, Intourist; Rose Donigian; Victor Gorskov, Amtorg Trading Corp.; Mrs. Faith Kaye, Russian Tea Room; Vera Kovarsky, TIME; Eleanor Lowenstein, Corner Book Shop; Boris Orekhov, Pravda; Mrs. Ada Parlin; Mrs. Penelope Roberts and August Burbiel, Radio Liberty Committee; Mrs. Nijole Salcius; Paul and Peter Schaffer, À La Vieille Russie; Theodore Shabad, The New York Times; Mr. and Mrs. Samuel Sweet; Alexis D. Tchenkeli-Thamys; Mrs. Kadi Tekkel; Dale R. Winkels; Abinit, Ltd.; Acutiques; American Gas Association; Baccarat & Porthault, Inc.; Bardith; Belgravia House; Bonniers Inc.; Central Book and Art Company; Christopher Chodoff; Country Floors Inc.; Cross Keys Antiques; Charles Deacon; Four Continents Book Corporation; Globe-Trotter Antiques; F. Gorevic & Son; Ned Baker, Alexander Hamilton Institute; House of Hite; Jean's Silversmiths; Georg Jensen; Hinda Kohn; H. J. Kratzer, Inc.; La Cuisinière Inc.; Léron; Le Roy Antiques; London Arcade; Nesle, Inc.; Podarogifts, Inc.; Elux C. Putting Antiques Corp.; Raphaelian Rug Co. Inc.; James Robinson, Inc.; Romanoff Caviar Co.; N. Sakiel & Son, Antiques; Frank Selby, Incorporated; Edward Sporar; Sylvia Tearston; J. Rochelle Thomas, Inc.; Tiffany & Company; Herbert Trigger.

Sources consulted in the production of this book include: Once a Grand Duke by Alexander, Grand Duke of Russia, Garden City Publishing Company; Central Asia, edited by Edward Allworth, Columbia University Press; The Romanovs by Martha Edith Almedingen, Holt, Rinehart and Winston; Armenian-American Cookbook by Rose Baboian, published by the author in Watertown, Mass.; Central Asia under Russian Rule by Elizabeth Bacon, Cornell University Press; Natural Regions of the U.S.S.R. by Lev Semenovich Berg, Macmillan Company; A History of Latvia by Alfred Bilmanis, Princeton University Press; Popular Lithuanian Recipes by Josephine Dauzvardis, Lithuanian Catholic Press; The Home Book of Russian Cookery by Nina and George Froud, Faber & Faber; The Balts by Marija Gimbutas, Frederick Praeger; Russian Cooking by Robin Howe, Roy Publishers; The Best of Russian Cooking by Alexandra Kropotkin, Charles Scribner's Sons; The People of the Soviet Union by Corliss Lamont, Harcourt, Brace & World; The Epicure in Imperial Russia by Marie Alexandre Markevitch, The Colt Press; Palmyra of the North by Christopher Marsden, Faber & Faber; Only in Russia by Howard Norton, D. Van Nostrand Co.; Russian Life in Town and Country by Francis H. E. Palmer, G. P. Putnam; The Russian Cook Book published by Russian War Relief, Inc.; Treasured Armenian Recipes compiled by the Armenian General Benevolent Union, Inc. (Detroit Women's Chapter); Daily Life in Russia under the Last Tsar by Henri Troyat, Macmillan Company; The Soviet Union by Sergei Tolstoi, Novosti Press, Moscow; Dining and Wining in Old Russia by Nina Nikolaevna Selivanova, E. P. Dutton & Co.; Ukraine: An Atlas of Its History and Geography by G. W. Simpson, Oxford University Press; Cooking the Russian Way by Musia Soper, Spring Books; Traditional Ukrainian Cookery by Savella Stechishin, Trident Press, Ltd., Winnipeg; Lost Splendor by Prince Felix Youssoupoff, G. P. Putnam's Sons; and the booklets on the individual Soviet Republics such as USSR: Georgia and USSR: Uzbekistan published by the Novosti Press Agency Publishing House, Moscow.

NOTE: Kits for decorating Easter eggs in the Ukrainian style, as shown on pages 60-61, may be bought for about $5 at folk-art stores in cities with Ukrainian communities. They can be ordered by mail from Arka Company, 48 East 7th Street, New York, N.Y. 10003. Some art supply stores also sell styluses of the kind shown in the diagrams.